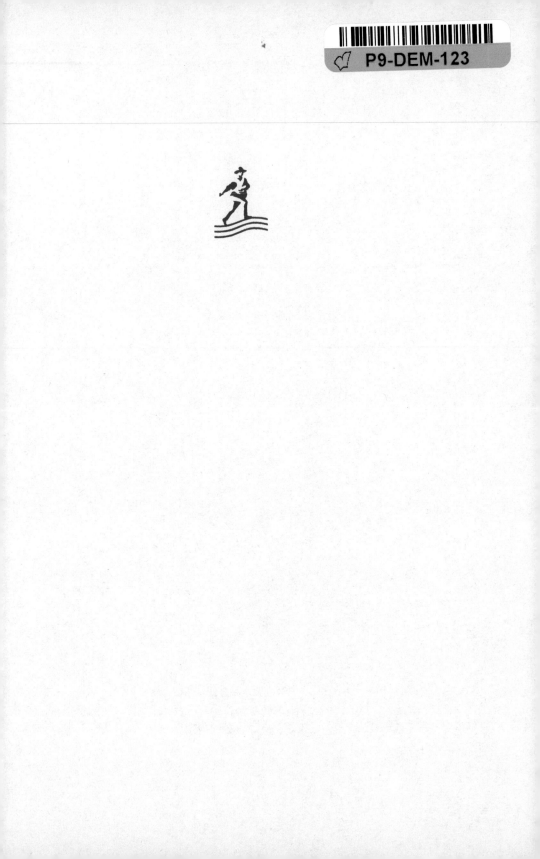

New, Revised and Expanded Third Edition

ON
DOCTOR⚕NG

STORIES, POEMS, ESSAYS

EDITED BY
RICHARD REYNOLDS, M.D.,
AND JOHN STONE, M.D.
*Lois LaCivita Nixon, Ph.D., M.P.H.,
and Delese Wear, Ph.D.,
Associate Editors*

Simon & Schuster

New York London Toronto Sydney

SIMON & SCHUSTER
Rockefeller Center
1230 Avenue of the Americas
New York, NY 10020

Designed by Barbara Marks

10 9 8 7
Library of Congress Cataloging-in-Publication Data
On doctor[i]ng: stories, poems, essays / edited by Richard Reynolds and John Stone;
Lois LaCivita Nixon and Delese Wear, associate editors.—New, rev., and expanded
3rd ed.
    p. cm.
    on t.p. "[i]" appears as a caduceus.
    1. Physicians—Literary collections.   2. Medicine—Literary collections.
    I. Reynolds, Richard C., date.   II. Stone, John, date.   III. Nixon, Lois LaCivita.
    IV. Wear, Delese.
PN6071.P45 05 2001
808.8'0356—dc21   2001020817
ISBN 978-1-4516-2412-0
Permissions begin on page 405.

For Our Teachers:
Our Students, Our Colleagues, Our Patients

CONTENTS

CONTENTS

CONTENTS

9

CONTENTS

CONTENTS

INTRODUCTION

*It's the humdrum, day-in, day-out, everyday work that is the
real satisfaction of the practice of medicine; the million and a
half patients a man has seen on his daily visits over a forty-year
period of weekdays and Sundays that make up his life. I have
never had a money practice; it would have been impossible for
me. But the actual calling on people, at all times and under all
conditions, the coming to grips with the intimate conditions of
their lives, when they were being born, when they were dying,
watching them die, watching them get well when they were ill,
has always absorbed me.*

In these few sentences from William Carlos Williams's autobiography,
he has captured very well the human splendor of medicine. We have
tried to do the same in compiling this anthology, which contains stories, poems, essays, excerpts, and memoirs. In the process of caring
for their patients, physicians have a unique—and privileged—window
on the full range of human emotions. Literature, too, is rich in its de-
scriptions of individual illnesses and plagues, in its capacity to reveal
patients' reactions to illness and doctors' dilemmas in providing care.
In its own way, literature defines the medical profession and its fit in
the larger society. Legacies and traditions, which are an important
part of medicine, are often best manifested in the literature of a given
period of history. Many of our selections were written by physicians.
Williams and Anton Chekhov, W. Somerset Maugham and Lewis
Thomas are only a few of the physician-writers who have relied on
their medical backgrounds to help them understand better the frailties
and strengths, the wonderment of the human condition. Some carried
on a lifelong practice of medicine while simultaneously achieving
literary recognition. Dr. Williams is a fine example—his work, it
seems fair to say, changed the face of American poetry, even as he
carried on a large medical practice (he delivered over three thousand
babies, for example). Somerset Maugham, although he discontinued
his medical practice after internship, gave full credit to the experience
in his autobiographical *The Summing Up:* "I do not know a better
training for a writer than to spend some years in the medical profession." Others, so well known for their writing, were also trained in
the medicine of their day. It is not generally known, for example, that
the Romantic poet John Keats did a five-year apprenticeship with a

surgeon. During those years he delivered so many babies that he was not required to take obstetrics and gynecology during the hospital phase of his training.

Of course, one need not be trained in medicine in order to make cogent and crucial observations about what it is like to be sick, hence vulnerable; to witness and record the isolation and alienation that comes eventually to all of us—finally, we are all patients. Consider the poems of the late Jane Kenyon and her husband, Donald Hall. Their writings poignantly describe the time before their ultimate separation by her death, in 1995. Their poems are human documents without parallel. In his compelling short story "The Immortals," Jorge Luis Borges (also not a physician) comments trenchantly and presciently on some of the major ethical dilemmas of our time, those centering on organ transplants and utilization of scarce medical resources.

We have included many poems in this anthology. Poems recommend themselves to the editors of such a work because of their economy of form: in a few words a poem can communicate a complete experience. Read aloud Margaret Atwood's "The Woman Who Could Not Live with Her Faulty Heart." In its rhythms one can hear the heart, first regular, then skipping. Or listen to the courage embodied in James Dickey's "The Cancer Match." Read Emily Dickinson's short poems, which transcend time and place to speak to us in completely modern—and human—terms. And share with Patricia Goedicke (in "One More Time") the universal experience of having an X ray taken: "When the technician says breathe / I breathe."

Nor have we neglected the wisdom gathered in essays from major clinical figures and teachers over the years; hence, Lewis Thomas's "House Calls" is included. We begin this book, in fact, with just such an essay, one that impressed us from the first time we encountered it in the pages of the *New England Journal of Medicine:* Carola Eisenberg's "It Is Still a Privilege to Be a Doctor." The reader will find his or her own favorites among the many others we have included.

This third edition of *On Doctoring* provided us with the chance to add other voices to those previously included: remarkable writing from physician-writers Mikhail Bulgakov and Susan Onthank Mates, for example. Many writers new to this anthology are well known and widely published: Rainer Maria Rilke, Mary Oliver, Paul Zimmer, Donald Justice, Derek Mahon, and Jenny Joseph. We note with pride that our youngest author ever is included in these pages: Gregory Edwards was ten years old when he wrote his insightful—and humorous—poem called "The Shot."

Each one of us, of course, has a vast and vested interest in what goes on in the myriad arenas of medicine—and in the nature of the individual doctor-patient encounters explored within the pages of this book. This is all to the good: physicians and patients must continue to talk and listen together—and literature can help in that exchange. As editors, we are pleased to have had some part in this dialogue: prior editions of *On Doctoring* have had a combined readership of two hundred thousand.

Henry David Thoreau wrote, "To affect the quality of the day— that is the highest of arts." Both medicine and literature have the capacity to affect the quality of the human day. Resonances between these two disciplines offer us a unique view of the human condition that neither one alone can provide. Read. And enjoy.

The Editors

One of the essential qualities of the clinician is interest in humanity, for the secret of the care of the patient is in caring for the patient.

—FRANCES WELD PEABODY

(1881–1927)

CAROLA EISENBERG

CAROLA EISENBERG (1917–). *American physician and educator. Born in Buenos Aires, Argentina, Dr. Eisenberg received her M.D. from the University of Buenos Aires, then did graduate training in psychiatry at that city's Hospicio de Las Mercedes and at Johns Hopkins Hospital. She has taught both at Johns Hopkins and at Harvard Medical School and was dean for student affairs for six years at Massachusetts Institute of Technology and for twelve years at Harvard Medical School.*

IT IS STILL A PRIVILEGE TO BE A DOCTOR

I have been dean for student affairs at Harvard Medical School for eight years. It is my responsibility and privilege to listen to medical students and to support their personal and professional development. What they have been telling me this year troubles me. It is exemplified by a recent encounter with a third-year student.

The student was distressed. What had sustained him through the preclinical years was the anticipation of learning patient care. Now he had earned the right to wear a white coat and enter the wards. What he had encountered had discouraged him profoundly. The problem was not the work; that was as exciting as he had hoped it would be. It was his interaction with his teachers. Once the formal teaching rounds were over, they talked only about the problems they faced. For some, the talk was about the malpractice crisis, the freeze on Medicare fees, the impact of diagnosis-related groups, and shrinking incomes. For others, it was the endless paperwork in applying for research funding, the competition for the declining number of grants, and the uncertainties of sustaining a research career. Medicine, they said, was no fun anymore. If students were included in the conversations, the faculty reminisced about the good old days, which neither they nor the students would ever see. They wondered aloud whether they would choose medicine if they had it to do all over again.

I have heard perhaps a dozen similar stories from students doing clerkships at some of Boston's leading teaching hospitals. But the lamentations about the woes afflicting medicine are hardly limited to teaching faculty. Almost every week, and sometimes daily, one or the other of the media quotes practitioners who threaten to close their offices if they are not granted relief from what they consider onerous restrictions on their income or their right to practice freely. All this hits students hard because they are already worried about the indebtedness they are incurring, particularly in view of the stories about the doctor glut, declining incomes, and the increasing competition for residency positions. They fear that their debts will force them to choose specialties on the basis of anticipated earnings rather than intrinsic interest. Indeed, some, in the role of tutors for premedical students, have begun to dissuade the college students they advise from choosing medicine, because they consider the prospects to be so bleak.

How absurd! It stands the world on its head to suggest that the liabilities of a career in medicine outweigh the assets. Of course there are major problems in the delivery of medical care, and we ought to be in the vanguard of those seeking solutions to them. But to lose sight of just how lucky we are to have a profession in which we do well for ourselves by doing well for others reflects a puzzling loss of perspective. The satisfaction of being able to relieve pain and restore function, the intellectual challenge of solving clinical problems, and the variety of human issues we confront in daily clinical practice will remain the essence of doctoring, whatever the changes in the organizational and economic structure of medicine.

Although physicians' incomes may have declined in real dollars in the 1980s, they remain in the upper decile of all U.S. incomes. Although the practice of medicine may be increasingly vexed by bureaucratic constraints, doctors still retain a degree of autonomy in their clinical activities that is rarely found in other occupations. Although research support may not have kept up with inflation, the opportunities for young investigators in this country exceed those to be found anywhere else in the world and are several orders of magnitude greater than they were forty years ago.

Let us put first things first. Medicine is still a great profession, one held in high esteem by the majority of the public, despite the increase in malpractice suits. Our students look to us as role models for their careers. What we must make sure they learn from us are the personal gratifications medicine brings and the obligation to public service it entails. Of course there are reasons for concern when cost controls are emphasized to the detriment of clinical care, when the untoward outcomes inevitable even with the best medical practice lead to charges of malpractice, and when false economies jeopardize the very research that can improve those outcomes.

But if we are to reverse these trends, we must mobilize our natural allies—our patients and the public at large. It is they who have the greatest stake in the battle to preserve excellence in medical care. Cutbacks in Medicaid and Medicare threaten the health of the poor and the elderly—far more than they do physician incomes. Given the promise of basic research, which has paid off so handsomely in better medicine, cutbacks in federal support penalize the ill whose suffering would have been prevented by the new knowledge—far more than they do research careers. If we focus on our primary responsibility to serve as advocates for our patients, we will both maintain our professional integrity and provide the leadership for a broad public coalition in defense of health care. As long as we emphasize self-serving complaints—threats to *our* incomes and to *our* freedom to practice as we see fit—we will remain isolated and impotent.

As physicians, we have a moral imperative to sustain the highest aspirations of the students we teach. In taking this position, I do not mean to be a Pollyanna. Our students need to know about the problems facing medicine. But those problems need to be seen in perspective. Medical education does not exist to provide doctors with an opportunity to earn a living, but to improve the health of the public. Let us enlist our students in the campaign for equity and quality in medical care. If that campaign is to succeed, it will need the efforts of the best and the brightest.

What we do as doctors, most of the time, is deeply gratifying, whatever the mix of patient care, research, and teaching in our individual careers. I cannot imagine a more satisfying calling. Let us make sure our students hear that message from us.

JOHN DONNE

JOHN DONNE (1572–1631). *English poet and clergyman. Donne's poetry is noted for its wit and its often startling images, drawn from varied realms of human thought and activity—geography, astronomy, law, alchemy, scripture, and even everyday life. His sermons are characterized by rich complexity of thought and spirit and imbued with the intellectual daring and passionate ingenuity he is best remembered for. Donne's works include the* Songs and Sonnets *and the* Holy Sonnets *(both poetry),* Devotions upon Emergent Occasions *(prose meditations on his own serious illness, from which he recovered), and stunning, sometimes bawdy individual poems such as "A Valediction Forbidding Mourning," "A Fever," "The Sun Rising," "The Flea," and "Elegy: Going to Bed."*

DEATH, BE NOT PROUD

Death, be not proud, though some have callèd thee
Mighty and dreadful, for thou art not so;
For those whom thou think'st thou dost overthrow
Die not, poor Death, nor yet canst thou kill me.
From rest and sleep, which but thy pictures be,
Much pleasure—then, from thee much more must flow;
And soonest our best men with thee do go,
Rest of their bones and soul's delivery.
Thou'rt slave to fate, chance, kings and desperate men,
And dost with poison, war, and sickness dwell;
And poppy or charms can make us sleep as well,
And better than thy stroke. Why swell'st thou then?
One short sleep past, we wake eternally,
And death shall be no more. Death, thou shalt die.

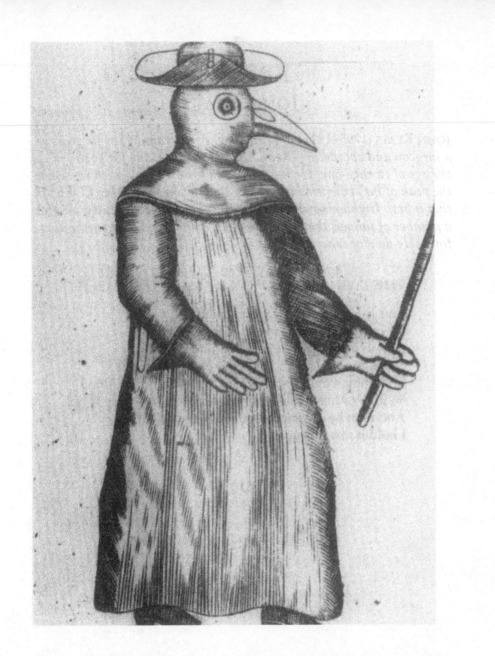

Seventeenth-century physicians caring for plague patients wore a strange, almost comical outfit that covered them completely. The gown was usually made of leather, as was the mask. The mask had glass windows over the eyes; its long beak was filled with antiseptics. In his gloved hand the plague doctor carried a wand to assess the pulse and to avoid direct contact.

JOHN KEATS

JOHN KEATS (1795–1821). *English poet. After training for six years as a surgeon and apothecary, Keats abandoned medicine for poetry at the age of twenty-one. He is best known for his odes, which represent the peak of his achievement; for "La Belle Dame Sans Merci," a work that is both frightening and magical in its apparent simplicity; and for a number of sonnets that mark him as a major Romantic poet in that form. He died of tuberculosis.*

THIS LIVING HAND, NOW WARM AND CAPABLE

This living hand, now warm and capable
Of earnest grasping, would, if it were cold
And in the icy silence of the tomb,
So haunt thy days and chill thy dreaming nights
That thou wouldst wish thine own heart dry of blood
So in my veins red life might stream again,
And thou be conscience-calmed—see here it is—
I hold it towards you.

OLIVER WENDELL HOLMES

OLIVER WENDELL HOLMES (1809–1894). *American physician, essayist, and poet. Holmes became the first dean of Harvard Medical School in 1842 and went on to become Parkman professor of anatomy and physiology there until his retirement, in 1882. He was a famous medical authority; his two important medical publications,* Homeopathy and Its Kindred Delusions *(1842) and* The Contagiousness of Puerperal Fever *(1843), were rivaled only by his frequent contributions to the* Atlantic Monthly, *which he helped found.*

Holmes's apparent delight in physiognomy is illustrated in such poetry as "The Living Temple" (1858), "La Griesette" (1863), and "The Stethoscope Song" (1849), given here.

THE STETHOSCOPE SONG,
A PROFESSIONAL BALLAD

There was a young man in Boston town,
    He bought him a *stethoscope* nice and new,
All mounted and finished and polished down,
    With an ivory cap and a stopper too.

It happened a spider within did crawl,
    And spun him a web of ample size,
Wherein there chanced one day to fall
    A couple of very imprudent flies.

Now being from Paris but recently,
    This fine young man would show his skill;
And so they gave him, his hand to try,
    A hospital patient extremely ill.

Then out his stethoscope he took,
    And on it placed his curious ear;
Mon Dieu! said he, with a knowing look,
    Why, here is a sound that's mighty queer!

There's *empyema* beyond a doubt;
    We'll plunge a *trocar* in his side.
The diagnosis was made out,—
    They tapped the patient; so he died.

Then six young damsels, slight and frail,
    Received this kind young doctor's cares;
They all were getting slim and pale,
    And short of breath on mounting stairs.

They all made rhymes with "sighs" and "skies,"
    And loathed their puddings and buttered rolls,
And dieted, much to their friends' surprise,
    On pickles and pencils and chalk and coals.

So fast their little hearts did bound,
    That frightened insects buzzed the more;
So over all their chests he found
    The *rale sifflant* and the *rale sonore.*

He shook his head. There's grave disease,—
    I greatly fear you all must die;
A slight *post-mortem,* if you please,
    Surviving friends would gratify.

The six young damsels wept aloud,
    Which so prevailed on six young men
That each his honest love avowed,
    Whereat they all got well again.

This poor young man was all aghast;
    The price of stethoscopes came down;
And so he was reduced at last
    To practice in a country town.

Now use your ears, all that you can,
    But don't forget to mind your eyes.
Or you may be cheated, like this young man.
    By a couple of silly, abnormal flies.

EMILY DICKINSON

EMILY DICKINSON (1830–1886). *American poet. Reclusive and idiosyncratic, Dickinson lived a retiring small-town life in Amherst, Massachusetts, where she composed more than seventeen hundred poems, only a few of which were published in her lifetime. Like her poems, her letters are illuminated by startlingly fresh imagery and intensely heartbreaking insights. Dickinson's voice is vigorous, direct, and wise with introspection; she is widely celebrated as one of America's greatest poets.*

THERE'S BEEN A DEATH

There's been a Death, in the Opposite House,
As lately as Today—
I know it, by the numb look
Such Houses have—alway—

The Neighbors rustle in and out—
The Doctor—drives away—
A Window opens like a Pod—
Abrupt—mechanically—

Somebody flings a Mattress out—
The Children hurry by—
They wonder if it died—on that—
I used to—when a Boy—

The Minister—goes stiffly in—
As if the House were His—
And He owned all the Mourners—now—
And little Boys—besides—

And then the Milliner—and the Man
Of the Appalling Trade—
To take the measure of the House—

There'll be that Dark Parade—

Of Tassels—and of Coaches—soon—
It's easy as a Sign—
The Intuition of the News—
In just a Country Town—

SURGEONS MUST BE VERY CAREFUL

Surgeons must be very careful
When they take the knife!
Underneath their fine incisions
Stirs the Culprit—*Life!*

I HEARD A FLY BUZZ

I heard a Fly buzz—when I died—
The Stillness in the Room
Was like the Stillness in the Air—
Between the Heaves of Storm—

The Eyes around—had wrung them dry—
And Breaths were gathering firm
For that last Onset—when the King
Be witnessed—in the Room—

I willed my Keepsakes—Signed away
What portion of me be
Assignable—and then it was
There interposed a Fly—

With Blue—uncertain stumbling Buzz—
Between the light—and me—
And then the Windows failed—and then
I could not see to see—

"HOPE" IS THE THING WITH FEATHERS

"Hope" is the thing with feathers—
That perches in the soul—
And sings the tune without the words—
And never stops—at all—

And sweetest—in the Gale—is heard—
And sore must be the storm—
That could abash the little Bird
That kept so many warm—

I've heard it in the chillest land—
And on the strangest Sea—
Yet, never, in Extremity,
It asked a crumb—of Me.

TELL ALL THE TRUTH

Tell all the Truth but tell it slant—
Success in Circuit lies
Too bright for our infirm Delight
The Truth's superb surprise

As Lightning to the Children eased
With explanation kind
The Truth must dazzle gradually
Or every man be blind—

BECAUSE I COULD NOT STOP FOR DEATH

Because I could not stop for Death—
He kindly stopped for me—
The Carriage held but just Ourselves—
And Immortality.

We slowly drove—He knew no haste
And I had put away
My labor and my leisure too,
For His Civility—

We passed the School, where Children strove
At Recess—in the Ring—
We passed the Fields of Gazing Grain—
We passed the Setting Sun—

Or rather—He passed Us—
The Dews drew quivering and chill—
For only Gossamer, my Gown—
My Tippet—only Tulle—

We paused before a House that seemed
A Swelling of the Ground—
The Roof was scarcely visible—
The Cornice—in the Ground—

Since then—'tis Centuries—and yet
Feels shorter than the Day
I first surmised the Horses' Heads
Were toward Eternity—

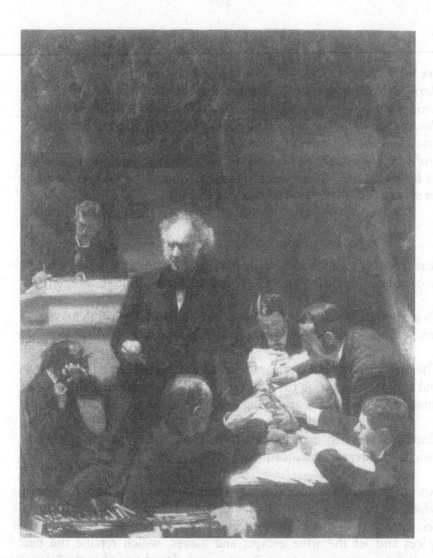

The Gross Clinic (1875) by Thomas Eakins. The American surgeon Samuel Gross, pictured here, did not believe in Lister's principles of antisepsis for the operating room. The surgeons wore no gowns or masks. A relative of the patient's, seated at the left, covers his face in dismay.

SIR WILLIAM OSLER

SIR WILLIAM OSLER (1849–1919). *Physician, writer, and educator. Born in Ontario, Canada, Osler received his M.D. from McGill University in Montreal. His career led him first to the University of Pennsylvania, then to the young Johns Hopkins University, where he organized the department of medicine. In 1904, he became Regius professor of medicine at Oxford University. Osler wrote extensively on both medical and nonmedical subjects, and had a great influence on medical education in America and England.*

APHORISMS

It is astonishing with how little reading a doctor can practice medicine, but it is not astonishing how badly he may do it.

To study the phenomena of disease without books is to sail an uncharted sea, while to study books without patients is not to go to sea at all.

The physician needs a clear head and a kind heart; his work is arduous and complex, requiring the exercise of the very highest faculties of the mind, while constantly appealing to the emotions and higher feelings.

Common sense in matters medical is rare, and is usually in inverse ratio to the degree of education.

An old writer says that there are four sorts of readers: "Sponges, which attract all without distinguishing; Howre-glasses, which receive and powre out as fast; Bagges, which retain the dregges of the spices and let the wine escape; and Sieves, which retaine the best onely." A man wastes a great many years before he reaches the "sieve" stage.

He who knows not, and knows not that he knows not, is a fool. Shun him.

He who knows not, and knows that he knows not, is simple. Teach him.

Professors may be divided into four classes. There is, first, the man who can think, but who has neither tongue nor technique. Though useless for the ordinary student, he may be the leaven of a faculty and the chief glory of his University. A second variety is the phonographic professor, who can talk, but who can neither think nor work. Under the old regime he repeated year by year the same lecture. A third is the man who has technique, but who can neither talk nor think; and a fourth is the rare professor who can do all three, think, talk, and work.

While medicine is to be your vocation or calling, see to it that you have also an avocation—some intellectual pastime which may serve to keep you in touch with the world of art, of science, or of letters. Begin at once the cultivation of some interest other than the purely professional. The difficulty is in a selection and the choice will be different according to your tastes and training. No matter what it is, have an outside hobby. For the hard-working medical student it is easier perhaps to keep up an interest in literature. Let each subject in your year's work have a corresponding outside author. When tired of anatomy refresh your minds with Oliver Wendell Holmes; after a worrying subject in physiology, turn to the great idealists, to Shelley or to Keats, for consolation; when chemistry distresses your soul, seek peace in the great pacifier, Shakespeare; ten minutes with Montaigne will lighten the burden.

No man is really happy or safe without a hobby, and it makes precious little difference what the outside interest may be—botany, beetles or butterflies, roses, tulips or irises: fishing, mountaineering or antiquities—anything will do so long as he straddles a hobby and rides it hard.

And, for the sake of what it brings, the grace of humility is a precious gift. When to the sessions of sweet silent thought you summon up the remembrance of your own imperfections, the faults of your brothers will seem less grievous, and in the quaint language of Sir Thomas Browne, you will "allow one eye for what is laudable in them."

The battle against polypharmacy, or the use of a large number of drugs (of the action of which we know little, yet we put them into bodies of the action of which we know less), has not been brought to a finish.

But know also, man has an inborn craving for medicine. Heroic dosing for several generations has given his tissues a thirst for drugs. As I once before remarked, the desire to take medicine is one feature which distinguishes man, the animal, from his fellow creatures. It is really one of the most serious difficulties with which we have to contend. Even in minor ailments, which would yield to dieting or to simple home remedies, the doctor's visit is not thought to be complete without the prescription.

Nothing will sustain you more potently in your humdrum routine, as perhaps it may be thought, than the power to recognize the true poetry of life—the poetry of the commonplace, of the ordinary man, of the plain, toil-worn woman, with their loves and their joys, their sorrows and their griefs.

It is a common error to think that the more a doctor sees the greater his experience and the more he knows. No one ever drew a more skillful distinction than Cowper in his oft-quoted lines, which I am never tired of repeating in a medical audience:

> "Knowledge and wisdom, far from being one,
> Have oft-times no connexion. Knowledge dwells
> In heads replete with thoughts of other men;
> Wisdom in minds attentive to their own.
> Knowledge is proud that he has learned so much;
> Wisdom is humble that he knows no more."

I wish I had time to speak of the value of note-taking. You can do nothing as a student in practice without it. Carry a small notebook which will fit into your waistcoat pocket, and never ask a new patient a question without notebook and pencil in hand.

For better or worse, there are few occupations of a more satisfying character than the practice of medicine, if a man can but once get *orientirt* and bring to it the philosophy of honest work, the philosophy that insists that we are here, not to get all we can out of life about us, but to see how much we can add to it. The discontent and grumblings which one hears have their source in the man more often than in the environment.

I have three personal ideals. One, to do the day's work well and not to bother about tomorrow . . . The second ideal has been to act the

Golden Rule, as far as in me lay, toward my professional brethren and toward the patients committed to my care. And the third has been to cultivate such a measure of equanimity as would enable me to bear success with humility, the affection of my friends without pride, and to be ready when the day of sorrow and grief came to meet it with the courage befitting a man.

The practice of medicine is an art, based on science.

Nothing in life is more wonderful than faith—the one great moving force which we can neither weigh in the balance nor test in the crucible.

Remember how much you do not know. Do not pour strange medicines into your patients.

In the physician or surgeon no quality takes rank with imperturbability.

Silence is a powerful weapon.

Medicine is learned by the bedside and not in the classroom.

Education is a lifelong process, in which the student can make only a beginning during his college course.

Undoubtedly the student tries to learn too much, and we teachers try to teach him too much—neither, perhaps, with great success.

Though a little one, the master-word looms large in meaning. It is the "Open Sesame" to every portal, the great equalizer in the world, the true philosopher's stone which transmutes all the base metals of humanity into gold. The stupid man among you it will make bright, the bright man brilliant, and the brilliant student steady. With the magic word in your heart, all things are possible, and without it all study is vanity and vexation. . . . And the master-word is WORK.

I desire no other epitaph than the statement that I taught medical students in the wards, as I regard this by far the most useful and important work I have been called upon to do.

ANTON CHEKHOV

ANTON CHEKHOV (1860–1904). *Russian playwright and fiction writer. Trained as a physician, Chekhov published many stories while still in medical school. His first collection,* The Fairy Tales of Melpomene, *was published in 1884, the year he got his degree. The second,* Motley Tales *(1886), brought him wide recognition, and soon after he was regarded as one of the great exponents of realism in Russian literature. Chekhov is considered one of the great modern dramatists, in large part for his acclaimed plays* The Sea Gull *(1896),* Uncle Vanya *(1899),* The Three Sisters *(1901), and* The Cherry Orchard *(1904); his hundreds of short stories and novellas have also established him as one of the great fiction writers of all time.*

MISERY
"To whom shall I tell my grief?"

The twilight of evening. Big flakes of wet snow are whirling lazily about the street lamps, which have just been lighted, and lying in a thin soft layer on roofs, horses' backs, shoulders, caps. Iona Potapov, the sledge-driver, is all white like a ghost. He sits on the box without stirring, bent as double as the living body can be bent. If a regular snowdrift fell on him it seems as though even then he would not think it necessary to shake it off.... His little mare is white and motionless too. Her stillness, the angularity of her lines, and the stick-like straightness of her legs make her look like a halfpenny gingerbread horse. She is probably lost in thought. Anyone who has been torn away from the plough, from the familiar gray landscapes, and cast into this slough, full of monstrous lights, of unceasing uproar and hurrying people, is bound to think.

It is a long time since Iona and his nag have budged. They came out of the yard before dinner-time and not a single fare yet. But now the shades of evening are falling on the town. The pale light of the street lamps changes to a vivid color, and the bustle of the street grows noisier.

"Sledge to Vyborgskaya!" Iona hears. "Sledge!"

Iona starts, and through his snow-plastered eyelashes sees an officer in a military overcoat with a hood over his head.

"To Vyborgskaya," repeats the officer. "Are you asleep? To Vyborgskaya!"

In token of assent Iona gives a tug at the reins which sends cakes of snow flying from the horse's back and shoulders. The officer gets into the sledge. The sledge-driver clicks to the horse, cranes his neck like a swan, rises in his seat, and more from habit than necessity brandishes his whip. The mare cranes her neck, too, crooks her stick-like legs, and hesitatingly sets off. . . .

"Where are you shoving, you devil?" Iona immediately hears shouts from the dark mass shifting to and fro before him. "Where the devil are you going? Keep to the r-right!"

"You don't know how to drive! Keep to the right," says the officer angrily.

A coachman driving a carriage swears at him; a pedestrian crossing the road and brushing the horse's nose with his shoulder looks at him angrily and shakes the snow off his sleeve. Iona fidgets on the box as though he were sitting on thorns, jerks his elbows, and turns his eyes about like one possessed, as though he did not know where he was or why he was there.

"What rascals they all are!" says the officer jocosely. "They are simply doing their best to run up against you or fall under the horse's feet. They must be doing it on purpose."

Iona looks at his fare and moves his lips. . . . Apparently he means to say something, but nothing comes but a sniff.

"What?" inquires the officer.

Iona gives a wry smile, and straining his throat, brings out huskily: "My son . . . er . . . my son died this week, sir."

"H'm! What did he die of?"

Iona turns his whole body round to his fare, and says:

"Who can tell! It must have been from fever. . . . He lay three days in the hospital and then he died. . . . God's will."

"Turn round, you devil!" comes out of the darkness. "Have you gone cracked, you old dog? Look where you are going!"

"Drive on! drive on! . . ." says the officer. "We shan't get there till to-morrow going on like this. Hurry up!"

The sledge-driver cranes his neck again, rises in his seat, and with heavy grace swings his whip. Several times he looks round at the officer, but the latter keeps his eyes shut and is apparently disinclined to listen. Putting his fare down at Vyborgskaya, Iona stops by a restaurant, and again sits huddled up on the box. . . . Again the wet snow paints him and his horse white. One hour passes, and then another. . . .

Three young men, two tall and thin, one short and hunchbacked, come up, railing at each other and loudly stamping on the pavement with their galoshes.

"Cabby, to the Police Bridge!" the hunchback cries in a cracked voice. "The three of us, ... twenty kopecks!"

Iona tugs at the reins and clicks to his horse. Twenty kopecks is not a fair price, but he has no thoughts for that. Whether it is a rouble or whether it is five kopecks does not matter to him now so long as he has a fare. . . . The three young men, shoving each other and using bad language, go up to the sledge, and all three try to sit down at once. The question remains to be settled: Which are to sit down and which one is to stand? After a long altercation, ill-temper, and abuse, they come to the conclusion that the hunchback must stand because he is the shortest.

"Well, drive on," says the hunchback in his cracked voice, settling himself and breathing down Iona's neck. "Cut along! What a cap you've got, my friend! You wouldn't find a worse one in all Petersburg. . . ."

"He-he! . . . he-he! . . ." laughs Iona. "It's nothing to boast of!"

"Well, then, nothing to boast of, drive on! Are you going to drive like this all the way? Eh? Shall I give you one in the neck?"

"My head aches," says one of the tall ones. "At the Dukmasovs' yesterday Vaska and I drank four bottles of brandy between us."

"I can't make out why you talk such stuff," says the other tall one angrily. "You lie like a brute."

"Strike me dead, it's the truth! . . ."

"It's about as true as that a louse coughs."

"He-he!" grins Iona. "Me-er-ry gentlemen!"

"Tfoo! the devil take you!" cries the hunchback indignantly. "Will you get on, you old plague, or won't you? Is that the way to drive? Give her one with the whip. Hang it all, give it her well."

Iona feels behind his back the jolting person and quivering voice of the hunchback. He hears abuse addressed to him, he sees people, and the feeling of loneliness begins little by little to be less heavy on his heart. The hunchback swears at him, till he chokes over some elaborately whimsical string of epithets and is overpowered by his cough. His tall companions begin talking of a certain Nadyezhda Petrovna. Iona looks round at them. Waiting till there is a brief pause, he looks round once more and says:

"This week . . . er . . . my . . . er . . . son died!"

"We shall all die, . . ." says the hunchback with a sigh, wiping his lips after coughing. "Come, drive on! drive on! My friends, I simply cannot stand crawling like this! When will he get us there?"

"Well, you give him a little encouragement . . . one in the neck!"

"Do you hear, you old plague? I'll make you smart. If one stands on ceremony with fellows like you one may as well walk. Do you hear, you old dragon? Or don't you care a hang what we say?"

And Iona hears rather than feels a slap on the back of his neck.

"He-he! . . ." he laughs. "Merry gentlemen. . . . God give you health!"

"Cabman, are you married?" asks one of the tall ones.

"I? He-he! Me-er-ry gentlemen. The only wife for me now is the damp earth. . . . He-ho-ho! . . . The grave that is! . . . Here my son's dead and I am alive. . . . It's a strange thing, death has come in at the wrong door. . . . Instead of coming for me it went for my son. . . ."

And Iona turns round to tell them how his son died, but at that point the hunchback gives a faint sigh and announces that, thank God! they have arrived at last. After taking his twenty kopecks, Iona gazes for a long while after the revelers, who disappear into a dark entry. Again he is alone and again there is silence for him. . . . The misery which has been for a brief space eased comes back again and tears his heart more cruelly than ever. With a look of anxiety and suffering Iona's eyes stray restlessly among the crowds moving to and fro on both sides of the street: can he not find among those thousands someone who will listen to him? But the crowds flit by heedless of him and his misery. . . . His misery is immense, beyond all bounds. If Iona's heart were to burst and his misery to flow out, it would flood the whole world, it seems, but yet it is not seen. It has found a hiding-place in such an insignificant shell that one would not have found it with a candle by daylight. . . .

Iona sees a house-porter with a parcel and makes up his mind to address him.

"What time will it be, friend?" he asks.

"Going on for ten. . . . Why have you stopped here? Drive on!"

Iona drives a few paces away, bends himself double, and gives himself up to his misery. He feels it is no good to appeal to people. But before five minutes have passed he draws himself up, shakes his head as though he feels a sharp pain, and tugs at the reins. . . . He can bear it no longer.

"Back to the yard!" he thinks. "To the yard!"

And his little mare, as though she knew his thoughts, falls to trotting. An hour and a half later Iona is sitting by a big dirty stove. On the stove, on the floor, and on the benches are people snoring. The air is full of smells and stuffiness. Iona looks at the sleeping figures, scratches himself, and regrets that he has come home so early. . . .

"I have not earned enough to pay for the oats, even," he thinks. "That's why I am so miserable. A man who knows how to do his work, . . . who has had enough to eat, and whose horse has had enough to eat, is always at ease. . . ."

In one of the corners a young cabman gets up, clears his throat sleepily, and makes for the water-bucket.

"Want a drink?" Iona asks him.

"Seems so."

"May it do you good. . . . But my son is dead, mate. . . . Do you hear? This week in the hospital. . . . It's queer business. . . ."

Iona looks to see the effect produced by his words, but he sees nothing. The young man has covered his head over and is already asleep. The old man sighs and scratches himself. . . . Just as the young man had been thirsty for water, he thirsts for speech. His son will soon have been dead a week, and he has not really talked to anybody yet. . . . He wants to talk of it properly, with deliberation. . . . He wants to tell how his son was taken ill, how he suffered, what he said before he died, how he died. . . . He wants to describe the funeral, and how he went to the hospital to get his son's clothes. He still has his daughter Anisya in the country. . . . And he wants to talk about her too. . . . Yes, he has plenty to talk about now. His listener ought to sigh and exclaim and lament. . . . It would be even better to talk to women. Though they are silly creatures, they blubber at the first word.

"Let's go out and have a look at the mare," Iona thinks. "There is always time for sleep. . . . You'll have sleep enough, no fear. . . ."

He puts on his coat and goes into the stables where his mare is standing. He thinks about oats, about hay, about the weather. . . . He cannot think about his son when he is alone. . . . To talk about him with someone is possible, but to think of him and picture him is insufferable anguish. . . .

"Are you munching?" Iona asks his mare, seeing her shining eyes. "There, munch away, munch away. . . . Since we have not earned enough for oats, we will eat hay. . . . Yes, . . . I have grown too old to drive. . . . My son ought to be driving, not I. . . . He was a real cabman. . . . He ought to have lived. . . ."

Iona is silent for a while, and then he goes on:

"That's how it is, old girl. . . . Kuzma Ionitch is gone. . . . He said good-bye to me. . . . He went and died for no reason. . . . Now, suppose you had a little colt, and you were mother to that little colt. . . . And all at once that same little colt went and died. . . . You'd be sorry, wouldn't you? . . ."

The little mare munches, listens, and breathes on her master's hands. Iona is carried away and tells her all about it.

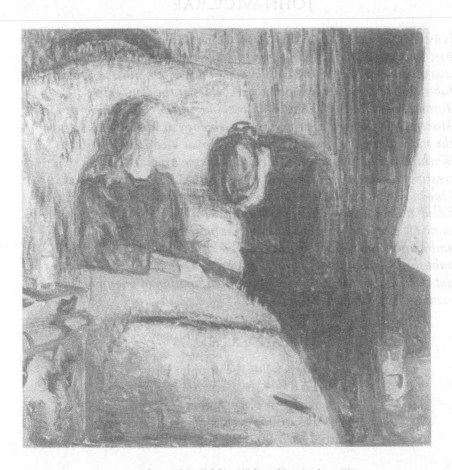

The Sick Child by Edvard Munch.

John McCrae

John McCrae (1872–1918). *Canadian physician, poet. One of the best-known poems to spring from the terrible losses of World War I was written by this prominent Canadian physician. Born in Ontario, John McCrae completed his medical studies at the University of Toronto, then took a fellowship in pathology at McGill University, in Montreal. He served as professor of pathology at McGill and was on the staffs of the Montreal General and Royal Victoria hospitals. As World War I began, in 1914, McCrae became brigade surgeon, treating the countless wounded, even serving on the guns as needed. One of his former students at McGill, Lieutenant Alexis Helmer, was killed at the battle of Ypres on May 2, 1915. The next day, McCrae came off duty early in the morning, sat on the step of a field ambulance, and wrote "In Flanders Fields." It was originally published (anonymously at first) in* Punch. *Dr. McCrae himself did not survive the war, succumbing to a combination of pneumonia and meningitis in January 1918.*

IN FLANDERS FIELDS

In Flanders fields the poppies blow
Between the crosses, row on row,
That mark our place; and in the sky
The larks, still bravely singing, fly
Scarce heard amid the guns below.

We are the Dead. Short days ago
We lived, felt dawn, saw sunset glow,
Loved, and were loved, and now we lie
In Flanders fields.

Take up our quarrel with the foe:
To you from failing hands we throw
The torch; be yours to hold it high.
If ye break faith with us who die
We shall not sleep, though poppies grow
In Flanders fields.

ROBERT FROST

ROBERT FROST (1874–1963). *American poet. Born in California, Frost studied first at Dartmouth College, then for two years at Harvard before abandoning formal education in 1900 to farm and teach in New Hampshire. In 1912, he and his family moved to England, where his first two collections of poetry were published:* A Boy's Will *(1913) and* North of Boston *(1914). Both were quickly republished in the United States; in 1915, Frost returned home to New Hampshire— and to critical acclaim which never abated. He became the most popular of poets, a sought-after speaker, and one of the great teachers and talkers of his age. Over the years, Frost won four Pulitzer Prizes for his work.*

"OUT, OUT—"

The buzz saw snarled and rattled in the yard
And made dust and dropped stove-length sticks of wood,
Sweet-scented stuff when the breeze drew across it.
And from there those that lifted eyes could count
Five mountain ranges one behind the other
Under the sunset far into Vermont.
And the saw snarled and rattled, snarled and rattled,
As it ran light, or had to bear a load.
And nothing happened: day was all but done.
Call it a day, I wish they might have said
To please the boy by giving him the half hour
That a boy counts so much when saved from work.
His sister stood beside them in her apron
To tell them "Supper." At the word, the saw,
As if to prove saws knew what supper meant,
Leaped out at the boy's hand, or seemed to leap—
He must have given the hand. However it was,
Neither refused the meeting. But the hand!
The boy's first outcry was a rueful laugh,
As he swung toward them holding up the hand,
Half in appeal, but half as if to keep
The life from spilling. Then the boy saw all—
Since he was old enough to know, big boy
Doing a man's work, though a child at heart—

He saw all spoiled. "Don't let him cut my hand off—
The doctor, when he comes. Don't let him, sister!"
So. But the hand was gone already.
The doctor put him in the dark of ether.
He lay and puffed his lips out with his breath.
And then—the watcher at his pulse took fright.
No one believed. They listened at his heart.
Little—less—nothing!—and that ended it.
No more to build on there. And they, since they
Were not the one dead, turned to their affairs.

W. SOMERSET MAUGHAM

W. SOMERSET MAUGHAM (1874–1965). *English novelist, short story writer, and playwright. Maugham was trained as a physician at St. Thomas's Hospital in London (where, seventy-five years earlier, John Keats was trained). He wrote more than sixty books, including the autobiographical novel* Of Human Bondage *(1915);* The Moon and Sixpence *(1919), based on the life of Paul Gauguin;* The Summing Up *(1938); and* A Writer's Notebook *(1949), a collection of personal reminiscences reflecting both his skepticism and his philosophy of life.*

Excerpt from THE SUMMING UP

I do not know a better training for a writer than to spend some years in the medical profession. I suppose that you can learn a good deal about human nature in a solicitor's office; but there on the whole you have to deal with men in full control of themselves. They lie perhaps as much as they lie to the doctor, but they lie more consistently, and it may be that for the solicitor it is not so necessary to know the truth. The interests he deals with, besides, are usually material. He sees human nature from a specialized standpoint. But the doctor, especially the hospital doctor, sees it bare. Reticences can generally be undermined; very often there are none. Fear for the most part will shatter every defence; even vanity is unnerved by it. Most people have a furious itch to talk about themselves and are restrained only by the disinclination of others to listen. Reserve is an artificial quality that is developed in most of us but as the result of innumerable rebuffs. The doctor is discreet. It is his business to listen and no details are too intimate for his ears.

But of course human nature may be displayed before you and if you have not the eyes to see you will learn nothing. If you are hidebound with prejudice, if your temper is sentimental, you can go through the wards of a hospital and be as ignorant of man at the end as you were at the beginning. If you want to get any benefit from such an experience you must have an open mind and an interest in human beings. I look upon myself as very fortunate in that though I have never much liked men I have found them so interesting that I am almost incapable of being bored by them. I do not particularly want to talk and I am very willing to listen. I do not care if people are interested in me or not. I have no desire to impart any knowledge I have to others nor do I feel the need to correct them if they are wrong. You can get a great deal of entertainment out of tedious people if you keep your head. I remember being taken for a drive in a foreign country by a kind lady who wanted to show me round. Her conversation was composed entirely of truisms and she had so large a vocabulary of hackneyed phrases that I despaired of remembering them. But one remark she made has stuck in my memory as have few witticisms; we passed a row of little houses by the sea and she said to me: "Those are week-end bungalows, if you understand what I mean; in other words they're bungalows that people go to on Saturdays and leave on Mondays." I should have been sorry to miss that.

I do not want to spend too long a time with boring people, but then I do not want to spend too long a time with amusing ones. I find social intercourse fatiguing. Most persons, I think, are both exhilarated and rested by conversation; to me it has always been an effort. When I was young and stammered, to talk for long singularly exhausted me, and even now that I have to some extent cured myself, it is a strain. It is a relief to me when I can get away and read a book.

I would not claim for a moment that those years I spent at St. Thomas's Hospital gave me a complete knowledge of human nature. I do not suppose anyone can hope to have that. I have been studying it, consciously and subconsciously, for forty years and I still find men unaccountable; people I know intimately can surprise me by some action of which I never thought them capable or by the discovery of some trait exhibit a side of themselves that I never even suspected. It is possible that my training gave me a warped view, for at St. Thomas's the persons I came in contact with were for the most part sick and poor and ill-educated. I have tried to guard against this. I have tried also to guard against my own prepossessions. I have no natural trust in others. I am more inclined to expect them to do ill than to do good. This is the price one has to pay for having a sense of humour. A sense of humour leads you to take pleasure in the discrepancies of human nature; it leads you to mistrust great professions and look for the unworthy motive that they conceal; the disparity between appearance and reality diverts you and you are apt when you cannot find it to create it. You tend to close your eyes to truth, beauty and goodness because they give no scope to your sense of the ridiculous. The humorist has a quick eye for the humbug; he does not always recognize the saint. But if to see men one-sidedly is a heavy price to pay for a sense of humour there is a compensation that has a value too. You are not angry with people when you laugh at them. Humour teaches tolerance, and the humorist, with a smile and perhaps a sigh, is more likely to shrug his shoulders than to condemn. He does not moralize, he is content to understand; and it is true that to understand is to pity and forgive.

But I must admit that, with these reservations that I have tried always to remember, the experience of all the years that have followed has only confirmed the observations on human nature that I made, not deliberately, for I was too young, but unconsciously, in the out-patients' departments and in the wards of St. Thomas's Hospital. I have seen men since as I saw them then, and thus have I drawn them. It may not be a true picture and I know that many have thought it an unpleasant one. It is doubtless partial, for naturally I have seen men through my own idiosyncrasies. A buoyant, optimistic, healthy and sentimental person would have seen the same people quite differently. I can only claim to have seen them coherently. Many writers seem to me not to observe at all, but to create their characters in stock sizes from images in their own fancy. They are like draughtsmen who draw their figures from recollections of the antique and have never attempted to draw from the living model. At their best they can only give living shape to the fantasies of their own minds. If their minds are noble they can give you noble figures and perhaps it does not matter if they lack the infinite complication of common life.

I have always worked from the living model. I remember that once in the dissecting room when I was going over my "part" with the demonstrator, he asked me what some nerve was and I did not know. He told me; whereupon I remonstrated, for it was in the wrong place. Nevertheless he insisted that it was the nerve I had been in vain look-ing for. I complained of the abnormality and he, smiling, said that in anatomy it was the normal that was uncommon. I was only annoyed at the time, but the remark sank into my mind and since then it has been forced upon me that it was true of man as well as of anatomy. The normal is what you find but rarely. The normal is an ideal. It is a picture that one fabricates of the average characteristics of men, and to find them all in a single man is hardly to be expected. It is this false picture that the writers I have spoke of take as their model and it is because they describe what is so exceptional that they seldom achieve the effect of life. Selfishness and kindliness, idealism and sensuality, vanity, shyness, disinterestedness, courage, laziness, nervousness, obstinacy, and diffidence, they can all exist in a single person and form a plausible harmony. It has taken a long time to persuade readers of the truth of this.

I do not suppose men in past centuries were any different from the men we know, but they must surely have appeared to their contemporaries more of a piece than they do to us now, or writers would not have thus represented them. It seemed reasonable to describe every man in his humour. The miser was nothing but miserly, the fop foppish, and the glutton gluttonous. It never occurred to anyone that the miser might be foppish and gluttonous; and yet we see constantly people who are; still less, that he might be an honest and upright man with a disinterested zeal for public service and a genuine passion for art. When novelists began to disclose the diversity that they had found in themselves or seen in others they were accused of maligning the human race. So far as I know the first novelist who did this with deliberate intention was Stendhal in *Le Rouge et le Noir*. Contemporary criticism was outraged. Even Sainte-Beuve, who needed only to look into his own heart to discover what contrary qualities could exist side by side in some kind of harmony, took him to task. Julien Sorel is one of the most interesting characters that a novelist has ever created. I do not think that Stendhal has succeeded in making him entirely plausible, but that, I believe, is due to causes that I shall mention in another part of this book. For the first three quarters of the novel he is perfectly consistent. Sometimes he fills you with horror; sometimes he is entirely sympathetic; but he has an inner coherence, so that though you often shudder you accept.

But it was long before Stendhal's example bore fruit. Balzac, with all his genius, drew his characters after the old models. He gave them his own immense vitality so that you accept them as real; but in fact they are humours as definitely as are the characters of old comedy. His people are unforgettable, but they are seen from the standpoint of the ruling passion that affected those with whom they were brought in contact. I suppose it is a natural prepossession of mankind to take people as though they were homogeneous. It is evidently less trouble to make up one's mind about a man one way or the other and dismiss suspense with the phrase, he's one of the best or he's a dirty dog. It is disconcerting to find that the saviour of his country may be stingy or that the poet who has opened new horizons to our consciousness may be a snob. Our natural egoism leads us to judge people by their relations to ourselves. We want them to be certain things to us, and for us that is what they are; because the rest of them is no good to us, we ignore it.

These reasons perhaps explain why there is so great a disinclination to accept the attempts to portray man with his incongruous and diverse qualities and why people turn away with dismay when candid biographers reveal the truth about famous persons. It is distressing to think that the composer of the quintet in the *Meistersinger* was dishonest in money matters and treacherous to those who had benefited him. But it may be that he could not have had great qualities if he had not also had great failings. I do not believe they are right who say that the defects of famous men should be ignored; I think it is better that we should know them. Then, though we are conscious of having faults as glaring as theirs, we can believe that that is no hindrance to our achieving also something of their virtues.

Besides teaching me something about human nature my training in a medical school furnished me with an elementary knowledge of science and scientific method. Till then I had been concerned only with art and literature. It was a very limited knowledge, for the demands of the curriculum at that time were small, but at all events it showed me the road that led to a region of which I was completely ignorant. I grew familiar with certain principles. The scientific world of which I thus obtained a cursory glimpse was rigidly materialistic and because its conceptions coincided with my own prepossessions I embraced them with alacrity; "For men," as Pope observed, "let them say what they will, never approve any other's sense, but as it squares with their own." I was glad to learn that the mind of man (himself the product of natural causes) was a function of the brain subject like the rest of his body to the laws of cause and effect and that these laws were the same as those that governed the movements of star and atom. I exulted at the thought that the universe was no more than a vast machine in which every event was determined by a preceding event so that nothing could be other than it was. These conceptions not only appealed to my dramatic instinct; they filled me besides with a very delectable sense of liberation. With the ferocity of youth I welcomed the hypothesis of the Survival of the Fittest. It gave me much satisfaction to learn that the earth was a speck of mud whirling round a second-rate star which was gradually cooling; and that evolution, which had produced man, would by forcing him to adapt himself to his environment deprive him of all the qualities he had acquired but those that were necessary to enable him to combat the increasing cold till at last the planet, an icy cinder, would no longer support even a vestige of life. I believed that we were wretched puppets at the mercy of a ruthless fate; and that, bound by the inexorable laws of nature, we were doomed to take part in the ceaseless struggle for existence with nothing to look forward to but inevitable defeat. I learnt that men were moved by a savage egoism, that love was only the dirty trick nature played on us to achieve the continuation of the species, and I decided that, whatever aims men set themselves, they were deluded, for it was impossible for them to aim at anything but their own selfish pleasures. When once I happened to do a friend a good turn (for what reasons, since I knew that all our actions were purely selfish, I did not stop to think) and wanting to show his gratitude (which of course he had no business to feel, for my apparent kindness was rigidly determined) he asked me what I would like as a present, I answered without hesitation Herbert Spencer's *First Principles.* I read it with complacency. But I was impatient of Spencer's maudlin belief in progress: the world I knew was going from bad to worse and I was as pleased as Punch at the thought of my remote descendants, having long forgotten art and science and handicraft, cowering skin-clad in caverns as they watched the approach of the cold and eternal night. I was violently pessimistic. All the same, having abundant vitality, I was getting on the whole a lot of fun out of life. I was ambitious to make a name for myself as a writer. I exposed myself to every vicissitude that seemed to offer a chance of gaining the greater experience that I wanted and I read everything I could lay my hands on.

RAINER MARIA RILKE

RAINER MARIA RILKE (1875–1926). German poet. One of the most important figures in European literature. Born in Prague, Bohemia, he was the only son of a couple who divorced when he was still a child. Sent to boarding school, then military school, he began writing poetry early and published his first book in 1894. He traveled widely: Munich, Berlin, Russia (where he met Tolstoy), Bremen, Trieste, Paris (where he wrote a book about the sculptor Auguste Rodin), Italy, Switzerland, and Austria. His most famous works include the Duino Elegies *and the* Sonnets to Orpheus. *His* Letters to a Young Poet, *a transcription of letters about life and writing, have encouraged young writers through the decades.*

GOING BLIND

She sat just like the others at the table.
But on second glance, she seemed to hold her cup
a little differently as she picked it up.
She smiled once. It was almost painful.

And when they finished and it was time to stand
and slowly, as chance selected them, they left
and moved through many rooms (they talked and laughed),
I saw her. She was moving far behind

the others, absorbed, like someone who will soon
have to sing before a large assembly;
upon her eyes, which were radiant with joy,
light played as on the surface of a pool.

She followed slowly, taking a long time,
as though there were some obstacle in the way;
and yet: as though, once it was overcome,
she would be beyond all walking, and would fly.

WILLIAM CARLOS WILLIAMS

WILLIAM CARLOS WILLIAMS (1883–1963). *American poet, essayist, and short story writer. A practicing physician, Williams delivered more than three thousand babies in a working-class, ethnically mixed neighborhood of Rutherford, New Jersey, where he was born. He changed the face of American poetry with his emphasis on everyday life and speech and his insistence on "no ideas but in things": an exhortation to capture within poetry the physical things of this world. His most famous poem begins, "so much depends / upon / a red wheel / barrow . . ." He won the Bollingen Prize, the National Book Award, and posthumously, the Pulitzer Prize.*

THE PRACTICE

It's the humdrum, day-in, day-out, everyday work that is the real satisfaction of the practice of medicine; the million and a half patients a man has seen on his daily visits over a forty-year period of weekdays and Sundays that make up his life. I have never had a money practice; it would have been impossible for me. But the actual calling on people, at all times and under all conditions, the coming to grips with the intimate conditions of their lives, when they were being born, when they were dying, watching them die, watching them get well when they were ill, has always absorbed me.

I lost myself in the very properties of their minds: for the moment at least I actually became *them*, whoever they should be, so that when I detached myself from them at the end of a half-hour of intense concentration over some illness which was affecting them, it was as though I were reawakening from a sleep. For the moment I myself did not exist, nothing of myself affected me. As a consequence I came back to myself, as from any other sleep, rested.

Time after time I have gone out into my office in the evening feeling as if I couldn't keep my eyes open a moment longer. I would start out on my morning calls after only a few hours' sleep, sit in front of some house waiting to get the courage to climb the steps and push the front-door bell. But once I saw the patient all that would disappear. In a flash the details of the case would begin to formulate themselves into a recognizable outline, the diagnosis would unravel itself, or would refuse to make itself plain, and the hunt was on. Along with that the patient himself would shape up into something that called for attention, his peculiarities, her reticences or candors. And though I might be attracted or repelled, the professional attitude which every physician must call on would steady me, dictate the terms on which I was to proceed. Many a time a man must watch the patient's mind as it watches him, distrusting him, ready to fly off at a tangent at the first opportunity; sees himself distrusted, sees the patient turn to someone else, rejecting him.

More than once we have all seen ourselves rejected, seen some hard-pressed mother or husband go to some other adviser when we know that the advice we have given him has been correct. That too is part of the game. But in general it is the rest, the peace of mind that comes from adopting the patient's condition as one's own to be struggled with toward a solution during those few minutes or that hour or those trying days when we are searching for causes, trying to relate this to that to build a reasonable basis for action which really gives us our peace. As I say, often after I have gone into my office harassed by personal perplexities of whatever sort, fatigued physically and mentally, after two hours of intense application to the work, I came out at the finish completely rested (and I mean rested), ready to smile and to laugh as if the day were just starting.

That is why as a writer I have never felt that medicine interfered with me but rather that it was my very food and drink, the very thing which made it possible for me to write. Was I not interested in man? There the thing was, right in front of me. I could touch it, smell it. It was myself, naked, just as it was, without a lie telling itself to me in its own terms. Oh, I knew it wasn't for the most part giving me anything very profound, but it was giving me terms, basic terms with which I could spell out matters as profound as I cared to think of.

I knew it was an elementary world that I was facing, but I have always been amazed at the authenticity with which the simple-minded often face that world when compared with the tawdriness of the public viewpoint exhibited in reports from the world at large. The public view which affects the behavior of so many is a very shabby thing when compared with what I see every day in my practice of medicine. I can almost say it is the interference of the public view of their lives with what I see which makes the difficulty, in most instances, between sham and a satisfactory basis of thought.

I don't care much about that, however. I don't care a rap what people are or believe. They come to me. I care for them and either they become my friends or they don't. That is their business. My business, aside from the mere physical diagnosis, is to make a different sort of diagnosis concerning them as individuals, quite apart from anything for which they seek my advice. That fascinates me. From the very beginning that fascinated me even more than I myself knew. For no matter where I might find myself, every sort of individual that it is possible to imagine in some phase of his development, from the highest to the lowest, at some time exhibited himself to me. I am sure I have seen them all. And all have contributed to my pie. Let the successful carry off their blue ribbons; I have known the unsuccessful, far better persons than their more lucky brothers. One can laugh at them both, whatever the costumes they adopt. And when one is able to reveal them to themselves, high or low, they are always grateful as they are surprised that one can so have revealed the inner secrets of another's private motives. To do this is what makes a writer worth heeding: that somehow or other, whatever the source may be, he has gone to the base of the matter to lay it bare before us in terms which, try as we may, we cannot in the end escape. There is no choice then but to accept him and make him a hero.

All day long the doctor carries on this work, observing, weighing, comparing values of which neither he nor his patients may know the significance. He may be insensitive. But if in addition to actually being an accurate craftsman and a man of insight he has the added quality of—some distress of mind, a restless concern with the . . . If he is not satisfied with mere cures, if he lacks ambition, if he is content to . . . If there is no content in him and likely to be none; if in other words, without wishing to force it, since that would interfere with his lifelong observation, he allows himself to be called a name! What can one think of him?

He is half-ashamed to have people suspect him of carrying on a clandestine, a sort of underhand piece of spying on the public at large. They naively ask him, "How do you do it? How can you carry on an active business like that and at the same time find time to write? You must be superhuman. You must have at the very least the energy of two men." But they do not grasp that one occupation complements the other, that they are two parts of a whole, that it is not two jobs at all, that one rests the man when the other fatigues him. The only person to feel sorry for is his wife. She practically becomes a recluse. His only fear is that the source of his interest, his daily going about among human beings of all sorts, all ages, all conditions will be terminated. That he will be found out.

As far as the writing itself is concerned it takes next to no time at all. Much too much is written every day of our lives. We are overwhelmed by it. But when at times we see through the welter of evasive or interested patter, when by chance we penetrate to some moving detail of a life, there is always time to bang out a few pages. The thing isn't to find the time for it—we waste hours every day doing absolutely nothing at all—the difficulty is to catch the evasive life of the thing, to phrase the words in such a way that stereotype will yield a moment of insight. That is where the difficulty lies. We are lucky when that underground current can be tapped and the secret spring of all our lives will send up its pure water. It seldom happens. A thousand trivialities push themselves to the front, our lying habits of everyday speech and thought are foremost, telling us that *that* is what "they" want to hear. Tell them something else. You know you want to be a successful writer. This sort of chitchat the daily practice of medicine tends drastically to cure.

Forget writing, it's a trivial matter. But day in, day out, when the inarticulate patient struggles to lay himself bare for you, or with nothing more than a boil on his back is so caught off balance that he reveals some secret twist of a whole community's pathetic way of thought, a man is suddenly seized again with a desire to speak of the underground stream which for a moment has come up just under the surface. It is just a glimpse, an intimation of all that which the daily print misses or deliberately hides, but the excitement is intense and the rush to write is on again. It is then we see, by this constant feeling for a meaning, from the unselected nature of the material, just as it comes in over the phone or at the office door, that there is no better way to get an intimation of what is going on in the world.

We catch a glimpse of something, from time to time, which shows us that a presence has just brushed past us, some rare thing—just when the smiling little Italian woman has left us. For a moment we are dazzled. What was that? We can't name it; we know it never gets into any recognizable avenue of expression; men will be long dead before they can have so much as ever approached it. Whole lives are spent in the tremendous affairs of daily events without even approaching the great sights that I see every day. My patients do not know what is about them among their very husbands and children, their wives and acquaintances. But there is no need for us to be such strangers to each other, saving alone laziness, indifference and age-old besotted ignorance.

So for me the practice of medicine has become the pursuit of a rare element which may appear at any time, at any place, at a glance. It can be most embarrassing. Mutual recognition is likely to flare up at a moment's notice. The relationship between physician and patient, if it were literally followed, would give us a world of extraordinary fertil-

ity of the imagination which we can hardly afford. There's no use trying to multiply cases, it is there, it is magnificent, it fills my thoughts,
it reaches to the farthest limits of our lives.

What is the use of reading the common news of the day, the tragic
deaths and abuses of daily living, when for over half a lifetime we have
known that they must have occurred just as they have occurred given
the conditions that cause them? There is no light in it. It is trivial
fill-gap. We know the plane will crash, the train be derailed. And we
know why. No one cares, no one can care. We get the news and
discount it, we are quite right in doing so. It is trivial. But the hunted
news I get from some obscure patients' eyes is not trivial. It is profound: whole academies of learning, whole ecclesiastical hierarchies
are founded upon it and have developed what they call their dialectic
upon nothing else, their lying dialectics. A dialectic is any arbitrary
system, which, since all systems are mere inventions, is necessarily in
each case a false premise, upon which a closed system is built shutting
those who confine themselves to it from the rest of the world. All men
one way or another use a dialectic of some sort into which they are
shut, whether it be an Argentina or a Japan. So each group is maimed.
Each is enclosed in a dialectic cloud, incommunicado, and for that
reason we rush into wars and prides of the most superficial natures.

Do we not see that we are inarticulate? That is what defeats us. It is
our inability to communicate to another how we are locked within
ourselves, unable to say the simplest thing of importance to one
another, any of us, even the most valuable, that makes our lives like
those of a litter of kittens in a wood-pile. That gives the physician, and
I don't mean the high-priced psychoanalyst, his opportunity; psychoanalysis amounts to no more than another dialectic into which to be
locked.

The physician enjoys a wonderful opportunity actually to witness
the words being born. Their actual colors and shapes are laid before
him carrying their tiny burdens which he is privileged to take into his
care with their unspoiled newness. He may see the difficulty with
which they have been born and what they are destined to do. No one
else is present but the speaker and ourselves, we have been the words'
very parents. Nothing is more moving.

But after we have run the gamut of the simple meanings that come
to one over the years, a change gradually occurs. We have grown used
to the range of communication which is likely to reach us. The girl
who comes to me breathless, staggering into my office, in her underwear a still breathing infant, asking me to lock her mother out of
the room; the man whose mind is gone—all of them finally say the

same thing. And then a new meaning begins to intervene. For under the language to which we have been listening all our lives a new, a more profound language underlying all the dialectics offers itself. It is what they call poetry. That is the final phase.

It is that, we realize, which beyond all they have been saying is what they have been trying to say. They laugh (For are they not laughable?); they can think of nothing more useless (What else are they but the same?); something made of words (Have they not been trying to use words all their lives?). We begin to see that the underlying meaning of all they want to tell us and have always failed to communicate is the poem, the poem which their lives are being lived to realize. No one will believe it. And it is the actual words, as we hear them spoken under all circumstances, which contain it. It is actually there, in the life before us, every minute that we are listening, a rarest element—not in our imaginations but there, there in fact. It is that essence which is hidden in the very words which are going in at our ears and from which we must recover underlying meaning as realistically as we recover metal out of ore.

The poem that each is trying actually to communicate to us lies in the words. It is at least the words that make it articulate. It has always been so. Occasionally that named person is born who catches a rumor of it, a Homer, a Villon, and his race and the world perpetuates his memory. Is it not plain why? The physician, listening from day to day, catches a hint of it in his preoccupation. By listening to the minutest variations of the speech we begin to detect that today, as always, the essence is also to be found, hidden under the verbiage, seeking to be realized.

But one of the characteristics of this rare presence is that it is jealous of exposure and that it is shy and revengeful. It is not a name that is bandied about in the market place, no more than it is something that can be captured and exploited by the academy. Its face is a particular face, it is likely to appear under the most unlikely disguises. You cannot recognize it from past appearances—in fact it is always a new face. It knows all that we are in the habit of describing. It will not use the same appearance for any new materialization. And it is our very life. It is we ourselves, at our rarest moments, but inarticulate for the most part except when in the poem one man, every five or six hundred years, escapes to formulate a few gifted sentences.

The poem springs from the half-spoken words of such patients as the physician sees from day to day. He observes it in the peculiar, actual conformations in which its life is hid. Humbly he presents himself before it and by long practice he strives as best he can to interpret the manner of its speech. In that the secret lies. This, in the end, comes perhaps to be the occupation of the physician after a lifetime of careful listening.

THE ARTIST

Mr. T.
    bareheaded
       in a soiled undershirt
        his hair standing out
          on all sides
           stood on his toes
      heels together
        arms gracefully
          for the moment
        curled above his head.
        Then he whirled about
        bounded
    into the air
      and with an *entrechat*
        perfectly achieved
    completed the figure.
    My mother
      taken by surprise
  where she sat
      in her invalid's chair
      was left speechless.
Bravo! she cried at last
    and clapped her hands.
      The man's wife
came from the kitchen:
  What goes on here? she said.
    But the show was over.

BETWEEN WALLS

  the back wings
  of the

  hospital where
  nothing

will grow lie
cinders

in which shine
the broken

pieces of a green
bottle

LE MÉDECIN MALGRÉ LUI

Oh I suppose I should
wash the walls of my office
polish the rust from
my instruments and keep them
definitely in order
build shelves in the laboratory
empty out the old stains
clean the bottles
and refill them, buy
another lens, put
my journals on edge instead of
letting them lie flat
in heaps—then begin
ten years back and
gradually
read them to date
cataloguing important
articles for ready reference.
I suppose I should
read the new books.
If to this I added
a bill at the tailor's
and at the cleaner's
grew a decent beard
and cultivated a look
of importance—
Who can tell? I might be
a credit to my Lady Happiness
and never think anything
but a white thought!

THE BIRTH

A 40 odd year old Para 10
    Navarra
        or Navatta she didn't know
uncomplaining
    in the little room
        where we had been working all night long
dozing off
    by 10 or 15 minute intervals
        her great pendulous belly
marked
    by contraction rings
        under the skin.
No progress.
It was restfully quiet
    approaching dawn on Guinea Hill
        in those days.
Wha's a ma', Doc?
    It do'n wanna come.
That finally roused me.
I got me a strong sheet
    wrapped it
        tight
around her belly.
    When the pains seized her again
        the direction
was changed
    not
        against her own backbone
but downward
    toward the exit.
        It began to move—stupid
not to have thought of that earlier.
Finally
    without a cry out of her
        more than a low animal moaning
the head emerged
    up to the neck.
It took its own time
    rotating.

I thought of a good joke
    about an infant
        at that moment of its career
and smiled to myself quietly
    behind my mask.
        I am a feminist.
After a while
    I was able
        to extract the shoulders
one at a time
    a tight fit.
        Madonna!
13½ pounds!
    Not a man among us
        can have equaled
that.

THE LAST WORDS OF MY ENGLISH GRANDMOTHER

        There were some dirty plates
        and a glass of milk
        beside her on a small table
        near the rank, disheveled bed—

        Wrinkled and nearly blind
        she lay and snored
        rousing with anger in her tones
        to cry for food,

        Gimme something to eat—
        They're starving me—
        I'm all right I won't go
        to the hospital. No, no, no

        Give me something to eat
        Let me take you
        to the hospital, I said
        and after you are well

        you can do as you please.
        She smiled, Yes

you do what you please first
then I can do what I please—

Oh, oh, oh! she cried
as the ambulance men lifted
her to the stretcher—
Is this what you call

making me comfortable?
By now her mind was clear—
Oh you think you're smart
you young people,

she said, but I'll tell you
you don't know anything.
Then we started.
On the way

we passed a long row
of elms. She looked at them
awhile out of
the ambulance window and said,

What are all those
fuzzy-looking things out there?
Trees? Well, I'm tired
of them and rolled her head away.

THE GIRL WITH A PIMPLY FACE

One of the local druggists sent in the call: 50 Summer St., second floor, the door to the left. It's a baby they've just brought from the hospital. Pretty bad condition I should imagine. Do you want to make it? I think they've had somebody else but don't like him, he added as an afterthought.

It was half past twelve. I was just sitting down to lunch. Can't they wait till after office hours?

Oh I guess so. But they're foreigners and you know how they are. Make it as soon as you can. I guess the baby's pretty bad.

It was two-thirty when I got to the place, over a shop in the business part of town. One of those street doors between plate glass show windows. A narrow entry with smashed mail boxes on one side and a dark stair leading straight up. I'd been to the address a number of times during the past years to see various people who had lived there.

Going up I found no bell so I rapped vigorously on the wavy-glass door-panel to the left. I knew it to be the door to the kitchen, which occupied the rear of that apartment.

Come in, said a loud childish voice.

I opened the door and saw a lank-haired girl of about fifteen standing chewing gum and eyeing me curiously from beside the kitchen table. The hair was coal black and one of her eyelids drooped a little as she spoke. Well, what do you want? she said. Boy, she was tough and no kidding but I fell for her immediately. There was that hard, straight thing about her that in itself gives an impression of excellence.

I'm the doctor, I said.

Oh, you're the doctor. The baby's inside. She looked at me. Want to see her?

Sure, that's what I came for. Where's your mother?

She's out. I don't know when she's coming back. But you can take a look at the baby if you want to.

All right. Let's see her.

She led the way into the bedroom, toward the front of the flat, one of the unlit rooms, the only windows being those in the kitchen and along the facade of the building.

There she is.

I looked on the bed and saw a small face, emaciated but quiet, unnaturally quiet, sticking out of the upper end of a tightly rolled bundle made by the rest of the baby encircled in a blue cotton blanket. The whole wasn't much larger than a good sized loaf of rye bread. Hands and everything were rolled up. Just the yellowish face showed, tightly hatted and framed around by a corner of the blanket.

What's the matter with her, I asked.

I dunno, said the girl as fresh as paint and seeming about as indifferent as though it had been no relative of hers instead of her sister. I looked at my informer very much amused and she looked back at me, chewing her gum vigorously, standing there her feet well apart. She cocked her head to one side and gave it to me straight in the eye, as much as to say, Well? I looked back at her. She had one of those small, squeezed up faces, snub nose, overhanging eyebrows, low brow and a terrible complexion, pimply and coarse.

When's your mother coming back do you *think*, I asked again.

Maybe in an hour. But maybe you'd better come some time when my father's here. He talks English. He ought to come in around five I guess.

But can't you tell me something about the baby? I hear it's been sick. Does it have a fever?

I dunno.

But has it diarrhoea, are its movements green?

Sure, she said, I guess so. It's been in the hospital but it got worse so my father brought it home today.

What are they feeding it?

A bottle. You can see that yourself. There it is.

There was a cold bottle of half finished milk lying on the coverlet the nipple end of it fallen behind the baby's head.

How old is she? It's a girl, did you say?

Yeah, it's a girl.

Your sister?

Sure. Want to examine it?

No thanks, I said. For the moment at least I had lost all interest in the baby. This young kid in charge of the house did something to me that I liked. She was just a child but nobody was putting anything over on her if she knew it, yet the real thing about her was the complete lack of the rotten smell of a liar. She wasn't in the least presumptive. Just straight.

But after all she wasn't such a child. She had breasts you knew would be like small stones to the hand, good muscular arms and fine hard legs. Her bare feet were stuck into broken down leather sandals such as you see worn by children at the beach in summer. She was heavily tanned too, wherever her skin showed. Just one of the kids you'll find loafing around the pools they have outside towns and cities everywhere these days. A tough little nut finding her own way in the world.

What's the matter with your legs? I asked. They were bare and covered with scabby sores.

Poison ivy, she answered, pulling up her skirts to show me.

Gee, but you ought to seen it two days ago. This ain't nothing. You're a doctor. What can I do for it?

Let's see, I said.

She put her leg up on a chair. It had been badly bitten by mosquitoes, as I saw the thing, but she insisted on poison ivy. She had torn at the affected places with her finger nails and that's what made it look worse.

Oh that's not so bad, I said, if you'll only leave it alone and stop scratching it.

Yeah, I know that but I can't. Scratching's the only thing makes it feel better.

What's that on your foot?

Where? looking.

That big brown spot there on the back of your foot.

Dirt I guess. Her gum chewing never stopped and her fixed defensive non-expression never changed.

Why don't you wash it?

I do. Say, what could I do for my face?

I looked at it closely. You have what they call acne, I told her. All those blackheads and pimples you see there, well, let's see, the first thing you ought to do, I suppose, is to get some good soap.

What kind of soap? Lifebuoy?

No. I'd suggest one of those cakes of Lux. Not the flakes but the cake.

Yeah, I know, she said. Three for seventeen.

Use it. Use it every morning. Bathe your face in very hot water. You know, until the skin is red from it. That's to bring the blood up to the skin. Then take a piece of ice. You have ice, haven't you?

Sure, we have ice.

Hold it in a face cloth—or whatever you have—and rub that all over your face. Do that right after you've washed it in the very hot water—before it has cooled. Rub the ice all over. And do it every day—for a month. Your skin will improve. If you like, you can take some cold cream once in a while, not much, just a little and rub that in last of all, if your face feels too dry.

Will that help me?

If you stick to it, it'll help you.

All right.

There's a lotion I could give you to use along with that. Remind me of it when I come back later. Why aren't you in school?

Agh, I'm not going any more. They can't make me. Can they?

They can try.

How can they? I know a girl thirteen that don't go and they can't make her either.

Don't you want to learn things?

I know enough already.

Going to get a job?

I got a job. Here. I been helping the Jews across the hall. They give me three fifty a week—all summer.

Good for you, I said. Think your father'll be here around five?

Guess so. He ought to be.

I'll come back then. Make it all the same call.

All right, she said, looking straight at me and chewing her gum as vigorously as ever.

Just then a little blond-haired thing of about seven came in through the kitchen and walked to me looking curiously at my satchel and then at the baby.

What are you, a doctor?

See you later, I said to the older girl and went out.

At five-thirty I once more climbed the wooden stairs after passing two women at the street entrance who looked me up and down from where they were leaning on the brick wall of the building talking.

This time a woman's voice said, Come in, when I knocked on the kitchen door.

It was the mother. She was impressive, a bulky woman, growing toward fifty, in a black dress, with lank graying hair and a long seamed face. She stood by the enameled kitchen table. A younger, plumpish woman with blond hair, well cared for and in a neat house dress—as if she had dolled herself up for the occasion—was standing beside her. The small blank child was there too and the older girl, behind the others, overshadowed by her mother, the two older women at least a head taller than she. No one spoke.

Hello, I said to the girl I had been talking to earlier. She didn't answer me.

Doctor, began the mother, save my baby. She very sick. The woman spoke with a thick, heavy voice and seemed overcome with grief and apprehension. Doctor! Doctor! she all but wept.

All right, I said to cut the woman short, let's take a look at her first.

So everybody headed toward the front of the house, the mother in the lead. As they went I lagged behind to speak to the second woman, the interpreter. What happened?

The baby was not doing so well. So they took it to the hospital to see if the doctors there could help it. But it got worse. So her husband took it out this morning. It looks bad to me.

Yes, said the mother who had overheard us. Me got seven children. One daughter married. This my baby, pointing to the child on the bed. And she wiped her face with the back of her hand. This baby no do good. Me almost crazy. Don't know who can help. What doctor, I don't know. Somebody tell me take to hospital. I think maybe do some good. Five days she there. Cost me two dollar every day. Ten dollar. I no got money. And when I see my baby, she worse. She look dead. I can't leave she there. No. No. I say to everybody, no. I take she home. Doctor, you save my baby. I pay you. I pay you every-thing—

Wait a minute, wait a minute, I said. Then I turned to the other woman. What happened?

The baby got like a diarrhoea in the hospital. And she was all dirty when they went to see her. They got all excited—

All sore behind, broke in the mother—

The younger woman said a few words to her in some language that sounded like Russian but it didn't stop her—

No. No. I send she to hospital. And when I see my baby like that I can't leave she there. My babies no that way. Never, she emphasized. Never! I take she home.

Take your time, I said. Take off her clothes. Everything off. This is a regular party. It's warm enough in here. Does she vomit?

She no eat. How she can vomit? said the mother.

But the other woman contradicted her. Yes, she was vomiting in the hospital, the nurse said.

It happens that this September we had been having a lot of such cases in my hospital also, an infectious diarrhoea which practically all the children got when they came in from any cause. I supposed that this was what happened to this child. No doubt it had been in a bad way before that, improper feeding, etc., etc. And then when they took it in there, for whatever had been the matter with it, the diarrhoea had developed. These things sometimes don't turn out so well. Lucky, no doubt, that they had brought it home when they did. I told them so, explaining at the same time: One nurse for ten or twenty babies, they do all they can but you can't run and change the whole ward every five minutes. But the infant looked too lifeless for that only to be the matter with it.

You want all clothes off, asked the mother again, hesitating and trying to keep the baby covered with the cotton blanket while undressing it.

Everything off, I said.

There it lay, just skin and bones with a round fleshless head at the top and the usual pot belly you find in such cases.

Look, said the mother, tilting the infant over on its right side with her big hands so that I might see the reddened buttocks. What kind of nurse that. My babies never that way.

Take your time, take your time, I told her. That's not bad. And it wasn't either. Any child with loose movements might have had the same half an hour after being cared for. Come on. Move away, I said and give me a chance. She kept hovering over the baby as if afraid I might expose it.

It had no temperature. There was no rash. The mouth was in reasonably good shape. Eyes, ears negative. The moment I put my stethoscope to the little bony chest, however, the whole thing became clear. The infant had a severe congenital heart defect, a roar when you listened over the heart that meant, to put it crudely, that she was no good, never would be.

The mother was watching me. I straightened up and looking at her told her plainly: She's got a bad heart.

That was the sign for tears. The big woman cried while she spoke. Doctor, she pleaded in blubbering anguish, save my baby.

I'll help her, I said, but she's got a bad heart. That will never be any better. But I knew perfectly well she wouldn't pay the least attention to what I was saying.

I give you anything, she went on. I pay you. I pay you twenty dollar. Doctor, you fix my baby. You good doctor. You fix.

All right, all right, I said. What are you feeding it?

They told me and it was a ridiculous formula, unboiled besides. I regulated it properly for them and told them how to proceed to make it up. Have you got enough bottles, I asked the young girl.

Sure, we got bottles, she told me.

O.K., then go ahead.

You think you cure she? The mother with her long, tearful face was at me again, so different from her tough female fifteen-year-old.

You do what I tell you for three days, I said, and I'll come back and see how you're getting on.

Tank you, doctor, so much. I pay you. I got today no money. I pay ten dollar to hospital. They cheat me. I got no more money. I pay you Friday when my husband get pay. You save my baby.

Boy! what a woman. I couldn't get away.

She my baby, doctor. I no want to lose. Me got seven children—

Yes, you told me.

But this my baby. You understand. She very sick. You good doctor—

Oh my God! To get away from her I turned again to the kid. You better get going after more bottles before the stores close. I'll come back Friday morning.

How about that stuff for my face you were gonna give me.

That's right. Wait a minute. And I sat down on the edge of the bed to write out a prescription for some lotio alba comp. such as we use in acne. The two older women looked at me in astonishment—wondering, I suppose, how I knew the girl. I finished writing the thing and handed it to her. Sop it on your face at bedtime, I said, and let it dry on. Don't get it into your eyes.

No, I won't.

I'll see you in a couple of days, I said to them all.

Doctor! the old woman was still after me. You come back. I pay you. But all a time short. Always tomorrow come milk man. Must pay rent, must pay coal. And no got money. Too much work. Too much wash. Too much cook. Nobody help. I don't know what's a matter. This door, doctor, this door. This house make sick. Make sick.

Do the best I can, I said as I was leaving.

The girl followed on the stairs. How much is this going to cost, she asked shrewdly holding the prescription.

Not much, I said, and then started to think. Tell them you only got half a dollar. Tell them I said that's all it's worth.

Is that right, she said.

Absolutely. Don't pay a cent more for it.

Say, you're all right, she looked at me appreciatively.

Have you got half a dollar?

Sure. Why not.

What's it all about, my wife asked me in the evening. She had heard about the case. Gee! I sure met a wonderful girl, I told her.

What! another?

Some tough baby. I'm crazy about her. Talk about straight stuff . . . And I recounted to her the sort of case it was and what I had done. The mother's an odd one too. I don't quite make her out.

Did they pay you?

No. I don't suppose they have any cash.

Going back?

Sure. Have to.

Well, I don't see why you have to do all this charity work. Now that's a case you should report to the Emergency Relief. You'll get at least two dollars a call from them.

But the father has a job, I understand. That counts me out.

What sort of a job?

I dunno. Forgot to ask.

What's the baby's name so I can put it in the book?

Damn it. I never thought to ask them that either. I think they must have told me but I can't remember it. Some kind of a Russian name—

You're the limit. Dumbbell, she laughed. Honestly— Who are they anyhow?

You know, I think it must be that family Kate was telling us about. Don't you remember. The time the little kid was playing there one afternoon after school, fell down the front steps and knocked herself senseless.

I don't recall.

Sure you do. That's the family. I get it now. Kate took the brat down there in a taxi and went up with her to see that everything was all right. Yop, that's it. The old woman took the older kid by the hair, because she hadn't watched her sister. And what a beating she gave her. Don't you remember Kate telling us afterward. She thought the old woman was going to murder the child she screamed and threw her around so. Some old gal. You can see they're all afraid of her. What a world. I suppose the damned brat drives her cuckoo. But boy, how she clings to that baby.

The last hope, I suppose, said my wife.

Yeah, and the worst bet in the lot. There's a break for you.

She'll love it just the same.

More, usually.

Three days later I called at the flat again. Come in. This time a resonant male voice. I entered, keenly interested.

By the same kitchen table stood a short, thickset man in baggy working pants and a heavy cotton undershirt. He seemed to have the stability of a cube placed on one of its facets, a smooth, highly colored Slavic face, long black moustaches and widely separated, perfectly candid blue eyes. His black hair, glossy and profuse, stood out carelessly all over his large round head. By his look he reminded me at once of his blond-haired daughter, absolutely unruffled. The shoulders of an ox. You the doctor, he said. Come in.

The girl and the small child were beside him, the mother was in the bedroom.

The baby no better. Won't eat, said the man in answer to my first question.

How are its bowels?

Not so bad.

Does it vomit?

No.

Then it is better, I objected. But by this time the mother had heard us talking and came in. She seemed worse than the last time. Absolutely inconsolable. Doctor! Doctor! She came up to me.

Somewhat irritated I put her aside and went in to the baby. Of course it was better, much better. So I told them. But the heart, naturally, was the same.

How she heart? the mother pressed me eagerly. Today little better?

I started to explain things to the man who was standing back giving his wife precedence but as soon as she got the drift of what I was saying she was all over me again and the tears began to pour. There was no use my talking. Doctor, you good doctor. You do something fix my baby. And before I could move she took my left hand in both hers and kissed it through her tears. As she did so I realized finally that she had been drinking.

I turned toward the man, looking a good bit like the sun at noonday and as indifferent, then back to the woman and I felt deeply sorry for her.

Then, not knowing why I said it nor of whom, precisely, I was speaking, I felt myself choking inwardly with the words: Hell! God damn it. The sons of bitches. Why do these things have to be?

The next morning as I came into the coat room at the hospital there were several of the visiting staff standing there with their cigarettes, talking. It was about a hunting dog belonging to one of the doctors. It had come down with distemper and seemed likely to die.

I called up half a dozen vets around here, one of them was saying. I even called up the one in your town, he added turning to me as I came in. And do you know how much they wanted to charge me for giving the serum to that animal?

Nobody answered.

They had the nerve to want to charge me five dollars a shot for it. Can you beat that? Five dollars a shot.

Did you give them the job, someone spoke up facetiously.

Did I? I should say I did not, the first answered. But can you beat that. Why we're nothing but a lot of slop-heels compared to those guys. We deserve to starve.

Get it out of them, someone rasped, kidding. That's the stuff.

Then the original speaker went on, buttonholing me as some of the others faded from the room. Did you ever see practice so rotten. By the way, I was called over to your town about a week ago to see a kid I delivered up here during the summer. Do you know anything about the case?

I probably got them on my list, I said. Russians?

Yeah, I thought as much. Has a job as a road worker or something. Said they couldn't pay me. Well, I took the trouble of going up to your court house and finding out what he was getting. Eighteen dollars a week. Just the type. And they had the nerve to tell me they couldn't pay me.

She told me ten.

She's a liar.

Natural maternal instinct, I guess.

Whisky appetite, if you should ask me.

Same thing.

O.K., buddy. Only I'm telling you. And did I tell *them*. They'll never call me down there again, believe me. I had that much satisfaction out of them anyway. You make 'em pay you. Don't you do anything for them unless they do. He's paid by the county. I tell you if I had taxes to pay down there I'd go and take it out of his salary.

You and how many others?

Say, they're bad actors, that crew. Do you know what they really do with their money? Whisky. Now I'm telling you. That old woman is the slickest customer you ever saw. She's drunk all the time. Didn't you notice it?

Not while I was there.

Don't you let them put any of that sympathy game over on you. Why they tell me she leaves that baby lying on the bed all day long screaming its lungs out until the neighbors complain to the police about it. I'm not lying to you.

Yeah, the old skate's got nerves, you can see that. I can imagine she's a bugger when she gets going.

But what about the young girl, I asked weakly. She seems like a pretty straight kid.

My confrere let out a wild howl. That thing! You mean that pimply-faced little bitch. Say, if I had my way I'd run her out of the town tomorrow. There's about a dozen wise guys on her trail every night in the week. Ask the cops. Just ask them. They know. Only nobody wants to bring in a complaint. They say you'll stumble over her on the roof, behind the stairs, anytime at all. Boy, they sure took you in.

Yes, I suppose they did, I said.

But the old woman's the ringleader. She's got the brains. Take my advice and make them pay.

The last time I went I heard the Come in! from the front of the house. The fifteen-year-old was in there at the window in a rocking chair with the tightly wrapped baby in her arms. She got up. Her legs were bare to the hips. A powerful little animal.

What are you doing? Going swimming? I asked.

Naw, that's my gym suit. What the kids wear for Physical Training in school.

How's the baby?

She's all right.

Do you mean it?

Sure, she eats fine now.

Tell your mother to bring it to the office some day so I can weigh it. The food'll need increasing in another week or two anyway.

I'll tell her.

How's your face?

Gettin' better.

My God, it *is*, I said. And it was much better. Going back to school now?

Yeah, I had tuh.

THE USE OF FORCE

They were new patients to me, all I had was the name, Olson. Please come down as soon as you can, my daughter is very sick.

When I arrived I was met by the mother, a big startled looking woman, very clean and apologetic who merely said, Is this the doctor? and let me in. In the back, she added. You must excuse us, doctor, we have her in the kitchen where it is warm. It is very damp here sometimes.

The child was fully dressed and sitting on her father's lap near the kitchen table. He tried to get up, but I motioned for him not to bother, took off my overcoat and started to look things over. I could see that they were all very nervous, eyeing me up and down distrustfully. As often, in such cases, they weren't telling me more than they had to, it was up to me to tell them; that's why they were spending three dollars on me.

The child was fairly eating me up with her cold, steady eyes, and no expression to her face whatever. She did not move and seemed, inwardly, quiet; an unusually attractive little thing, and as strong as a heifer in appearance. But her face was flushed, she was breathing rapidly, and I realized that she had a high fever. She had magnificent blond hair, in profusion. One of those picture children often reproduced in advertising leaflets and the photogravure sections of the Sunday papers.

She's had a fever for three days, began the father, and we don't know what it comes from. My wife has given her things, you know, like people do, but it don't do no good. And there's been a lot of sickness around. So we tho't you'd better look her over and tell us what is the matter.

As doctors often do I took a trial shot at it as a point of departure. Has she had a sore throat?

Both parents answered me together, No . . . No, she says her throat don't hurt her.

Does your throat hurt you? added the mother to the child. But the little girl's expression didn't change nor did she move her eyes from my face.

Have you looked?

I tried to, said the mother, but I couldn't see.

As it happens we had been having a number of cases of diphtheria in the school to which this child went during that month and we were all, quite apparently, thinking of that, though no one had as yet spoken of the thing.

Well, I said, suppose we take a look at the throat first. I smiled in my best professional manner and asking for the child's first name I said, come on, Mathilda, open your mouth and let's take a look at your throat.

Nothing doing.

Aw, come on, I coaxed, just open your mouth wide and let me take a look. Look, I said opening both hands wide, I haven't anything in my hands. Just open up and let me see.

Such a nice man, put in the mother. Look how kind he is to you. Come on, do what he tells you to. He won't hurt you.

At that I ground my teeth in disgust. If only they wouldn't use the word "hurt" I might be able to get somewhere. But I did not allow myself to be hurried or disturbed but speaking quietly and slowly I approached the child again.

As I moved my chair a little nearer suddenly with one cat-like movement both her hands clawed instinctively for my eyes and she almost reached them too. In fact she knocked my glasses flying and they fell, though unbroken, several feet away from me on the kitchen floor.

Both the mother and father almost turned themselves inside out in embarrassment and apology. You bad girl, said the mother, taking her and shaking her by one arm. Look what you've done. The nice man ...

For heaven's sake, I broke in. Don't call me a nice man to her. I'm here to look at her throat on the chance that she might have diphtheria and possibly die of it. But that's nothing to her. Look here, I said to the child, we're going to look at your throat. You're old enough to understand what I'm saying. Will you open it now by yourself or shall we have to open it for you?

Not a move. Even her expression hadn't changed. Her breaths however were coming faster and faster. Then the battle began. I had to do it. I had to have a throat culture for her own protection. But first I told the parents that it was entirely up to them. I explained the danger but said that I would not insist on a throat examination so long as they would take the responsibility.

If you don't do what the doctor says you'll have to go to the hospital, the mother admonished her severely.

Oh yeah? I had to smile to myself. After all, I had already fallen in love with the savage brat, the parents were contemptible to me. In the ensuing struggle they grew more and more abject, crushed, exhausted while she surely rose to magnificent heights of insane fury of effort bred of her terror of me.

The father tried his best, and he was a big man but the fact that she was his daughter, his shame at her behavior and his dread of hurting her made him release her just at the critical moment several times when I had almost achieved success, till I wanted to kill him. But his dread also that she might have diphtheria made him tell me to go on, go on though he himself was almost fainting, while the mother moved back and forth behind us raising and lowering her hands in an agony of apprehension.

Put her in front of you on your lap, I ordered, and hold both her wrists.

But as soon as he did the child let out a scream. Don't, you're hurting me. Let go of my hands. Let them go I tell you. Then she shrieked terrifyingly, hysterically. Stop it! Stop it! You're killing me!

Do you think she can stand it, doctor! said the mother.

You get out, said the husband to his wife. Do you want her to die of diphtheria?

Come on now, hold her, I said.

Then I grasped the child's head with my left hand and tried to get the wooden tongue depressor between her teeth. She fought, with clenched teeth, desperately! But now I also had grown furious—at a child. I tried to hold myself down but I couldn't. I know how to expose a throat for inspection. And I did my best. When finally I got the wooden spatula behind the last teeth and just the point of it into the mouth cavity, she opened up for an instant but before I could see anything she came down again and gripping the wooden blade between her molars she reduced it to splinters before I could get it out again.

Aren't you ashamed, the mother yelled at her. Aren't you ashamed to act like that in front of the doctor?

Get me a smooth-handled spoon of some sort, I told the mother. We're going through with this. The child's mouth was already bleeding. Her tongue was cut and she was screaming in wild hysterical shrieks. Perhaps I should have desisted and come back in an hour or more. No doubt it would have been better. But I have seen at least two children lying dead in bed of neglect in such cases, and feeling that I must get a diagnosis now or never I went at it again. But the worst of it was that I too had got beyond reason. I could have torn the child apart in my own fury and enjoyed it. It was a pleasure to attack her. My face was burning with it.

The damned little brat must be protected against her own idiocy, one says to one's self at such times. Others must be protected against her. It is social necessity. And all these things are true. But a blind fury, a feeling of adult shame, bred of a longing for muscular release are the operatives. One goes on to the end.

In a final unreasoning assault I overpowered the child's neck and jaws. I forced the heavy silver spoon back of her teeth and down her throat till she gagged. And there it was—both tonsils covered with membrane. She had fought valiantly to keep me from knowing her secret. She had been hiding that sore throat for three days at least and lying to her parents in order to escape just such an outcome as this.

Now truly she *was* furious. She had been on the defensive before but now she attacked. Tried to get off her father's lap and fly at me while tears of defeat blinded her eyes.

COMPLAINT

They call me and I go.
It is a frozen road
past midnight, a dust
of snow caught
in the rigid wheeltracks.
The door opens.
I smile, enter and
shake off the cold.
Here is a great woman
on her side in the bed.
She is sick,
perhaps vomiting,
perhaps laboring
to give birth to
a tenth child. Joy! Joy!
Night is a room
darkened for lovers,
through the jalousies the sun
has sent one gold needle!
I pick the hair from her eyes
and watch her misery
with compassion.

FRANCES CORNFORD

FRANCES CORNFORD (1886–1960). *English poet. The granddaughter of Charles Darwin, Frances Cornford lived most of her life in Cambridge, England, where she spent her time writing delicate poems of an intensely personal nature; she is best remembered for her sublime illumination of the emotions. Her* Collected Poems *was published in 1956.*

THE WATCH

I wakened on my hot, hard bed,
Upon the pillow lay my head;
Beneath the pillow I could hear
My little watch was ticking clear.
I thought the throbbing of it went
Like my continual discontent.
I thought it said in every tick:
I am so sick, so sick, so sick.
O death, come quick, come quick, come quick,
Come quick, come quick, come quick, come quick!

MIKHAIL BULGAKOV

MIKHAIL BULGAKOV (1891–1940). *Russian physician, novelist, playwright, journalist, and short story writer. Bulgakov was born in Russia (Kiev), the eldest of six children of a theology professor. He studied medicine at Kiev University and for eighteen demanding months worked as a general physician in truly frontline-district medical outposts (usually one-doctor hospitals of about forty beds). The two stories here, from this period of Bulgakov's life, may summon up the feelings of inadequacy many young physicians feel in their early clinical encounters. He specialized in venereology in Kiev for a time, but then gave up medicine for writing. Like many Russian artists, Bulgakov encountered political problems from Stalin and the authorities during the years before World War II. His works, including masterpieces such as* The Master and Margarita, *were not all published in Russia until the 1980s.*

THE STEEL WINDPIPE

So I was alone, surrounded by November gloom and whirling snow; the house was smothered in it and there was a moaning in the chimneys. I had spent all twenty-four years of my life in a huge city and thought that blizzards only howled in novels. It appeared that they howled in real life. The evenings here are unusually long, and I fell to daydreaming, staring at the reflection on the window of the lamp with its dark green shade. I dreamed of the nearest town, thirty-two miles away. I longed to leave my country clinic and go there. They had electricity, and there were four doctors whom I could consult. At all events it would be less frightening than this place. But there was no chance of running away, and at times I realised that it would be cowardly. It was for precisely this, after all, that I had been studying medicine.

'Yes, but suppose they bring me a woman in labour and there are complications? Or, say, a patient with a strangulated hernia? What shall I do then? Kindly tell me that. Forty-eight days ago I qualified "with distinction"; but distinction is one thing and hernia is another. Once I watched a professor operating on a strangulated hernia. He did it, while I sat in the amphitheatre. And I only just managed to survive . . .'

More than once I broke out in a cold sweat down my spine at the thought of hernia. Every evening, as I drank my tea, I would sit in the same attitude: by my left hand lay all the manuals on obstetrical surgery, on top of them the small edition of Döderlein. To my right were ten different illustrated volumes on operative surgery. I groaned, smoked and drank cold tea without milk.

Once I fell asleep. I remember that night perfectly—it was 29 November, and I was woken by someone banging on the door. Five minutes later I was pulling on my trousers, my eyes glued imploringly to those sacred books on operative surgery. I could hear the creaking of sleigh-runners in the yard—my ears had become unusually sensitive. The case turned out to be, if anything, even more terrifying than a hernia or a transverse foetus. At eleven o'clock that night a little girl was brought to the Muryovo hospital. The nurse said tonelessly to me:

'The little girl's weak, she's dying . . . Would you come over to the hospital, please, doctor . . .'

I remember crossing the yard towards the hospital porch, mesmerised by the flickering light of a kerosene lamp. The lights were on in the surgery, and all my assistants were waiting for me, already dressed in their overalls: the *feldsher* Demyan Lukich, young but very capable, and two experienced midwives, Anna Nikolaevna and Pelagea Ivanovna. Only twenty-four years old, having qualified a mere two months ago, I had been placed in charge of the Muryovo hospital.

The *feldsher* solemnly flung open the door and the mother came in—or rather she seemed to fly in, slithering on her ice-covered felt boots, unmelted snow still on her shawl. In her arms she carried a bundle, from which came a steady hissing, whistling sound. The mother's face was contorted with noiseless weeping. When she had thrown off her sheepskin coat and shawl and unwrapped the bundle, I saw a little girl of about three years old. For a while the sight of her made me forget operative surgery, my loneliness, the load of useless knowledge acquired at university: it was all completely effaced by the beauty of this baby girl. What can I liken her to? You only see children like that on chocolate boxes—hair curling naturally into big ringlets the colour of ripe rye, enormous dark blue eyes, doll-like cheeks. They used to draw angels like that. But in the depths of her eyes was a strange cloudiness and I recognised it as terror—the child could not breathe. 'She'll be dead in an hour,' I thought with absolute certainty, feeling a sharp twinge of pity for the child.

Her throat was contracting into hollows with each breath, her veins were swollen and her face was turning from pink to a pale lilac. I immediately realised what this colouring meant. I made my first diagnosis, which was not only correct but, more important, was given at the same moment as the midwives' with all their experience: 'The little girl has diphtherial croup. Her throat is already choked with membrane and soon it will be blocked completely.'

'How long has she been ill?' I asked, breaking the tense silence of my assistants.

'Five days now,' the mother answered, staring hard at me with dry eyes.

'Diphtheria,' I said to the *feldsher* through clenched teeth, and turned to the mother:

'Why have you left it so long?'

At that moment I heard a tearful voice behind me:

'Five days, sir, five days!'

I turned round and saw that a round-faced old woman had silently come in. 'I wish these old women didn't exist,' I thought to myself. With an aching presentiment of trouble I said:

'Quiet, woman, you're only in the way,' and repeated to the mother: 'Why have you left it so long? Five days? Hmm?'

Suddenly with an automatic movement the mother handed the little girl to the grandmother and sank to her knees in front of me.

'Give her some medicine,' she said and banged her forehead on the floor. 'I'll kill myself if she dies.'

'Get up at once,' I replied, 'or I won't even talk to you.'

The mother stood up quickly with a rustle of her wide skirt, took the baby from the grandmother and started rocking it. The old woman turned to the doorpost and began praying, while the little girl continued to breathe with a snake-like hiss. The *feldsher* said:

'That's what they're all like. These people!' And he gave a twitch of his moustache.

'Does that mean she's going to die?' the mother asked, staring at me with what looked like black fury.

'Yes, she'll die,' I said quietly and firmly.

The grandmother picked up the hem of her skirt and wiped her eyes. The mother shouted in an ugly voice:

'Give her something! Help her! Give her some medicine!'

I could see what was in store for me and remained firm.

'What medicine can I give her? Go on, you tell me. The little girl is suffocating, her throat is already blocked up. For five days you kept her ten miles away from me. Now what do you want me to do?'

'You're the one who's supposed to know,' the old woman whined by my left shoulder in an affected voice which made me immediately detest her.

'Shut up!' I said to her. I turned to the *feldsher* and ordered the little girl to be taken away. The mother handed her to the midwife and the child started to struggle, evidently trying to cry, but her voice could no longer make itself heard. The mother made a protective move towards her, but we kept her away and I managed to look into the little girl's throat by the light of the pressure-lamp. I had never seen diphtheria before except for mild, forgettable cases. Her throat was full of ragged, pulsating, white substance. The little girl suddenly breathed out and spat in my face, but I was so absorbed that I did not flinch.

'Well now,' I said, astonished at my own calm. 'This is the situation: it's late, and the little girl is dying. Nothing will help her except one thing—an operation.'

I was appalled, wondering why I had said this, but I could not help saying it. The thought flashed through my mind: 'What if she agrees to it?'

'How do you mean?' the mother asked.

'I'll have to cut open her throat near the bottom of her neck and put in a silver pipe so that she can breathe, and then maybe we can save her,' I explained.

The mother looked at me as if I was mad and shielded the little girl from me with her arms, while the old woman started muttering again:

'The idea! Don't you let them cut her open! What—cut her throat?'

'Go away, old woman,' I said to her with hatred. 'Inject the camphor!' I ordered the *feldsher*.

The mother refused to hand over the little girl when she saw the syringe, but we explained to her that there was nothing terrible about it.

'Perhaps that will cure her?' she asked.

'No, it won't cure her at all.'

Then the mother burst into tears.

'Stop it,' I said. I took out my watch, and added: 'I'm giving you five minutes to think it over. If you don't agree in five minutes, I shall refuse to do it.'

'I don't agree!' the mother said sharply.

'No, we won't agree to it,' the grandmother put in.

'It's up to you,' I said in a hollow voice, and thought: 'Well, that's that. It makes it easier for me. I've said my piece and given them a chance. Look how dumbfounded the midwives are. They've refused and I'm saved.' No sooner had I thought this than some other being spoke for me in a voice that was not mine:

'Look, have you gone mad? What do you mean by not agreeing? You're condemning the baby to death. You must consent. Have you no pity?'

'No!' the mother shouted once more.

I thought to myself: 'What am I doing? I shall only kill the child.' But I said:

'Come on, come on—you've got to agree! You must! Look, her nails are already turning blue.'

'No, no!'

'All right, take them to the ward. Let them sit there.'

They were led away down the half-lit passage. I could hear the weeping of the women and the hissing of the little girl. The *feldsher* returned almost at once and said:

'They've agreed!'

I felt my blood run cold, but I said in a clear voice:

'Sterilise a scalpel, scissors, hooks and a probe at once.'

A minute later I was running across the yard, through a swirling, blinding snowstorm. I rushed to my room and, counting the minutes, grabbed a book, leafed through it and found an illustration of a tracheotomy. Everything about it was clear and simple: the throat was laid open and the knife plunged into the windpipe. I started reading the text, but could take none of it in—the words seemed to jump before my eyes. I had never seen a tracheotomy performed. 'Ah well, it's a bit late now,' I said to myself, and looked miserably at the green lamp and the clear illustration. Feeling that I had suddenly been burdened with a most fearful and difficult task, I went back to the hospital, oblivious of the snowstorm.

In the surgery a dim figure in full skirts clung to me and a voice whined:

'Oh, sir, how can you cut a little girl's throat? How can you? She's agreed to it because she's stupid. But you haven't got my permission—no you haven't. I agree to giving her medicine, but I shan't allow her throat to be cut.'

'Get this woman out!' I shouted, and added vehemently: 'You're the stupid one! Yes, you are. And she's the clever one. Anyway, nobody asked you! Get her out of here!'

A midwife took a firm hold of the old woman and pushed her out of the room.

'Ready!' the *feldsher* said suddenly.

We went into the small operating theatre; the shiny instruments, blinding lamplight and oilcloth seemed to belong to another world ... for the last time I went out to the mother, and the little girl could scarcely be torn from her arms. She just said in a hoarse voice: 'My husband's away in town. When he comes back and finds out what I've done, he'll kill me!'

'Yes, he'll kill her,' the old woman echoed, looking at me in horror. 'Don't let them into the operating theatre!' I ordered.

So we were left in the operating theatre, my assistants, myself, and Lidka, the little girl. She sat naked and pathetic on the table and wept soundlessly. They laid her on the table, strapped her down, washed her throat and painted it with iodine. I picked up the scalpel, still wondering what on earth I was doing. It was very quiet. With the scalpel I made a vertical incision down the swollen white throat. Not one drop of blood emerged. Again I drew the knife along the white strip which protruded between the slit skin. Again not a trace of blood. Slowly, trying to remember the illustrations in my textbooks, I started to part the delicate tissues with the blunt probe. At once dark blood gushed out from the lower end of the wound, flooding it instantly and pouring down her neck. The *feldsher* started to stanch it with swabs but could not stop the flow. Calling to mind everything I had seen at university, I set about clamping the edges of the wound with forceps, but this did no good either.

I went cold and my forehead broke out in a sweat. I bitterly regretted having studied medicine and having landed myself in this wilderness. In angry desperation I jabbed the forceps haphazardly into the region of the wound, snapped them shut and the flow of blood stopped immediately. We swabbed the wound with pieces of gauze; now it faced me clean and absolutely incomprehensible. There was no windpipe anywhere to be seen. This wound of mine was quite unlike any illustration. I spent the next two or three minutes aimlessly poking about in the wound, first with the scalpel and then with the probe, searching for the windpipe. After two minutes of this, I despaired of finding it. 'This is the end,' I thought. 'Why did I ever do this? I needn't have offered to do the operation, and Lidka could have died quietly in the ward. As it is she will die with her throat slit open and I can never prove that she would have died anyway, that I couldn't have made it any worse ...' The midwife wiped my brow in silence. 'I ought to put down my scalpel and say: I don't know what to do next.' As I thought this I pictured the mother's eyes. I picked up the knife again and made a deep, undirected slash into Lidka's neck. The tissues parted and to my surprise the windpipe appeared before me.

'Hooks!' I croaked hoarsely.

The *feldsher* handed them to me. I pierced each side with a hook and handed one of them to him. Now I could see one thing only: the greyish ringlets of the windpipe. I thrust the sharp knife into it—and froze in horror. The windpipe was coming out of the incision and the *feldsher* appeared to have taken leave of his wits: he was tearing it out.

Behind me the two midwives gasped. I looked up and saw what was the matter: the *feldsher* had fainted from the oppressive heat and, still holding the hook, was tearing at the windpipe. 'It's fate,' I thought, 'everything's against me. We've certainly murdered Lidka now.' And I added grimly to myself: 'As soon as I get back to my room, I'll shoot myself.' Then the older midwife, who was evidently very experienced, pounced on the *feldsher* and tore the hook out of his hand, saying through her clenched teeth:

'Go on, doctor . . .'

The *feldsher* collapsed to the floor with a crash but we did not turn to look at him. I plunged the scalpel into the trachea and then inserted a silver tube. It slid in easily but Lidka remained motionless. The air did not flow into her windpipe as it should have done. I sighed deeply and stopped: I had done all I could. I felt like begging someone's forgiveness for having been so thoughtless as to study medicine. Silence reigned. I could see Lidka turning blue. I was just about to give up and weep, when the child suddenly gave a violent convulsion, expelled a fountain of disgusting clotted matter through the tube, and the air whistled into her windpipe. As she started to breathe, the little girl began to howl. That instant the *feldsher* got to his feet, pale and sweaty, looked at her throat in stupefied horror and helped me to sew it up.

Dazed, my vision blurred by a film of sweat, I saw the happy faces of the midwives and one of them said to me:

'You did the operation brilliantly, doctor.'

I thought she was making fun of me and glowered at her. Then the doors were opened and a gust of fresh air blew in. Lidka was carried out wrapped in a sheet and at once the mother appeared in the doorway. Her eyes had the look of a wild beast. She asked me:

'Well?'

When I heard the sound of her voice, I felt a cold sweat run down my back as I realised what it would have been like if Lidka had died on the table. But I answered her in a very calm voice:

'Don't worry, she's alive. And she'll stay alive, I hope. Only she won't be able to talk until we take the pipe out, so don't let that upset you.'

Just then the grandmother seemed to materialise from nowhere and crossed herself, bowing to the doorhandle, to me, and to the ceiling. This time I did not lose my temper with her, I turned away and ordered Lidka to be given a camphor injection and for the staff to take turns at watching her. Then I went across the yard to my quarters. I remember the green lamp burning in my study, Döderlein lying there and books scattered everywhere. I walked over to the couch fully dressed, lay down and was immediately lost to the world in a dreamless sleep.

A month passed, then another. I grew more experienced and some of the things I saw were rather more frightening than Lidka's throat, which passed out of my mind. Snow lay all around, and the size of my practice grew daily. Early in the new year, a woman came to my surgery holding by the hand a little girl wrapped in so many layers that she looked as round as a little barrel. The woman's eyes were shining. I took a good look and recognised them.

'Ah, Lidka! How are things?'

'Everything's fine.'

The mother unwound the scarves from Lidka's neck. Though she was shy and resisted I managed to raise her chin and took a look. Her pink neck was marked with a brown vertical scar crossed by two fine stitch marks.

'All's well,' I said. 'You needn't come any more.'

'Thank you, doctor, thank you,' the mother said, and turned to Lidka: 'Say thank you to the gentleman!'

But Lidka had no wish to speak to me.

I never saw her again. Gradually I forgot about her. Meanwhile my practice still grew. The day came when I had a hundred and ten patients. We began at nine in the morning and finished at eight in the evening. Reeling with fatigue, I was taking off my overall when the senior midwife said to me:

'It's the tracheotomy that has brought you all these patients. Do you know what they're saying in the villages? The story goes that when Lidka was ill a steel throat was put into her instead of her own and then sewn up. People go to her village especially to look at her. There's fame for you, doctor. Congratulations.'

'So they think she's living with a steel one now, do they?' I enquired.

'That's right. But you were wonderful, doctor. You did it so coolly, it was marvellous to watch.'

'Hm, well, I never allow myself to worry, you know,' I said, not knowing why. I was too tired even to feel ashamed, so I just looked away. I said goodnight and went home. Snow was falling in large flakes, covering everything, the lantern was lit and my house looked silent, solitary and imposing. As I walked I had only one desire—sleep.

BAPTISM BY ROTATION

As time passed in my country hospital, I gradually got used to the new way of life.

They were braking flax in the villages as they had always done, the roads were still impassable, and no more than five patients came to my daily surgery. My evenings were entirely free, and I spent them sorting out the library, reading surgical manuals and spending long hours drinking tea alone with the gently humming samovar.

For whole days and nights it poured with rain, the drops pounded unceasingly on the roof and the water cascaded past my window, swirling along the gutter and into a tub. Outside was slush, darkness and fog, through which the windows of the *feldsher*'s house and the kerosene lantern over the gateway were no more than faint, blurred patches of light.

On one such evening I was sitting in my study with an atlas of topographical anatomy. The absolute silence was only disturbed by the occasional gnawing of mice behind the sideboard in the dining-room.

I read until my eyelids grew so heavy that they began to stick together. Finally I yawned, put the atlas aside and decided to go to bed. I stretched in pleasant anticipation of sleeping soundly to the accompaniment of the noisy pounding of the rain, then went across to my bedroom, undressed and lay down.

No sooner had my head touched the pillow than there swam hazily before me the face of Anna Prokhorova, a girl of seventeen from the village of Toropovo. She had needed a tooth extracting. Demyan Lukich, the *feldsher*, floated silently past holding a gleaming pair of pincers. Remembering how he always said 'suchlike' instead of 'such' because he was fond of a high-falutin' style, I smiled and fell asleep.

About half an hour later, however, I suddenly woke up as though I had been pinched, sat up, stared fearfully into the darkness and listened.

Someone was drumming loudly and insistently on the outer door and I immediately sensed that those knocks boded no good.

Then came a knock on the door of my quarters.

The noise stopped, there was a grating of bolts, the sound of the cook talking, an indistinct voice in reply, then someone came creaking up the stairs, passed quietly through the study and knocked on my bedroom door.

'Who is it?'

'It's me,' came the reply in a respectful whisper. 'Me, Aksinya, the nurse.'

'What's the matter?'

'Anna Nikolaevna has sent for you. They want you to come to the hospital as quickly as possible.'

'What's happened?' I asked, feeling my heart literally miss a beat.

'A woman has been brought in from Dultsevo. She's having a difficult labour.'

'Here we go!' I thought to myself, quite unable to get my feet into my slippers. 'Hell, the matches won't light. Ah well, it had to happen sooner or later. You can't expect to get nothing but cases of laryngitis or abdominal catarrh all your life.'

'All right, go and tell them I'm coming at once!' I shouted as I got out of bed. Aksinya's footsteps shuffled away from the door and the bolt grated again. Sleep vanished in a moment. Hurriedly, with shaking fingers, I lit the lamp and began dressing. Half past eleven . . . What could be wrong with this woman who was having a difficult birth? Malpresentation? Narrow pelvis? Or perhaps something worse. I might even have to use forceps. Should I send her straight into town? Out of the question! A fine doctor he is, they'll all say. In any case, I have no right to do that. No, I really must do it myself. But do what? God alone knows. It would be disastrous if I lost my head—I might disgrace myself in front of the midwives. Anyway, I must have a look first; no point in getting worried prematurely . . .

I dressed, threw an overcoat over my shoulders, and hoping that all would be well, ran to the hospital through the rain across the creaking duckboards. At the entrance I could see a cart in the semi-darkness, the horse pawing at the rotten boards under its hooves.

'Did you bring the woman in labour?' I asked the figure lurking by the horse.

'Yes, that's right . . . we did, sir,' a woman's voice replied dolefully.

Despite the hour, the hospital was alive and bustling. A flickering pressure-lamp was burning in the surgery. In the little passage leading to the delivery room Aksinya slipped past me carrying a basin. A faint moan came through the door and died away again. I opened the door and went into the delivery room. The small, whitewashed room was brightly lit by a lamp in the ceiling. On a bed alongside the operating table, covered with a blanket up to her chin, lay a young woman. Her face was contorted in a grimace of pain and wet strands of hair were sticking to her forehead. Holding a large thermometer, Anna Nikolaevna was preparing a solution in a graduated jug, while Pelagea

Ivanovna was getting clean sheets out of the cupboard. The *feldsher* was leaning against the wall in a Napoleonic pose. Seeing me, they all jerked into life. The pregnant woman opened her eyes, wrung her hands and renewed her pathetic, long drawn-out groaning.

'Well now, what seems to be the trouble?' I asked, sounding confident.

'Transverse lie,' Anna Nikolaevna answered promptly as she went on pouring water into the solution.

'I see-ee,' I drawled, and added, frowning: 'Well, let's have a look . . .'

'Aksinya! Wash the doctor's hands!' snapped Anna Nikolaevna. Her expression was solemn and serious.

As the water flowed, rinsing away the lather from my hands, reddened from scrubbing, I asked Anna Nikolaevna a few trivial questions, such as when the woman had been brought in, where she was from . . . Pelagea Ivanovna's hand turned back the blanket, I sat down on the edge of the bed and began gently feeling the swollen belly. The woman groaned, stretched, dug her fingers into her flesh and crumpled the sheet.

'There, there, relax . . . it won't take long,' I said as I carefully put my hands to the hot, dry, distended skin.

The fact was that once the experienced Anna Nikolaevna had told me what was wrong, this examination was quite pointless. I could examine the woman as much as I liked, but I would not find out any more than Anna Nikolaevna knew already. Her diagnosis was, of course, correct: transverse lie. It was obvious. Well, what next?

Frowning, I continued palpating the belly on all sides and glanced sidelong at the midwives' faces. Both were watching with intense concentration and their looks registered approval of what I was doing. But although my movements were confident and correct, I did my best to conceal my unease as thoroughly as possible.

'Very well,' I said with a sigh, standing up from the bed, as there was nothing more to be seen from an external examination. 'Let's examine her internally.'

Another look of approval from Anna Nikolaevna.

'Aksinya!'

More water flowed.

'Oh, if only I could consult Döderlein now!' I thought miserably as I soaped my hands. Alas, this was quite impossible. In any case, how could Döderlein help me at a moment like this? I washed off the thick lather and painted my fingers with iodine. A clean sheet rustled in Pelagea Ivanovna's hands and, bending down over the expectant mother, I began cautiously and timidly to carry out an internal examination. Into my mind came an involuntary recollection of the operating theatre in the maternity hospital. Gleaming electric lights in frosted-glass globes, a shining tiled floor, taps and instruments a-glitter everywhere. A junior registrar in a snow-white coat is manipulating the woman, surrounded by three intern assistants, probationers, and a crowd of students doing their practicals. Everything bright, well ordered and safe.

And there was I, all on my own, with a woman in agony on my hands and I was responsible for her. I had no idea, however, what I was supposed to do to help her, because I had seen childbirth at close quarters only twice in my life in a hospital, and both occasions were completely normal. The fact that I was conducting an examination was of no value to me or to the woman; I understood absolutely nothing and could feel nothing of what was inside her.

It was time to make some sort of decision.

'Transverse lie . . . since it's a transverse lie I must . . . I must . . .'

'Turn it round by the foot,' muttered Anna Nikolaevna as though thinking aloud, unable to restrain herself.

An older, more experienced doctor would have looked askance at her for butting in, but I am not the kind to take offence.

'Yes,' I concurred gravely, 'a podalic version.'

The pages of Döderlein flickered before my eyes. Internal method . . . Combined method . . . External method . . . Page after page, covered in illustrations. A pelvis; twisted, crushed babies with enormous heads . . . a little dangling arm with a loop on it.

Indeed I had read it not long ago and had underlined it, soaking up every word, mentally picturing the interrelationship of every part of the whole and every method. And as I read it I imagined that the entire text was being imprinted on my brain for ever.

Yet now only one sentence of it floated back into my memory:

'A transverse lie is a wholly unfavourable position.'

Too true. Wholly unfavourable both for the woman and for a doctor who only qualified six months ago.

'Very well, we'll do it,' I said as I stood up.

Anna Nikolaevna's expression came to life.

'Demyan Lukich,' she turned to the *feldsher*, 'get the chloroform ready.'

It was a good thing that she had said so, because I was still not certain whether the operation was supposed to be done under anaesthesia or not! Of course, under anaesthesia—how else?

Still, I must have a look at Döderlein . . .

As I washed my hands I said:

'All right, then . . . prepare her for anaesthesia and make her comfortable. I'll be back in a moment; I must just go to my room and fetch some cigarettes.'

'Very good, doctor, we'll be ready by the time you come back,' replied Anna Nikolaevna.

I dried my hands, the nurse threw my coat over my shoulders and without putting my arms into the sleeves I set off for home at a run.

In my study I lit the lamp and, forgetting to take off my cap, rushed straight to the bookcase.

There it was—Döderlein's *Operative Obstetrics*. I began hastily to leaf through the glossy pages.

'. . . version is always a dangerous operation for the mother . . .'

A cold shiver ran down my spine.

'The chief danger lies in the possibility of a spontaneous rupture of the uterus . . .'

Spon-tan-e-ous . . .

'If in introducing his hand into the uterus the obstetrician encounters any hindrances to penetrating to the foot, whether from lack of space or as a result of a contraction of the uterine wall, he should refrain from further attempts to carry out the version . . .'

Good. Provided I am able, by some miracle, to recognise these 'hindrances' and I refrain from 'further attempts,' what, might I ask, am I then supposed to do with an anaesthetised woman from the village of Dultsevo?

Further:

'It is absolutely impermissible to attempt to reach the feet by penetrating behind the back of the foetus . . .'

Noted.

'It must be regarded as erroneous to grasp the upper leg, as doing so may easily result in the foetus being revolved too far; this can cause the foetus to suffer a severe blow, which can have the most deplorable consequences . . .'

'Deplorable consequences.' Rather a vague phrase, but how sinister. What if the husband of the woman from Dultsevo is left a widower? I wiped the sweat from my brow, rallied my strength and disregarded all the terrible things that could go wrong, trying only to remember the absolute essentials: what I had to do, where and how to put my hands. But as I ran my eye over the lines of black print, I kept encountering new horrors. They leaped out at me from the page.

'. . . in view of the extreme danger of rupture . . .'

'. . . the internal and combined methods must be classified as among the most dangerous obstetric operations to which a mother can be subjected . . .'

And as a grand finale:

'. . . with every hour of delay the danger increases . . .'

That was enough. My reading had borne fruit: my head was in a complete muddle. For a moment I was convinced that I understood nothing, and above all that I had no idea what sort of version I was going to perform: combined, bi-polar, internal, external . . .

I abandoned Döderlein and sank into an armchair, struggling to reduce my random thoughts to order. Then I glanced at my watch. Hell! I had already spent twenty minutes in my room, and they were waiting for me.

'. . . with every hour of delay . . .'

Hours are made up of minutes, and at times like this the minutes fly past at insane speed. I threw Döderlein aside and ran back to the hospital.

Everything there was ready. The *feldsher* was standing over a little table preparing the anaesthetic mask and the chloroform bottle. The expectant mother already lay on the operating table. Her ceaseless moans could be heard all over the hospital.

'There now, be brave,' Pelagea Ivanovna muttered consolingly as she bent over the woman, 'the doctor will help you in a moment.'

'Oh, no! I haven't the strength . . . No . . . I can't stand it!'

'Don't be afraid,' whispered the midwife. 'You'll stand it. We'll just give you something to sniff, and then you won't feel anything.'

Water gushed noisily from the taps as Anna Nikolaevna and I began washing and scrubbing our arms bared to the elbow. Against a background of groans and screams Anna Nikolaevna described to me how my predecessor, an experienced surgeon, had performed versions. I listened avidly to her, trying not to miss a single word. Those ten minutes told me more than everything I had read on obstetrics for my qualifying exams, in which I had actually passed the obstetrics paper 'with distinction.' From her brief remarks, unfinished sentences and passing hints I learned the essentials which are not to be found in any textbooks. And by the time I had begun to dry the perfect whiteness and cleanliness of my hands with sterile gauze, I was seized with confidence and a firm and absolutely definite plan had formed in my mind. There was simply no need to bother any longer over whether it was to be a combined or bi-polar version.

None of these learned words meant anything at that moment. Only one thing mattered: I had to put one hand inside, assist the version with the other hand from outside and without relying on books but on common sense, without which no doctor is any good, carefully but firmly bring one foot downwards and pull the baby after it.

I had to be calm and cautious yet at the same time utterly decisive and unfaltering.

'Right, off you go,' I instructed the *feldsher* as I began painting my fingers with iodine.

At once Pelagea Ivanovna folded the woman's arms and the *feldsher* clamped the mask over her agonised face. Chloroform slowly began to drip out of the dark yellow glass bottle, and the room started to fill with the sweet, nauseous odour. The expressions of the *feldsher* and midwives hardened with concentration, as though inspired . . .

'Haaa! Ah!' The woman suddenly shrieked. For a few seconds she writhed convulsively, trying to force away the mask.

'Hold her!'

Pelagea Ivanovna seized her by the arms and lay across her chest. The woman cried out a few more times, jerking her face away from the mask. Her movements slowed down, although she mumbled dully:

'Oh . . . let me go . . . . ah . . .'

She grew weaker and weaker. The white room was silent. The translucent drops continued to drip, drip, drip on to the white gauze.

'Pulse, Pelagea Ivanovna?'

'Firm.'

Pelagea Ivanovna raised the woman's arm and let it drop: as lifeless as a leather thong, it flopped on to the sheet. Removing the mask, the *feldsher* examined the pupil of her eye.

'She's asleep.'

A pool of blood. My arms covered in blood up to the elbows. Blood-stains on the sheets. Red clots and lumps of gauze. Pelagea Ivanovna shaking and slapping the baby, Aksinya rattling buckets as she poured water into basins.

The baby was dipped alternately into cold and hot water. He did not make a sound, his head flopping lifelessly from side to side as though on a thread. Then suddenly there came a noise somewhere between a squeak and a sigh, followed by the first weak, hoarse cry.

'He's alive . . . alive . . .' mumbled Pelagea Ivanovna as she laid the baby on a pillow.

And the mother was alive. Fortunately nothing had gone wrong. I felt her pulse. Yes, it was firm and steady; the *feldsher* gently shook her by the shoulder as he said:

'Wake up now, my dear.'

The bloodstained sheets were thrown aside and the mother hastily covered with a clean one before the *feldsher* and Aksinya wheeled her away to the ward. The swaddled baby was borne away on his pillow, the brown, wrinkled little face staring out from its white wrapping as he cried ceaselessly in a thin, pathetic whimper.

Water gushing from the taps of the sluice. Anna Nikolaevna coughed as she dragged hungrily at a cigarette.

'You did the version well, doctor. You seemed very confident.'

Scrubbing furiously at my hands, I glanced sidelong at her: was she being sarcastic? But no, her expression was a sincere one of pride and satisfaction. My heart was brimming with joy. I glanced round at the white and bloodstained disorder, at the red water in the basin and felt that I had won. But somewhere deep down there wriggled a worm of doubt.

'Let's wait and see what happens now,' I said.

Anna Nikolaevna turned to look at me in astonishment.

'What can happen? Everything's all right.'

I mumbled something vague in reply. What I had meant to say was to wonder whether the mother was really safe and sound, whether I might not have done her some harm during the operation . . . the thought nagged dully at my mind. My knowledge of obstetrics was so vague, so fragmentary and bookish. What about a rupture? How would it show? And when would it show—now or, perhaps, later? Better not talk about that.

'Well, almost anything,' I said. 'The possibility of infection cannot be ruled out,' I added, repeating the first sentence from some textbook that came into my mind.

'Oh, tha-at,' Anna Nikolaevna drawled complacently. 'Well, with luck nothing of that sort will happen. How could it, anyway? Everything here is clean and sterile.'

It was after one o'clock when I went back to my room. In a pool of light on the desk in my study lay Döderlein open at the page headed 'Dangers of Version.' For another hour after that, sipping my cooling tea, I sat over it, turning the pages. And an interesting thing happened: all the previously obscure passages became entirely comprehensible, as though they had been flooded with light; and there, at night, under the lamplight in the depth of the countryside I realised what real knowledge was.

'One can gain a lot of experience in a country practice,' I thought as I fell asleep, 'but even so one must go on and on reading, reading . . . more and more . . .'

ARCHIBALD MACLEISH

ARCHIBALD MACLEISH (1892–1982). *American poet, educator, public servant. MacLeish was born in Glencoe, Illinois, and educated at Yale, then Harvard Law School, from which he graduated first in his class. During this time he began to write poetry. He was an ambulance driver, then captain of artillery during World War I, afterward working as an editor at* Fortune. *In 1939, MacLeish accepted an appointment as librarian of Congress. He later worked as assistant secretary of state for cultural affairs. He wrote many books and won the Pulitzer Prize three times (twice for poetry, once for drama) and the Bollingen Prize. He served as Harvard's Boylston professor of rhetoric and oratory for many years.*

THE OLD GRAY COUPLE (I)

They have only to look at each other to laugh—
no one knows why, not even they:
something back in the lives they've lived,
something they both remember but no words can say.

They go off at an evening's end to talk
but they don't, or to sleep but they lie awake—
hardly a word, just a touch, just near,
just listening but not to hear.

Everything they know they know together—
everything, that is, but one:
their lives they've learned like secrets from each other;
their deaths they think of in the nights alone.

THE OLD GRAY COUPLE (II)

She: Love, says the poet, has no reasons.

He: Not even after fifty years?

She: Particularly after fifty years.

He: What was it, then, that lured us, that still teases?

She: You used to say my plaited hair!

He: And then you'd laugh.

She: Because it wasn't plaited.
Love had no reasons so you made one up
to laugh at. Look! The old, gray couple!

He: No, to prove the adage true:
Love has no reasons but old lovers do.

She: And they can't tell.

He: I can and so can you.
Fifty years ago we drew each other,
magnetized needle toward the longing north.
It was your naked presence that so moved me.
It was your absolute presence that was love.

She: Ah, *was!*

He: And now, years older, we begin to see
absence not presence: what the world would be
without your footstep in the world—the garden
empty of the radiance where you are.

She: And that's your reason?—that old lovers see
their love because they know now what its loss will be?

He: Because, like Cleopatra in the play,
they know there's nothing left once love's away . . .

She: Nothing remarkable beneath the visiting moon . . .

He: Ours is the late, last wisdom of the afternoon.
We know that love, like light, grows dearer toward the
dark.

JORGE LUIS BORGES

JORGE LUIS BORGES (1899–1986). *Argentinean poet, essayist, and fiction writer. Educated in Europe, Borges returned to Buenos Aires in 1921 and became the leader of a South American literary movement known as magic realism. During the regime of Juan Perón, he was removed from his directorship of the National Library for political reasons and made a chicken inspector. He is best known for the short story collection* Ficciones *(tr. 1962),* The Aleph and Other Stories *(tr. 1970), and* Dreamtigers *(tr. 1964), a collection of poems and short parables, of which the title piece is an account of Homer's blindness. (Borges himself was nearly blind by 1960, when the collection was first published in Spanish.) His last works were* Dr. Brodie's Report *(tr. 1972) and* The Book of Sand *(tr. 1977).*

THE IMMORTALS

And see, no longer blinded by our eyes.

—RUPERT BROOKE

Whoever could have foreseen, way back in that innocent summer of 1923, that the novelette *The Chosen One* by Camilo N. Huergo, presented to me by the author with his personal inscription on the flyleaf (which I had the decorum to tear out before offering the volume for sale to successive men of the book trade), hid under the thin varnish of fiction a prophetic truth. Huergo's photograph, in an oval frame, adorns the cover. Each time I look at it, I have the impression that the snapshot is about to cough, a victim of that lung disease which nipped in the bud a promising career. Tuberculosis, in short, denied him the happiness of acknowledging the letter I wrote him in one of my characteristic outbursts of generosity.

The epigraph prefixed to this thoughtful essay has been taken from the aforementioned novelette; I requested Dr. Montenegro, of the Academy, to render it into Spanish, but the results were negative. To give the unprepared reader the gist of the matter, I shall now sketch, in condensed form, an outline of Huergo's narrative, as follows:

The storyteller pays a visit, far to the south in Chubut, to the English rancher don Guillermo Blake, who devotes his energies not only to the breeding of sheep but also to the ramblings of the world-famous Plato and to the latest and more freakish experiments in the

97

field of surgical medicine. On the basis of his reading, don Guillermo concludes that the five senses obstruct or deform the apprehension of reality and that, could we free ourselves of them, we would see the world as it is—endless and timeless. He comes to think that the eternal models of things lie in the depths of the soul and that the organs of perception with which the Creator has endowed us are, *grosso modo,* hindrances. They are no better than dark spectacles that blind us to what exists outside, diverting our attention at the same time from the splendor we carry within us.

Blake begets a son by one of the farm girls so that the boy may one day become acquainted with reality. To anesthetize him for life, to make him blind and deaf and dumb, to emancipate him from the senses of smell and taste, were the father's first concerns. He took, in the same way, all possible measures to make the chosen one unaware of his own body. As to the rest, this was arranged with contrivances designed to take over respiration, circulation, nourishment, digestion, and elimination. It was a pity that the boy, fully liberated, was cut off from all human contact.

Owing to the press of practical matters, the narrator goes away. After ten years, he returns. Don Guillermo has died; his son goes on living after his fashion, with natural breathing, heart regular, in a dusty shack cluttered with mechanical devices. The narrator, about to leave for good, drops a cigarette butt that sets fire to the shack and he never quite knows whether this act was done on purpose or by pure chance. So ends Huergo's story, strange enough for its time but now, of course, more than outstripped by the rockets and astronauts of our men of science.

Having dashed off this disinterested compendium of the tale of a now dead and forgotten author—from whom I have nothing to gain—I steer back to the heart of the matter. Memory restores to me a Saturday morning in 1964 when I had an appointment with the eminent gerontologist Dr. Raúl Narbondo. The sad truth is that we young bloods of yesteryear are getting on; the thick mop begins to thin, one or another ear stops up, the wrinkles collect grime, molars grow hollow, a cough takes root, the backbone hunches up, the foot trips on a pebble, and, to put it plainly, the paterfamilias falters and withers. There was no doubt about it, the moment had come to see Dr. Narbondo for a general checkup, particularly considering the fact that he specialized in the replacement of malfunctioning organs.

Sick at heart because that afternoon the Palermo Juniors and the Spanish Sports were playing a return match and maybe I could not occupy my place in the front row to bolster my team, I betook myself to the clinic on Corrientes Avenue near Pasteur. The clinic, as its fame betrays, occupies the fifteenth floor of the Adamant Building. I went up by elevator (manufactured by the Electra Company). Eye to eye with Narbondo's brass shingle, I pressed the bell, and at long last, taking my courage in both hands, I slipped through the partly open door and entered into the waiting room proper. There, alone with the latest issues of *Ladies' Companion* and *Jumbo,* I whiled away the passing hours until a cuckoo clock struck twelve and sent me leaping from my armchair. At once, I asked myself, What happened? Planning my every move now like a sleuth, I took a step or two toward the next room, peeped in, ready, admittedly, to fly the coop at the slightest sound. From the streets far below came the noise of horns and traffic, the cry of a newspaper hawker, the squeal of brakes sparing some pedestrian, but, all around me, a reign of silence. I crossed a kind of laboratory, or pharmaceutical back room, furnished with instruments and flasks of all sorts. Stimulated by the aim of reaching the men's room, I pushed open a door at the far end of the lab.

Inside, I saw something that my eyes did not understand. The small enclosure was circular, painted white, with a low ceiling and neon lighting, and without a single window to relieve the sense of claustrophobia. The room was inhabited by four personages, or pieces of furniture. Their color was the same as the walls, their material wood, their form cubic. On each cube was another small cube with a latticed opening and below it a slot as in a mailbox. Carefully scrutinizing the grilled opening, you noted with alarm that from the interior you were being watched by something like eyes. The slots emitted, from time to time, a chorus of sighs or whisperings that the good Lord himself could not have made head or tail of. The placement of these cubes was such that they faced each other in the form of a square, composing a kind of conclave. I don't know how many minutes lapsed. At this point, the doctor came in and said to me, "My pardon, Bustos, for having kept you waiting. I was just out getting myself an advance ticket for today's match between the Palermo Juniors and the Spanish Sports." He went on, indicating the cubes, "Let me introduce you to Santiago Silberman, to retired clerk-of-court Ludueña, to Aquiles Molinari, and to Miss Bugard."

Out of the furniture came faint rumbling sounds. I quickly reached out a hand and, without the pleasure of shaking theirs, withdrew in good order, a frozen smile on my lips. Reaching the vestibule as best I could, I managed to stammer, "A drink. A stiff drink."

Narbondo came out of the lab with a graduated beaker filled with water and dissolved some effervescent drops into it. Blessed concoction—the wretched taste brought me to my senses. Then, the door to the small room closed and locked tight, came the explanation:

"I'm glad to see, my dear Bustos, that my immortals have made quite an impact on you. Whoever would have thought that *Homo sapiens*, Darwin's barely human ape, could achieve such perfection? This, my house, I assure you, is the only one in all Indo-America where Dr. Eric Stapledon's methodology has been fully applied. You recall, no doubt, the consternation that the death of the late lamented doctor, which took place in New Zealand, occasioned in scientific circles. I flatter myself, furthermore, for having implemented his precursory labors with a few Argentinean touches. In itself, the thesis—Newton's apple all over again—is fairly simple. The death of the body is a result, always, of the failure of some organ or other, call it the kidney, lungs, heart, or what you like. With the replacement of the organism's various components, in themselves perishable, with other corresponding stainless or polyethylene parts, there is no earthly reason whatever why the soul, why you yourself—Bustos Domecq—should not be immortal. None of your philosophical niceties here; the body can be vulcanized and from time to time recaulked, and so the mind keeps going. Surgery brings immortality to mankind. Life's essential aim has been attained— the mind lives on without fear of cessation. Each of our immortals is comforted by the certainty, backed by our firm's guarantee, of being a witness *in aeternum*. The brain, refreshed night and day by a system of electrical charges, is the last organic bulwark in which ball bearings and cells collaborate. The rest is Formica, steel, plastics. Respiration, alimentation, generation, mobility—elimination itself!—belong to the past. Our immortal is real estate. One or two minor touches are still missing, it's true. Oral articulation, dialogue, may still be improved. As for the costs, you need not worry yourself. By means of a procedure that circumvents legal red tape, the candidate transfers his property to us, and the Narbondo Company, Inc.—I, my son, his descendants— guarantees your upkeep, *in statu quo*, to the end of time. And, I might add, a money-back guarantee."

It was then that he laid a friendly hand on my shoulder. I felt his will taking power over me. "Ha-ha! I see I've whetted your appetite, I've tempted you, dear Bustos. You'll need a couple of months or so to get your affairs in order and to have your stock portfolio signed over to us. As far as the operation goes, naturally, as a friend, I want to save you a little something. Instead of our usual fee of ten thousand dollars, for you, ninety-five hundred—in cash, of course. The rest is yours. It goes to pay your lodging, care, and service. The medical procedure in itself is painless. No more than a question of amputation and replacement. Nothing to worry about. On the eve, just keep yourself calm, untroubled. Avoid heavy meals, tobacco, and alcohol, apart from your accustomed and imported, I hope, Scotch or two. Above all, refrain from impatience."

"Why two months?" I asked him. "One's enough, and then some. I come out of the anesthesia and I'm one more of your cubes. You have my address and phone number. We'll keep in touch. I'll be back next Friday at the latest."

At the escape hatch he handed me the card of Nemirovski, Nemirovski & Nemirovski, Counsellors at Law, who would put themselves at my disposal for all the details of drawing up the will. With perfect composure I walked to the subway entrance, then took the stairs at a run. I lost no time. That same night, without leaving the slightest trace behind, I moved to the New Impartial, in whose register I figure under the assumed name of Aquiles Silberman. Here, in my bedroom at the far rear of this modest hotel, wearing a false beard and dark spectacles, I am setting down this account of the facts.

TRANSLATED BY NORMAN THOMAS DI GIOVANNI

ERNEST HEMINGWAY

Ernest Hemingway (1899–1961). *American journalist and fiction writer. Son of a doctor, Hemingway went to Italy after graduating from high school to volunteer as an ambulance driver for the Red Cross. He then served in the Italian army and was seriously wounded; this experience later inspired one of his finest novels,* A Farewell to Arms *(1929). Success had already come, with* The Sun Also Rises *(1926), followed by the short story collection* Men Without Women *(1927). Among Hemingway's most notable works was* The Old Man and the Sea, *which won the 1953 Pulitzer Prize and helped him win the Nobel Prize for literature in 1954.*

INDIAN CAMP

At the lake shore there was another rowboat drawn up. The two Indians stood waiting.

Nick and his father got in the stern of the boat and the Indians shoved it off and one of them got in to row. Uncle George sat in the stern of the camp rowboat. The young Indian shoved the camp boat off and got in to row Uncle George.

The two boats started off in the dark. Nick heard the oarlocks of the other boat quite a way ahead of them in the mist. The Indians rowed with quick choppy strokes. Nick lay back with his father's arm around him. It was cold on the water. The Indian who was rowing them was working very hard, but the other boat moved further ahead in the mist all the time.

"Where are we going, Dad?" Nick asked.

"Over to the Indian camp. There is an Indian lady very sick."

"Oh," said Nick.

Across the bay they found the other boat beached. Uncle George was smoking a cigar in the dark. The young Indian pulled the boat way up on the beach. Uncle George gave both the Indians cigars.

They walked up from the beach through a meadow that was soaking wet with dew, following the young Indian who carried a lantern. Then they went into the woods and followed a trail that led to the logging road that ran back into the hills. It was much lighter on the logging road as the timber was cut away on both sides. The young Indian stopped and blew out his lantern and they all walked on along the road.

They came around a bend and a dog came out barking. Ahead were the lights of the shanties where the Indian bark-peelers lived. More dogs rushed out at them. The two Indians sent them back to the shanties. In the shanty nearest the road there was a light in the window. An old woman stood in the doorway holding a lamp.

Inside on a wooden bunk lay a young Indian woman. She had been trying to have her baby for two days. All the old women in the camp had been helping her. The men had moved off up the road to sit in the dark and smoke out of range of the noise she made. She screamed just as Nick and the two Indians followed his father and Uncle George into the shanty. She lay in the lower bunk, very big under a quilt. Her head was turned to one side. In the upper bunk was her husband. He had cut his foot very badly with an ax three days before. He was smoking a pipe. The room smelled very bad.

Nick's father ordered some water to be put on the stove, and while it was heating he spoke to Nick.

"This lady is going to have a baby, Nick," he said.

"I know," said Nick.

"You don't know," said his father. "Listen to me. What she is going through is called being in labor. The baby wants to be born and she wants it to be born. All her muscles are trying to get the baby born. That is what is happening when she screams."

"I see," Nick said.

Just then the woman cried out.

"Oh, Daddy, can't you give her something to make her stop screaming?" asked Nick.

"No. I haven't any anæsthetic," his father said. "But her screams are not important. I don't hear them because they are not important."

The husband in the upper bunk rolled over against the wall.

The woman in the kitchen motioned to the doctor that the water was hot. Nick's father went into the kitchen and poured about half of the water out of the big kettle into a basin. Into the water left in the kettle he put several things he unwrapped from a handkerchief.

"Those must boil," he said, and began to scrub his hands in the basin of hot water with a cake of soap he had brought from the camp. Nick watched his father's hands scrubbing each other with the soap. While his father washed his hands very carefully and thoroughly, he talked.

"You see, Nick, babies are supposed to be born head first but sometimes they're not. When they're not they make a lot of trouble for everybody. Maybe I'll have to operate on this lady. We'll know in a little while."

When he was satisfied with his hands he went in and went to work.

"Pull back that quilt, will you, George?" he said. "I'd rather not touch it."

Later when he started to operate Uncle George and three Indian men held the woman still. She bit Uncle George on the arm and Uncle George said, "Damn squaw bitch!" and the young Indian who had rowed Uncle George over laughed at him. Nick held the basin for his father. It all took a long time.

His father picked the baby up and slapped it to make it breathe and handed it to the old woman.

"See, it's a boy, Nick," he said. "How do you like being an interne?"

Nick said, "All right." He was looking away so as not to see what his father was doing.

"There. That gets it," said his father and put something into the basin.

Nick didn't look at it.

"Now," his father said, "there's some stitches to put in. You can watch this or not, Nick, just as you like. I'm going to sew up the incision I made."

Nick did not watch. His curiosity had been gone for a long time.

His father finished and stood up. Uncle George and the three Indian men stood up. Nick put the basin out in the kitchen.

Uncle George looked at his arm. The young Indian smiled reminiscently.

"I'll put some peroxide on that, George," the doctor said.

He bent over the Indian woman. She was quiet now and her eyes were closed. She looked very pale. She did not know what had become of the baby or anything.

"I'll be back in the morning," the doctor said, standing up. "The nurse should be here from St. Ignace by noon and she'll bring everything we need."

He was feeling exalted and talkative as football players are in the dressing room after a game.

"That's one for the medical journal, George," he said. "Doing a Cæsarian with a jack-knife and sewing it up with nine-foot, tapered gut leaders."

Uncle George was standing against the wall, looking at his arm.

"Oh, you're a great man, all right," he said.

"Ought to have a look at the proud father. They're usually the worst sufferers in these little affairs," the doctor said. "I must say he took it all pretty quietly."

He pulled back the blanket from the Indian's head. His hand came away wet. He mounted on the edge of the lower bunk with the lamp in one hand and looked in. The Indian lay with his face toward the wall. His throat had been cut from ear to ear. The blood had flowed down into a pool where his body sagged the bunk. His head rested on his left arm. The open razor lay, edge up, in the blankets.

"Take Nick out of the shanty, George," the doctor said.

There was no need of that. Nick, standing in the door of the kitchen, had a good view of the upper bunk when his father, the lamp in one hand, tipped the Indian's head back.

It was just beginning to be daylight when they walked along the logging road back toward the lake.

"I'm terribly sorry I brought you along, Nickie," said his father, all his post-operative exhilaration gone. "It was an awful mess to put you through."

"Do ladies always have such a hard time having babies?" Nick asked.

"No, that was very, very exceptional."

"Why did he kill himself, Daddy?"

"I don't know, Nick. He couldn't stand things, I guess."

"Do many men kill themselves, Daddy?"

"Not very many, Nick."

"Do many women?"

"Hardly ever."

"Don't they ever?"

"Oh, yes. They do sometimes."

"Daddy?"

"Yes."

"Where did Uncle George go?"

"He'll turn up all right."

"Is dying hard, Daddy?"

"No, I think it's pretty easy, Nick. It all depends."

They were seated in the boat, Nick in the stern, his father rowing. The sun was coming up over the hills. A bass jumped, making a circle in the water. Nick trailed his hand in the water. It felt warm in the sharp chill of the morning.

In the early morning on the lake sitting in the stern of the boat with his father rowing, he felt quite sure that he would never die.

HILLS LIKE WHITE ELEPHANTS

The hills across the valley of the Ebro were long and white. On this side there was no shade and no trees and the station was between two lines of rails in the sun. Close against the side of the station there was the warm shadow of the building and a curtain, made of strings of bamboo beads, hung across the open door into the bar, to keep out flies. The American and the girl with him sat at a table in the shade, outside the building. It was very hot and the express from Barcelona would come in forty minutes. It stopped at this junction for two minutes and went on to Madrid.

"What should we drink?" the girl asked. She had taken off her hat and put it on the table.

"It's pretty hot," the man said.

"Let's drink beer."

"Dos cervezas," the man said into the curtain.

"Big ones?" a woman asked from the doorway.

"Yes. Two big ones."

The woman brought two glasses of beer and two felt pads. She put the felt pads and the beer glasses on the table and looked at the man and the girl. The girl was looking off at the line of hills. They were white in the sun and the country was brown and dry.

"They look like white elephants," she said.

"I've never seen one," the man drank his beer.

"No, you wouldn't have."

"I might have," the man said. "Just because you say I wouldn't have doesn't prove anything."

The girl looked at the bead curtain. "They've painted something on it," she said. "What does it say?"

"Anis del Toro. It's a drink."

"Could we try it?"

The man called "Listen" through the curtain. The woman came out from the bar.

"Four reales."

"We want two Anis del Toro."

"With water?"

"Do you want it with water?"

"I don't know," the girl said. "Is it good with water?"

"It's all right."

"You want them with water?" asked the woman.

"Yes, with water."

"It tastes like licorice," the girl said and put the glass down.

"That's the way with everything."

"Yes," said the girl. "Everything tastes of licorice. Especially all the things you've waited so long for, like absinthe."

"Oh, cut it out."

"You started it," the girl said. "I was being amused. I was having a fine time."

"Well, let's try and have a fine time."

"All right. I was trying. I said the mountains looked like white elephants. Wasn't that bright?"

"That was bright."

"I wanted to try this new drink. That's all we do, isn't it—look at things and try new drinks?"

"I guess so."

The girl looked across at the hills.

"They're lovely hills," she said. "They don't really look like white elephants. I just meant the coloring of their skin through the trees."

"Should we have another drink?"

"All right."

The warm wind blew the bead curtain against the table.

"The beer's nice and cool," the man said.

"It's lovely," the girl said.

"It's really an awfully simple operation, Jig," the man said. "It's not really an operation at all."

The girl looked at the ground the table legs rested on.

"I know you wouldn't mind it, Jig. It's really not anything. It's just to let the air in."

The girl did not say anything.

"I'll go with you and I'll stay with you all the time. They just let the air in and then it's all perfectly natural."

"Then what will we do afterward?"

"We'll be fine afterward. Just like we were before."

"What makes you think so?"

"That's the only thing that bothers us. It's the only thing that's made us unhappy."

The girl looked at the bead curtain, put her hand out and took hold of two of the strings of beads.

"And you think then we'll be all right and be happy."

"I know we will. You don't have to be afraid. I've known lots of people that have done it."

"So have I," said the girl. "And afterward they were all so happy."

"Well," the man said, "if you don't want to you don't have to. I wouldn't have you do it if you didn't want to. But I know it's perfectly simple."

"And you really want to?"

"I think it's the best thing to do. But I don't want you to do it if you don't really want to."

"And if I do it you'll be happy and things will be like they were and you'll love me?"

"I love you now. You know I love you."

"I know. But if I do it, then it will be nice again if I say things are like white elephants, and you'll like it?"

"I'll love it. I love it now but I just can't think about it. You know how I get when I worry."

"If I do it you won't ever worry?"

"I won't worry about that because it's perfectly simple."

"Then I'll do it. Because I don't care about me."

"What do you mean?"

"I don't care about me."

"Well, I care about you."

"Oh, yes. But I don't care about me. And I'll do it and then everything will be fine."

"I don't want you to do it if you feel that way."

The girl stood up and walked to the end of the station. Across, on the other side, were fields of grain and trees along the banks of the Ebro. Far away, beyond the river, were mountains. The shadow of a cloud moved across the field of grain and she saw the river through the trees.

"And we could have all this," she said. "And we could have everything and every day we make it more impossible."

"What did you say?"

"I said we could have everything."

"We can have everything."

"No, we can't."

"We can have the whole world."

"No, we can't."

"We can go everywhere."

"No, we can't. It isn't ours any more."

"It's ours."

"No, it isn't. And once they take it away, you never get it back."

"But they haven't taken it away."

"We'll wait and see."

"Come on back in the shade," he said. "You mustn't feel that way."

"I don't feel any way," the girl said. "I just know things."

"I don't want you to do anything that you don't want to do—"

"Nor that isn't good for me," she said. "I know. Could we have another beer?"

"All right. But you've got to realize—"

"I realize," the girl said. "Can't we maybe stop talking?"

They sat down at the table and the girl looked across at the hills on the dry side of the valley and the man looked at her and at the table.

"You've got to realize," he said, "that I don't want you to do it if you don't want to. I'm perfectly willing to go through with it if it means anything to you."

"Doesn't it mean anything to you? We could get along."

"Of course it does. But I don't want anybody but you. I don't want any one else. And I know it's perfectly simple."

"Yes, you know it's perfectly simple."

"It's all right for you to say that, but I do know it."

"Would you do something for me now?"

"I'd do anything for you."

"Would you please please please please please please please stop talking?"

He did not say anything but looked at the bags against the wall of the station. There were labels on them from all the hotels where they had spent nights.

"But I don't want you to," he said, "I don't care anything about it."

"I'll scream," the girl said.

The woman came out through the curtains with two glasses of beer and put them down on the damp felt pads. "The train comes in five minutes," she said.

"What did she say?" asked the girl.

"That the train is coming in five minutes."

The girl smiled brightly at the woman, to thank her.

"I'd better take the bags over to the other side of the station," the man said. She smiled at him.

"All right. Then come back and we'll finish the beer."

He picked up the two heavy bags and carried them around the station to the other tracks. He looked up the tracks but could not see the train. Coming back, he walked through the barroom, where people waiting for the train were drinking. He drank an Anis at the bar and looked at the people. They were all waiting reasonably for the train. He went out through the bead curtains. She was sitting at the table and smiled at him.

"Do you feel better?" he asked.

"I feel fine," she said. "There's nothing wrong with me. I feel fine."

ARNA BONTEMPS

ARNA BONTEMPS (1902–1974). *African-American novelist. Bontemps's work focused on the black experience in the United States and in Haiti. His novels include* God Sends Sunday (*1931; later dramatized, with Countee Cullen, as* St. Louis Woman), Black Thunder (*1935*), *and* Drums at Dusk (*1939*).

A SUMMER TRAGEDY

Old Jeff Patton, the black share farmer, fumbled with his bow tie. His fingers trembled and the high stiff collar pinched his throat. A fellow loses his hand for such vanities after thirty or forty years of simple life. Once a year, or maybe twice if there's a wedding among his kinfolks, he may spruce up; but generally fancy clothes do nothing but adorn the wall of the big room and feed the moths. That had been Jeff Patton's experience. He had not worn his stiff-bosomed shirt more than a dozen times in all his married life. His swallowtailed coat lay on the bed beside him, freshly brushed and pressed, but it was as full of holes as the overalls in which he worked on weekdays. The moths had used it badly. Jeff twisted his mouth into a hideous tooth-less grimace as he contended with the obstinate bow. He stamped his good foot and decided to give up the struggle.

"Jennie," he called.

"What's that, Jeff?" His wife's shrunken voice came out of the adjoining room like an echo. It was hardly bigger than a whisper.

"I reckon you'll have to help me wid this heah bow tie, baby," he said meekly. "Dog if I can hitch it up."

Her answer was not strong enough to reach him, but presently the old woman came to the door, feeling her way with a stick. She had a wasted, dead-leaf appearance. Her body, as scrawny and gnarled as a string bean, seemed less than nothing in the ocean of frayed and faded petticoats that surrounded her. These hung an inch or two above the tops of her heavy unlaced shoes and showed little grotesque piles where the stockings had fallen down from her negligible legs.

"You oughta could do a heap mo' wid a thing like that'n me—beingst as you got yo' good sight."

"Looks like I oughta could," he admitted. "But ma fingers is gone democrat on me. I get all mixed up in the looking glass and can't tell wicha way to twist the devilish thing."

Jennie sat on the side of the bed and old Jeff Patton got down on one knee while she tied the bow knot. It was a slow and painful ordeal for each of them in this position. Jeff's bones cracked, his knee ached, and it was only after a half dozen attempts that Jennie worked a semblance of a bow into the tie.

"I got to dress maself now," the old woman whispered. "These is ma old shoes and stockings, and I ain't so much as unwrapped ma dress."

"Well, don't worry 'bout me no mo', baby," Jess said. "That 'bout finishes me. All I gotta do now is slip on that old coat 'n ves' an' I'll be fixed to leave."

Jennie disappeared again through the dim passage into the shed room. Being blind was no handicap to her in that black hole. Jeff heard the cane placed against the wall beside the door and knew that his wife was on easy ground. He put on his coat, took a battered top hat from the bedpost and hobbled to the front door. He was ready to travel. As soon as Jennie could get on her Sunday shoes and her old black silk dress, they would start.

Outside the tiny log house, the day was warm and mellow with sunshine. A host of wasps were humming with busy excitement in the trunk of a dead sycamore. Gray squirrels were searching through the grass for hickory nuts and blue jays were in the trees, hopping from branch to branch. Pine woods stretched away to the left like a black sea. Among them were scattered scores of log houses like Jeff's, houses of black share farmers. Cows and pigs wandered freely among the trees. There was no danger of loss. Each farmer knew his own stock and knew his neighbor's as well as he knew his neighbor's children.

Down the slope to the right were the cultivated acres on which the colored folks worked. They extended to the river, more than two miles away, and they were today green with the unmade cotton crop. A tiny thread of a road, which passed directly in front of Jeff's place, ran through these green fields like a pencil mark.

Jeff, standing outside the door, with his absurd hat in his left hand, surveyed the wide scene tenderly. He had been forty-five years on these acres. He loved them with the unexplained affection that others have for the countries to which they belong.

The sun was hot on his head, his collar still pinched his throat, and the Sunday clothes were intolerably hot. Jeff transferred the hat to his right hand and began fanning with it. Suddenly the whisper that was Jennie's voice came out of the shed room.

"You can bring the car round front whilst you's waitin'," it said feebly. There was a tired pause; then it added, "I'll soon be fixed to go."

"A'right, baby," Jeff answered. "I'll get it in a minute."

But he didn't move. A thought struck him that made his mouth fall open. The mention of the car brought to his mind, with new intensity, the trip he and Jennie were about to take. Fear came into his eyes; excitement took his breath. Lord, Jesus!

"Jeff . . . O Jeff," the old woman's whisper called.

He awakened with a jolt. "Hunh, baby?"

"What you doin'?"

"Nuthin'. Jes studyin'. I jes been turnin' things round 'n round in ma mind."

"You could be gettin' the car," she said.

"Oh yes, right away, baby."

He started round to the shed, limping heavily on his bad leg. There were three frizzly chickens in the yard. All his other chickens had been killed or stolen recently. But the frizzly chickens had been saved somehow. That was fortunate indeed, for these curious creatures had a way of devouring "Poison" from the yard and in that way protecting against conjure and black luck and spells. But even the frizzly chickens seemed now to be in a stupor. Jeff thought they had some ailment; he expected all three of them to die shortly.

The shed in which the old T-model Ford stood was only a grass roof held up by four corner poles. It had been built by tremulous hands at a time when the little rattletrap car had been regarded as a peculiar treasure. And, miraculously, despite wind and downpour, it still stood.

Jeff adjusted the crank and put his weight upon it. The engine came to life with a sputter and bang that rattled the old car from radiator to taillight. Jeff hopped into the seat and put his foot on the accelerator. The sputtering and banging increased. The rattling became more violent. That was good. It was good banging, good sputtering and rattling, and it meant that the aged car was still in running condition. She could be depended on for this trip.

Again Jeff's thought halted as if paralyzed. The suggestion of the trip fell into the machinery of his mind like a wrench. He felt dazed and weak. He swung the car out into the yard, made a half turn and drove around to the front door. When he took his hands off the wheel, he noticed that he was trembling violently. He cut off the motor and climbed to the ground to wait for Jennie.

A few minutes later she was at the window, her voice rattling against the pane like a broken shutter.

"I'm ready, Jeff."

He did not answer, but limped into the house and took her by the arm. He led her slowly through the big room, down the step and across the yard.

"You reckon I'd oughta lock the do'?" he asked softly.

They stopped and Jennie weighed the question. Finally she shook her head.

"Ne' mind the do'," she said. "I don't see no cause to lock up things."

"You right," Jeff agreed. "No cause to lock up."

Jeff opened the door and helped his wife into the car. A quick shudder passed over him. Jesus! Again he trembled.

"How come you shaking so?" Jennie whispered.

"I don't know," he said.

"You mus' be scairt, Jeff."

"No, baby, I ain't scairt."

He slammed the door after her and went around to crank up again. The motor started easily. Jeff wished that it had not been so responsive. He would have liked a few more minutes in which to turn things around in his head. As it was, with Jennie chiding him about being afraid, he had to keep going. He swung the car into the little pencil-mark road and started off toward the river, driving very slowly, very cautiously.

Chugging across the green countryside, the small battered Ford seemed tiny indeed. Jeff felt a familiar excitement, a thrill, as they came down the first slope to the immense levels on which the cotton was growing. He could not help reflecting that the crops were good. He knew what that meant, too; he had made forty-five of them with his own hands. It was true that he had worn out nearly a dozen mules, but that was the fault of old man Stevenson, the owner of the land. Major Stevenson had the odd notion that one mule was all a share farmer needed to work a thirty-acre plot. It was an expensive notion, the way it killed mules from overwork, but the old man held to it. Jeff thought it killed a good many share farmers as well as mules, but he had no sympathy for them. He had always been strong, and he had been taught to have no patience with weakness in men. Women or children might be tolerated if they were puny, but a weak man was a curse. Of course, his own children—

Jeff's thought halted there. He and Jennie never mentioned their dead children any more. And naturally he did not wish to dwell upon them in his mind. Before he knew it, some remark would slip out of his mouth and that would make Jennie feel blue. Perhaps she would cry. A woman like Jennie could not easily throw off the grief that comes from losing five grown children within two years. Even Jeff was still staggered by the blow. His memory had not been much good recently. He frequently talked to himself. And, although he had kept it a secret, he knew that his courage had left him. He was terrified by the least unfamiliar sound at night. He was reluctant to venture far from home in the daytime. And that habit of trembling when he felt fearful was now far beyond his control. Sometimes he became afraid and trembled without knowing what had frightened him. The feeling would just come over him like a chill.

The car rattled slowly over the dusty road. Jennie sat erect and silent, with a little absurd hat pinned to her hair. Her useless eyes seemed very large, very white in their deep sockets. Suddenly Jeff heard her voice, and he inclined his head to catch the words.

"Is we passed Delia Moore's house yet?" she asked.

"Not yet," he said.

"You must be drivin' mighty slow, Jeff."

"We might just as well take our time, baby."

There was a pause. A little puff of steam was coming out of the radiator of the car. Heat wavered above the hood. Delia Moore's house was nearly half a mile away. After a moment Jennie spoke again.

"You ain't really scairt, is you, Jeff?"

"Nah, baby, I ain't scairt."

"You know how we agreed—we gotta keep on goin'."

Jewels of perspiration appeared on Jeff's forehead. His eyes rounded, blinked, becamed fixed on the road.

"I don't know," he said with a shiver. "I reckon it's the only thing to do."

"Hm."

A flock of guinea fowls, pecking in the road, were scattered by the passing car. Some of them took to their wings; others hid under bushes. A blue jay, swaying on a leafy twig, was annoying a roadside squirrel. Jeff held an even speed till he came near Delia's place. Then he slowed down noticeably.

Delia's house was really no house at all, but an abandoned store building converted into a dwelling. It sat near a crossroads, beneath a single black cedar tree. There Delia, a catish old creature of Jennie's age, lived alone. She had been there more years than anybody could remember, and long ago had won the disfavor of such women as Jennie. For in her young days Delia had been gayer, yellower and saucier than seemed proper in those parts. Her ways with menfolks had been dark and suspicious. And the fact that she had had as many husbands as children did not help her reputation.

"Yonder's old Delia," Jeff said as they passed.

"What she doin'?"

"Jes sittin' in the do'," he said.

"She see us?"

"Hm," Jeff said. "Musta did."

That relieved Jennie. It strengthened her to know that her old enemy had seen her pass in her best clothes. That would give the old she-devil something to chew her gums and fret about, Jennie thought. Wouldn't she have a fit if she didn't find out? Old evil Delia! This would be just the thing for her. It would pay her back for being so evil. It would also pay her, Jennie thought, for the way she used to grin at Jeff—long ago when her teeth were good.

The road became smooth and red, and Jeff could tell by the smell of the air that they were nearing the river. He could see the rise where the road turned and ran along parallel to the stream. The car chugged on monotonously. After a long silent spell, Jennie leaned against Jeff and spoke.

"How many bale o' cotton you think we got standin'?" she said.

Jeff wrinkled his forehead as he calculated.

"'Bout twenty-five, I reckon."

"How many you make las' year?"

"Twenty-eight," he said. "How come you ask that?"

"I's jes thinkin'," Jennie said quietly.

"It don't make a speck o' difference though," Jeff reflected. "If we get much or if we get little, we still gonna be in debt to old man Stevenson when he gets through counting up agin us. It's took us a long time to learn that."

Jennie was not listening to these words. She had fallen into a trance-like meditation. Her lips twitched. She chewed her gums and rubbed her gnarled hands nervously. Suddenly she leaned forward, buried her face in the nervous hands and burst into tears. She cried aloud in a dry cracked voice that suggested the rattle of fodder on dead stalks. She cried aloud like a child, for she had never learned to suppress a genuine sob. Her slight old frame shook heavily and seemed hardly able to sustain such violent grief.

"What's the matter, baby?" Jeff asked awkwardly. "Why you cryin' like all that?"

"I's jes thinkin'," she said.

"So you the one what's scairt now, hunh?"

"I ain't scairt, Jeff. I's jes thinkin' 'bout leavin' eve'thing like this—eve'thing we been used to. It's right sad-like."

Jeff did not answer, and presently Jennie buried her face again and cried.

The sun was almost overhead. It beat down furiously on the dusty wagon-path road, on the parched roadside grass and the tiny battered car. Jeff's hands, gripping the wheel, became wet with perspiration; his forehead sparkled. Jeff's lips parted. His mouth shaped a hideous grimace. His face suggested the face of a man being burned. But the torture passed and his expression softened again.

"You mustn't cry, baby," he said to his wife. "We gotta be strong. We can't break down."

Jennie waited a few seconds, then said, "You reckon we oughta do it, Jeff? You reckon we oughta go 'head an' do it, really?"

Jeff's voice choked; his eyes blurred. He was terrified to hear Jennie say the thing that had been in his mind all morning. She had egged him on when he had wanted more than anything in the world to wait, to reconsider, to think things over a little longer. Now she was getting cold feet. Actually there was no need of thinking the question through again. It would only end in making the same painful decision once more. Jeff knew that. There was no need of fooling around longer.

"We jes as well to do like we planned," he said. "They ain't nothin' else for us now—it's the bes' thing."

Jeff thought of the handicaps, the near impossibility, of making another crop with his leg bothering him more and more each week. Then there was always the chance that he would have another stroke, like the one that had made him lame. Another one might kill him. The least it could do would be to leave him helpless. Jeff gasped—Lord, Jesus! He could not bear to think of being helpless, like a baby, on Jennie's hands. Frail, blind Jennie.

The little pounding motor of the car worked harder and harder. The puff of steam from the cracked radiator became larger. Jeff realized that they were climbing a little rise. A moment later the road turned abruptly and he looked down upon the face of the river.

"Jeff."

"Hunh?"

"Is that the water I hear?"

"Hm. Tha's it."

"Well, which way you goin' now?"

"Down this a way," he said. "The road runs 'longside o' the water a lil piece."

She waited a while calmly. Then she said, "Drive faster."

"A'right, baby," Jeff said.

The water roared in the bed of the river. It was fifty or sixty feet below the level of the road. Between the road and the water there was a long smooth slope, sharply inclined. The slope was dry, the clay hardened by prolonged summer heat. The water below, roaring in a narrow channel, was noisy and wild.

"Jeff."

"Hunh?"

"How far you goin'?"

"Jes a lil piece down the road."

"You ain't scairt, is you, Jeff?"

"Nah, baby," he said trembling. "I ain't scairt."

"Remember how we planned it, Jeff. We gotta do it like we said. Brave-like."

"Hm."

Jeff's brain darkened. Things suddenly seemed unreal, like figures in a dream. Thoughts swam in his mind foolishly, hysterically, like little blind fish in a pool within a dense cave. They rushed, crossed one another, jostled, collided, retreated and rushed again. Jeff soon became dizzy. He shuddered violently and turned to his wife.

"Jennie, I can't do it. I can't." His voice broke pitifully.

She did not appear to be listening. All the grief had gone from her face. She sat erect, her unseeing eyes wide open, strained and frightful. Her glossy black skin had become dull. She seemed as thin, as sharp and bony, as a starved bird. Now, having suffered and endured the sadness of tearing herself away from beloved things, she showed no anguish. She was absorbed with her own thoughts, and she didn't even hear Jeff's voice shouting in her ear.

Jeff said nothing more. For an instant there was light in his cavernous brain. The great chamber was, for less than a second, peopled by characters he knew and loved. They were simple, healthy creatures, and they behaved in a manner that he could understand. They had quality. But since he had already taken leave of them long ago, the remembrance did not break his heart again. Young Jeff Patton was among them, the Jeff Patton of fifty years ago who went down to New Orleans with a crowd of country boys to the Mardi Gras doings. The gay young crowd, boys with candy-striped shirts and rouged-brown girls in noisy silks, was like a picture in his head. Yet it did not make him sad. On that very trip Slim Burns had killed Joe Beasley—the crowd had been broken up. Since then Jeff Patton's world had been the Greenbriar Plantation. If there had been other Mardi Gras carnivals, he had not heard of them. Since then there had been no time; the years had fallen on him like waves. Now he was old, worn out. Another paralytic stroke (like the one he had already suffered) would put him on his back for keeps. In that condition, with a frail blind woman to look after him, he would be worse off than if he were dead.

Suddenly Jeff's hands became steady. He actually felt brave. He slowed down the motor of the car and carefully pulled off the road. Below, the water of the stream boomed, a soft thunder in the deep channel. Jeff ran the car onto the clay slope, pointed it directly toward the stream and put his foot heavily on the accelerator. The little car leaped furiously down the steep incline toward the water. The movement was nearly as swift and direct as a fall. The two old black folks, sitting quietly side by side, showed no excitement. In another instant the car hit the water and dropped immediately out of sight.

A little later it lodged in the mud of a shallow place. One wheel of the crushed and upturned little Ford became visible above the rushing water.

ZORA NEALE HURSTON

ZORA NEALE HURSTON (1903–1960). *African-American anthropologist and writer. Hurston graduated from Barnard College in 1928 with a specialty in anthropological research. Very much a woman before her time, Zora Neale Hurston is now more than ever being recognized and appreciated for the multitalented genius she was. Among her novels, short stories, and anthropological studies are the recently republished* Mules and Men; Their Eyes Were Watching God; Moses, Man of the Mountain; *and* Tell My Horse. *Also reissued are her* Complete Stories.

MY MOST HUMILIATING
JIM CROW EXPERIENCE

My most humiliating Jim Crow experience came in New York instead of the South as one would have expected. It was in 1931 when Mrs. R. Osgood Mason was financing my researches in anthropology. I returned to New York from the Bahama Islands ill with some disturbances of the digestive tract.

Godmother (Mrs. Mason liked for me to call her Godmother) became concerned about my condition and suggested a certain white specialist at her expense. His office was in Brooklyn.

Mr. Paul Chapin called up and made the appointment for me. The doctor told the wealthy and prominent Paul Chapin that I would get the best of care.

So two days later I journeyed to Brooklyn to submit myself to the care of the great specialist.

His reception room was more than swanky, with a magnificent hammered copper door and other decor on the same plane as the door.

But his receptionist was obviously embarrassed when I showed up. I mentioned the appointment and got inside the door. She went into the private office and stayed a few minutes, then the doctor appeared in the door all in white, looking very important, and also very unhappy from behind his rotund stomach.

He did not approach me at all, but told one of his nurses to take me into a private examination room.

The room was private all right, but I would not rate it highly as an examination room. Under any other circumstances, I would have sworn it was a closet where the soiled towels and uniforms were tossed until called for by the laundry. But I will say this for it, there was a chair in there wedged in between the wall and the pile of soiled linen.

The nurse took me in there, closed the door quickly, and disappeared. The doctor came in immediately and began in a desultory manner to ask me about my symptoms. It was evident he meant to get me off the premises as quickly as possible. Being the sort of objective person I am, I did not get up and sweep out angrily as I was first disposed to do. I stayed to see just what would happen, and further to torture him more. He went through some motions, stuck a tube down my throat to extract some bile from my gall bladder, wrote a prescription and asked for twenty dollars as fee.

I got up, set my hat at a reckless angle and walked out, telling him that I would send him a check, which I never did. I went away feeling the pathos of Anglo-Saxon civilization.

And I still mean pathos, for I know that anything with such a false foundation cannot last. Whom the gods would destroy, they first made mad.

PABLO NERUDA

PABLO NERUDA *(1904–1973). Chilean writer of poetry and fiction, social observer, and political leader. Neruda received the Lenin and Stalin Peace Prize in 1953 and the Nobel Prize in literature in 1971, though he has always been cherished as dearly for the earthy sensuality and eroticism of his love poetry as for his statements of political belief. His works have been translated into many languages and include* Un Canto para Bolívar *(1941),* Alturas de Macchu-Picchu *(1948),* Obras Completas *(1957), and* Cien Sonetas de Amor *(1960).*

LARYNX

Now this is it, said Death,
and as far as I could see
Death was looking at me, at me.

This all happened in hospital,
in washed out corridors,
and the doctor peered at me
with periscopic eyes.
He stuck his head in my mouth,
scratched away at my larynx—
perhaps a small seed
of death was stuck there.

At first, I turned into smoke
so that the cindery one
would pass and not recognize me.
I played the fool, I grew thin,
pretended to be simple or transparent—
I wanted to be a cyclist
to pedal out of death's range.

Then rage came over me
and I said, "Death, you bastard,
must you always keep butting in?
Haven't you enough with all those bones?
I'll tell you exactly what I think:
you have no discrimination, you're deaf
and stupid beyond belief.

"Why are you following me?
What do you want with my skeleton?
Why don't you take the miserable one,
the cataleptic, the smart one,
the bitter, the unfaithful, the ruthless,
the murderer, the adulterers,
the two-faced judge,
the deceiving journalist,
tyrants from islands,
those who set fire to mountains,
the chiefs of police,
jailers and burglars?
Why do you have to take me?
What business have I with Heaven?
Hell doesn't suit me—
I feel fine on the earth."

With such internal mutterings
I kept myself going
while the restless doctor
went tramping through my lungs,
from bronchea to bronchea
like a bird from branch to branch.
I couldn't feel my throat;
my mouth was open like the jaws of a suit of armor,
and the doctor ran up and down
my larynx on his bicycle,
till, serious and certain,
he looked at me through his telescope
and pried me loose from death.

It wasn't what they had thought.
It wasn't my turn.

If I tell you I suffered a lot,
and really loved the mystery,
that Our Lord and Our Lady
were waiting for me in their oasis,
if I talk of enchantment,
and being eaten up by distress
at not being close to dying,
if I say like a stupid chicken
that I die by not dying,
give me a boot in the butt,
fit punishment for a liar.

TRANSLATED BY ALASTAIR REID

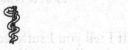

W. H. AUDEN

W. H. AUDEN (1907–1973). English poet and dramatist. As a youth, Auden specialized in biology, but by the time he was fifteen he had discovered his vocation as a poet. Earning his living as a schoolmaster, Auden published poetry widely throughout the 1930s; he became known as the leading radical, antifascist poet of that decade, as much of his writing served as social criticism in verse form without ever becoming mere propaganda. In 1939, he left England with the intention of residing permanently in the United States, but spent the latter years of his life in both Kirchstetten, Austria, and New York City. His later verse, collected in New Year Letter *(1941),* The Age of Anxiety *(1947),* Homage to Clio *(1960), and* About the House *(1965), lost its radical political bent and became overtly Christian. Today, Auden is recognized as one of the major figures in twentieth-century Anglo-American poetry.*

MUSÉE DES BEAUX ARTS

About suffering they were never wrong,
The Old Masters: how well they understood
Its human position; how it takes place
While someone else is eating or opening a window or just walking
    dully along;
How, when the aged are reverently, passionately waiting
For the miraculous birth, there always must be
Children who did not specially want it to happen, skating
On a pond at the edge of the wood:
They never forgot
That even the dreadful martyrdom must run its course
Anyhow in a corner, some untidy spot
Where the dogs go on with their doggy life and the torturer's horse
Scratches its innocent behind on a tree.

In Brueghel's *Icarus*, for instance: how everything turns away
Quite leisurely from the disaster; the ploughman may
Have heard the splash, the forsaken cry,
But for him it was not an important failure; the sun shone
As it had to on the white legs disappearing into the green
Water; and the expensive delicate ship that must have seen
Something amazing, a boy falling out of the sky,
Had somewhere to get to and sailed calmly on.

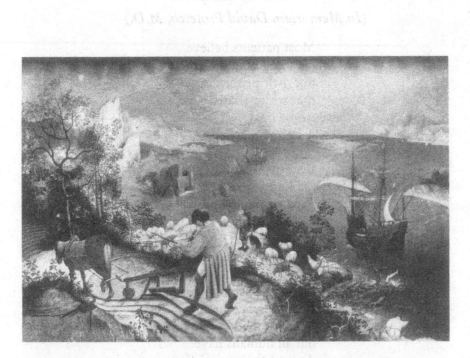

Landscape with the Fall of Icarus by Pieter Brueghel. In mythology, Icarus and his father, Daedalus, escaped from captivity by flying on wings made of feathers held together with wax. But ignoring his father's admonitions, the exuberant Icarus flew too near the sun; its heat melted the wax on his wings, and he fell into the ocean and drowned. In Brueghel's painting, Icarus is seen in the right foreground, his "white legs disappearing into the green water."

THE ART OF HEALING
(In Memoriam David Protetch, M.D.)

Most patients believe
dying is something they do,
    not their physician,
    that white-coated sage,
never to be imagined
    naked or married.

Begotten by one,
I should know better. 'Healing,'
    Papa would tell me,
    'is not a science,
but the intuitive art
    of wooing Nature.

Plants, beasts, may react
according to the common
    whim of their species,
    but all humans have
prejudices of their own
    which can't be foreseen.

To some, ill-health is
a way to be important,
    others are stoics,
    a few fanatics,
who won't feel happy until
    they are cut open.'

Warned by him to shun
the sadist, the nod-crafty,
    and the fee-conscious,
    I knew when we met,
I had found a consultant
    who thought as he did,

yourself a victim
of medical engineers
    and their arrogance,
    when they atom-bombed
your sick pituitary
    and over-killed it.

    'Every sickness
is a musical problem,'
    so said Novalis,
    'and every cure
a musical solution':
    You knew that also.

    Not that in my case
you heard any shattering
    discords to resolve:
    to date my organs
still seem pretty sure of their
    self-identity.

    For my small ailments
you, who were mortally sick,
    prescribed with success:
    my major vices,
my mad addictions, you left
    to my own conscience.

    Was it your very
predicament that made me
    sure I could trust you,
    if I were dying,
to say so, not insult me
    with soothing fictions?

    Must diabetics
all contend with a nisus
    to self-destruction?
    One day you told me:
'It is only bad temper
    that keeps me going.'

But neither anger
nor lust are omnipotent,
nor should we even
want our friends to be
superhuman. Dear David,
dead one, rest in peace,

having been what all
doctors should be, but few are,
and, even when most
difficult, condign
of our biassed affection
and objective praise.

STOP ALL THE CLOCKS

Stop all the clocks, cut off the telephone,
Prevent the dog from barking with a juicy bone,
Silence the pianos and with muffled drum
Bring out the coffin, let the mourners come.

Let aeroplanes circle moaning overhead
Scribbling on the sky the message He Is Dead,
Put crêpe bows round the white necks of the public doves,
Let the traffic policemen wear black cotton gloves.

He was my North, my South, my East and West,
My working week and my Sunday rest,
My noon, my midnight, my talk, my song;
I thought that love would last for ever: I was wrong.

The stars are not wanted now: put out every one;
Pack up the moon and dismantle the sun;
Pour away the ocean and sweep up the wood;
For nothing now can ever come to any good.

W. H. AUDEN

GIVE ME A DOCTOR

Give me a doctor, partridge-plump,
Short in the leg and broad in the rump,
An endomorph with gentle hands,
Who'll never make absurd demands
That I abandon all my vices,
Nor pull a long face in a crisis,
But with a twinkle in his eye
Will tell me that I have to die.

EUDORA WELTY

*EUDORA WELTY (1909–). American fiction writer. Although her early
ambition was to be a painter, Welty devoted her life to writing after
the success of her first book of stories,* A Curtain of Green *(1941). She
is widely admired as a writer who values and records the richness of
her home region (the South, especially Mississippi) and comments
perceptively on the inward awareness of the individual. Her
collections of stories are many, including* The Wide Net *(1943),* The
Golden Apples *(1949),* The Bride Innisfallen *(1955),* Thirteen Stories
(1965), and Collected Stories of Eudora Welty *(1980). She won the
Pulitzer Prize in 1972 for* The Optimist's Daughter. *Welty's recent
works include* A Worn Path *(1991) and* The Shoe Bird *(1993).*

A WORN PATH

It was December—a bright frozen day in the early morning. Far
out in the country there was an old Negro woman with her head tied
in a red rag, coming along a path through the pinewoods. Her name
was Phoenix Jackson. She was very old and small and she walked
slowly in the dark pine shadows, moving a little from side to side in
her steps, with the balanced heaviness and lightness of a pendulum
in a grandfather clock. She carried a thin, small cane made from an
umbrella, and with this she kept tapping the frozen earth in front of
her. This made a grave and persistent noise in the still air, that seemed
meditative like the chirping of a solitary little bird.

She wore a dark striped dress reaching down to her shoe tops, and
an equally long apron of bleached sugar sacks, with a full pocket: all
neat and tidy, but every time she took a step she might have fallen
over her shoelaces, which dragged from her unlaced shoes. She looked
straight ahead. Her eyes were blue with age. Her skin had a pattern all
its own of numberless branching wrinkles and as though a whole little
tree stood in the middle of her forehead, but a golden color ran underneath, and the two knobs of her cheeks were illumined by a yellow
burning under the dark. Under the red rag her hair came down on her
neck in the frailest of ringlets, still black, and with an odor like copper.

Now and then there was a quivering in the thicket. Old Phoenix
said, "Out of my way, all you foxes, owls, beetles, jack rabbits, coons
and wild animals! . . . Keep out from under these feet, little bob-
whites. . . . Keep the big wild hogs out of my path. Don't let none of

EUDORA WELTY

those come running my direction. I got a long way." Under her small
black-freckled hand her cane, limber as a buggy whip, would switch
at the brush as if to rouse up any hiding things.

On she went. The woods were deep and still. The sun made the
pine needles almost too bright to look at, up where the wind rocked.
The cones dropped as light as feathers. Down in the hollow was the
mourning dove—it was not too late for him.

The path ran up a hill. "Seem like there is chains about my feet,
time I get this far," she said, in the voice of argument old people keep
to use with themselves. "Something always take a hold of me on this
hill—pleads I should stay."

After she got to the top she turned and gave a full, severe look behind her where she had come. "Up through pines," she said at length.
"Now down through oaks."

Her eyes opened their widest, and she started down gently. But
before she got to the bottom of the hill a bush caught her dress.

Her fingers were busy and intent, but her skirts were full and long,
so that before she could pull them free in one place they were caught
in another. It was not possible to allow the dress to tear. "I in the
thorny bush," she said. "Thorns, you doing your appointed work.
Never want to let folks pass, no sir. Old eyes thought you was a pretty
little *green* bush."

Finally, trembling all over, she stood free, and after a moment dared
to stoop for her cane.

"Sun so high!" she cried, leaning back and looking, while the thick
tears went over her eyes. "The time getting all gone here."

At the foot of this hill was a place where a log was laid across the
creek.

"Now comes the trail," said Phoenix.

Putting her right foot out, she mounted the log and shut her eyes.
Lifting her skirt, leveling her cane fiercely before her, like a festival
figure in some parade, she began to march across. Then she opened
her eyes and she was safe on the other side.

"I wasn't as old as I thought," she said.

But she sat down to rest. She spread her skirts on the bank around
her and folded her hands over her knees. Up above her was a tree in a
pearly cloud of mistletoe. She did not dare to close her eyes, and when
a little boy brought her a plate with a slice of marble-cake on it she
spoke to him. "That would be acceptable," she said. But when she
went to take it there was just her own hand in the air.

So she left that tree, and had to go through a barbed-wire fence.
There she had to creep and crawl, spreading her knees and stretching

131

her fingers like a baby trying to climb the steps. But she talked loudly to herself: she could not let her dress be torn now, so late in the day, and she could not pay for having her arm or her leg sawed off if she got caught fast where she was.

At last she was safe through the fence and risen up out in the clearing. Big dead trees, like black men with one arm, were standing in the purple stalks of the withered cotton field. There sat a buzzard.

"Who you watching?"

In the furrow she made her way along.

"Glad this not the season for bulls," she said, looking sideways, "and the good Lord made his snakes to curl up and sleep in the winter. A pleasure I don't see no two-headed snake coming around that tree, where it come once. It took a while to get by him, back in the summer."

She passed through the old cotton and went into a field of dead corn. It whispered and shook and was taller than her head. "Through the maze now," she said, for there was no path.

Then there was something tall, black, and skinny there, moving before her.

At first she took it for a man. It could have been a man dancing in the field. But she stood still and listened, and it did not make a sound. It was as silent as a ghost.

"Ghost," she said sharply, "who be you the ghost of? For I have heard of nary death close by."

But there was no answer—only the ragged dancing in the wind.

She shut her eyes, reached out her hand, and touched a sleeve. She found a coat and inside that an emptiness, cold as ice.

"You scarecrow," she said. Her face lighted. "I ought to be shut up for good," she said with laughter. "My senses is gone. I too old. I the oldest people I ever know. Dance, old scarecrow," she said, "while I dancing with you."

She kicked her foot over the furrow, and with mouth drawn down, shook her head once or twice in a little strutting way. Some husks blew down and whirled in streamers about her skirts.

Then she went on, parting her way from side to side with the cane, through the whispering field. At last she came to the end, to a wagon track where the silver grass blew between the red ruts. The quail were walking around like pullets, seeming all dainty and unseen.

"Walk pretty," she said. "This the easy place. This the easy going."

She followed the track, swaying through the quiet bare fields, through the little strings of trees silver in their dead leaves, past cabins silver from weather, with the doors and windows boarded shut, all like old women under a spell sitting there. "I walking in their sleep," she said, nodding her head vigorously.

In a ravine she went where a spring was silently flowing through a hollow log. Old Phoenix bent and drank. "Sweet-gum makes the water sweet," she said, and drank more. "Nobody know who made this well, for it was here when I was born."

The track crossed a swampy part where the moss hung as white as lace from every limb. "Sleep on, alligators, and blow your bubbles." Then the track went into the road.

Deep, deep the road went down between the high green-colored banks. Overhead the live-oaks met, and it was as dark as a cave.

A black dog with a lolling tongue came up out of the weeds by the ditch. She was meditating, and not ready, and when he came at her she only hit him a little with her cane. Over she went in the ditch, like a little puff of milkweed.

Down there, her sense drifted away. A dream visited her, and she reached her hand up, but nothing reached down and gave her a pull. So she lay there and presently went to talking. "Old woman," she said to herself, "that black dog come up out of the weeds to stall you off, and now there he sitting on his fine tail, smiling at you."

A white man finally came along and found her—a hunter, a young man, with his dog on a chain.

"Well, Granny!" he laughed. "What are you doing there?"

"Lying on my back like a June-bug waiting to be turned over, mister," she said, reaching up her hand.

He lifted her up, gave her a swing in the air, and set her down. "Anything broken, Granny?"

"No sir, them old dead weeds is springy enough," said Phoenix, when she had got her breath. "I thank you for your trouble."

"Where do you live, Granny?" he asked, while the two dogs were growling at each other.

"Away back yonder, sir, behind the ridge. You can't even see it from here."

"On your way home?"

"No sir, I going to town."

"Why, that's too far! That's as far as I walk when I come out myself, and I get something for my trouble." He patted the stuffed bag he carried, and there hung down a little closed claw. It was one of the bob-whites, with its beak hooked bitterly to show it was dead. "Now you go on home, Granny!"

"I bound to go to town, mister," said Phoenix. "The time come around."

He gave another laugh, filling the whole landscape. "I know you old colored people! Wouldn't miss going to town to see Santa Claus!"

But something held old Phoenix very still. The deep lines in her face went into a fierce and different radiation. Without warning, she had seen with her own eyes a flashing nickel fall out of the man's pocket onto the ground.

"How old are you, Granny?" he was saying.

"There is no telling, mister," she said, "no telling."

Then she gave a little cry and clapped her hands and said, "Git on away from here, dog! Look! Look at that dog!" She laughed as if in admiration. "He ain't scared of nobody. He a big black dog." She whispered, "Sic him!"

"Watch me get rid of that cur," said the man. "Sic him, Pete! Sic him!"

Phoenix heard the dogs fighting, and heard the man running and throwing sticks. She even heard a gunshot. But she was slowly bending forward by that time, further and further forward, the lids stretched down over her eyes, as if she were doing this in her sleep. Her chin was lowered almost to her knees. The yellow palm of her hand came out from the fold of her apron. Her fingers slid down and along the ground under the piece of money with the grace and care they would have in lifting an egg from under a setting hen. Then she slowly straightened up, she stood erect, and the nickel was in her apron pocket. A bird flew by. Her lips moved. "God watching me the whole time. I come to stealing."

The man came back, and his own dog panted about them. "Well, I scared him off that time," he said, and then he laughed and lifted his gun and pointed it at Phoenix.

She stood straight and faced him.

"Doesn't the gun scare you?" he said, still pointing it.

"No, sir, I seen plenty go off closer by, in my day, and for less than what I done," she said, holding utterly still.

He smiled, and shouldered the gun. "Well, Granny," he said, "you must be a hundred years old, and scared of nothing. I'd give you a dime if I had any money with me. But you take my advice and stay home, and nothing will happen to you."

"I bound to go on my way, mister," said Phoenix. She inclined her head in the red rag. Then they went in different directions, but she could hear the gun shooting again and again over the hill.

She walked on. The shadows hung from the oak trees to the road like curtains. Then she smelled wood-smoke, and smelled the river, and she saw a steeple and the cabins on their steep steps. Dozens of little black children whirled around her. There ahead was Natchez shining. Bells were ringing. She walked on.

In the paved city it was Christmas time. There were red and green electric lights strung and criss-crossed everywhere, and all turned on in the daytime. Old Phoenix would have been lost if she had not distrusted her eyesight and depended on her feet to know where to take her.

She paused quietly on the sidewalk where people were passing by. A lady came along in the crowd, carrying an armful of red-, green- and silver-wrapped presents; she gave off perfume like the red roses in hot summer, and Phoenix stopped her.

"Please, missy, will you lace up my shoe?" She held up her foot.

"What do you want, Grandma?"

"See my shoe," said Phoenix. "Do all right for out in the country, but wouldn't look right to go in a big building."

"Stand still then, Grandma," said the lady. She put her packages down on the sidewalk beside her and laced and tied both shoes tightly.

"Can't lace 'em with a cane," said Phoenix. "Thank you, missy. I doesn't mind asking a nice lady to tie up my shoe, when I gets out on the street."

Moving slowly and from side to side, she went into the big building, and into a tower of steps, where she walked up and around and around until her feet knew to stop.

She entered a door, and there she saw nailed up on the wall the document that had been stamped with the gold seal and framed in the gold frame, which matched the dream that was hung up in her head.

"Here I be," she said. There was a fixed and ceremonial stiffness over her body.

"A charity case, I suppose," said an attendant who sat at the desk before her.

But Phoenix only looked above her head. There was sweat on her face, the wrinkles in her skin shone like a bright net.

"Speak up, Grandma," the woman said. "What's your name? We must have your history, you know. Have you been here before? What seems to be the trouble with you?"

Old Phoenix only gave a twitch to her face as if a fly were bothering her.

"Are you deaf?" cried the attendant.

But then the nurse came in.

"Oh, that's just old Aunt Phoenix," she said. "She doesn't come for herself—she has a little grandson. She makes these trips just as regular as clockwork. She lives away back off the Old Natchez Trace." She bent down. "Well, Aunt Phoenix, why don't you just take a seat? We won't keep you standing after your long trip." She pointed.

The old woman sat down, bolt upright in the chair.

"Now, how is the boy?" asked the nurse.

Old Phoenix did not speak.

"I said, how is the boy?"

But Phoenix only waited and stared straight ahead, her face very solemn and withdrawn into rigidity.

"Is his throat any better?" asked the nurse. "Aunt Phoenix, don't you hear me? Is your grandson's throat any better since the last time you came for the medicine?"

With her hands on her knees, the old woman waited, silent, erect and motionless, just as if she were in armor.

"You mustn't take up our time this way, Aunt Phoenix," the nurse said. "Tell us quickly about your grandson, and get it over. He isn't dead, is he?"

At last there came a flicker and then a flame of comprehension across her face, and she spoke.

"My grandson. It was my memory had left me. There I sat and forgot why I made my long trip."

"Forgot?" The nurse frowned. "After you came so far?"

Then Phoenix was like an old woman begging a dignified forgiveness for waking up frightened in the night. "I never did go to school, I was too old at the Surrender," she said in a soft voice. "I'm an old woman without an education. It was my memory fail me. My little grandson, he is just the same, and I forgot it in the coming."

"Throat never heals, does it?" said the nurse, speaking in a loud, sure voice to old Phoenix. By now she had a card with something written on it, a little list. "Yes. Swallowed lye. When was it?—January— two–three years ago—"

Phoenix spoke unasked now. "No, missy, he not dead, he just the same. Every little while his throat begin to close up again, and he not able to swallow. He not get his breath. He not able to help himself. So the time come around, and I go on another trip for the soothing medicine."

"All right. The doctor said as long as you came to get it, you could have it," said the nurse. "But it's an obstinate case."

"My little grandson, he sit up there in the house all wrapped up, waiting by himself," Phoenix went on. "We is the only two left in the world. He suffer and it don't seem to put him back at all. He got a sweet look. He going to last. He wear a little patch quilt and peep out holding his mouth open like a little bird. I remembers so plain now. I not going to forget him again, no, the whole enduring time. I could tell him from all the others in creation."

"All right." The nurse was trying to hush her now. She brought her a bottle of medicine. "Charity," she said, making a check mark in a book.

Old Phoenix held the bottle close to her eyes, and then carefully put it into her pocket.

"I thank you," she said.

"It's Christmas time, Grandma," said the attendant. "Could I give you a few pennies out of my purse?"

"Five pennies is a nickel," said Phoenix stiffly.

"Here's a nickel," said the attendant.

Phoenix rose carefully and held out her hand. She received the nickel and then fished the other nickel out of her pocket and laid it beside the new one. She stared at her palm closely, with her head on one side.

Then she gave a tap with her cane on the floor.

"This is what come to me to do," she said. "I going to the store and buy my child a little windmill they sells, made out of paper. He going to find it hard to believe there such a thing in the world. I'll march myself back where he waiting, holding it straight up in this hand."

She lifted her free hand, gave a little nod, turned around, and walked out of the doctor's office. Then her slow step began on the stairs, going down.

JOSEPHINE MILES

JOSEPHINE MILES (1911–1985). *American poet, scholar, and teacher. Born in Chicago, Miles spent most of her professional life at the University of California, Berkeley. She published ten volumes of poetry, culminating in her* Collected Poems.

SHEEP

Led by Johns Hopkins on a trip through the heart
To the uttermost reaches of the body,
I was disappointed by X-ray and camera
At what was to be found there.

Mostly I missed the green pastures
Which I knew lay on either side of the path,
The running streams of tears in their salty waters,
Their crystal waters, and the steadfast sheep.

Sheep of my heart, where do you nibble,
At the pump of the ventricle, course of the artery,
That you do not look up into the camera
To tell on what you feed?

CONCEPTION

Death did not come to my mother
Like an old friend.
She was a mother, and she must
Conceive him.

Up and down the bed she fought crying
Help me, but death
Was a slow child
Heavy. He

Waited. When he was born
We took and tired him, now he is ready
To do his good in the world.

He has my mother's features.
He can go among strangers
To save lives.

MAY SARTON

MAY SARTON (1912–1995). *American poet and writer. Sarton's prolific writings in poetry, fiction, and autobiography have provided thoughtful examinations of love, loss, solitude, and dying. Although a world traveler, Sarton's life and fictional world are associated with New England, especially Boston, New Hampshire, and Maine. Frequently her work explores difficulties faced by women trying to balance careers, families, and lifestyles. Having survived a stroke as well as cancer, she recounts the emotional and physical experiences of such illnesses in* After the Stroke; Recovering; Endgame; *and* Encore. *Sarton, who regarded herself primarily as a poet, has received wide acclaim for the poignancy of personal reflections about aging in the volumes* Halfway to Silence *and* Coming into Eighty.

THE TIDES

I pretend
To live in the present.
Now is what I crave,
Finches at the feeder,
Sunlight on a rose.

But memory
The relentless tide
Suddenly brings alive
A forgotten moment
With such a freight
Of passionate grief in it
I cry out
Alone.

The past is Now.
The tide rises and falls.
There is no shutting it out.

WANTING TO DIE

Sometimes
I want to die,
To be done with it all
At last,
Never make my bed again,
Never answer another letter
Or water the plants,
None of those efforts
I must make
Every day
To keep alive.

But then
I do not want to die.
The leaves are turning
And I must see
The scarlet and gold
One more time,
A single yellow leaf
Tumbling through
The sunlit air
One last time.

THE ENDER, THE BEGINNER

Becoming eighty
Might be nothing much
If I could be well,
But it feels weighty

Because I am in touch
Because I have been ill
With Heaven and with Hell,
Unbalanced on that crutch,

A place of no return
And of no mending
With a long life to burn
And its long ending.

The ender, the beginner,
The child and the old soul,
The mystic and the sinner
At eighty remain whole.

I am still whole and merry
And when all's said and done
Rejoice in my strange story,
Ardent and alone.

EDWARD LOWBURY

EDWARD LOWBURY (1913–). *English physician, microbiologist, and poet. Lowbury has been much honored for his work on hospital infection control and the treatment of burns. Born in London, he earned degrees in physiology and medicine at Oxford University (where he also won the Newdigate Prize for poetry and the Matthew Arnold Prize for a critical essay). His poetry has appeared in more than twenty books and pamphlets, including* Collected Poems *(1993). Now retired from the practice of medicine, Dr. Lowbury lives near Birmingham, England.*

GLAUCOMA

Shadows are creeping in
From a grey perimeter:
My blinkered years begin—

Not blindness, but a smear
On the landscape, where once
The outlines were clear.

I curse this whim of chance
That monkeyed with my sight
And led my steps a dance;

Then think how Milton might
Have cried for joy if his
Perpetual black night

Had given way to this
Imperfect light of mine:
Its touch would be a kiss,

Its taste a heady wine,
While field, flock, herd,
Bloom, human face divine,

Once lost, now disinterred,
Would bring back his lyric youth;
And yet, the last word,—

The dazzling epic truth,
He gleaned by *inner* light.
That memory can soothe

My nerves, as I recite
This catalogue of moans
About my blinkered sight:

I'll give up picking bones.

LEWIS THOMAS

LEWIS THOMAS (1913–1993). American physician and essayist. Dr. Thomas was a professor, dean, and chairman of pathology departments at several medical schools. He was for many years president of Memorial Sloan-Kettering Cancer Center, and in 1992 he retired from Cornell University Medical Center in New York City, where he served as scholar in residence. His many books include The Lives of a Cell *(which won the National Book Award);* The Medusa and the Snail; Late Night Thoughts on Listening to Mahler's Ninth Symphony; The Youngest Science: Notes of a Medicine Watcher; *and* Et Cetera, Et Cetera, *an exploration of the vagaries of word origins.*

HOUSE CALLS

My father took me along on house calls whenever I was around the house, all through my childhood. He liked company, and I liked watching him and listening to him. This must have started when I was five years old, for I remember riding in the front seat from one house to another, and back and forth from the hospital, when my father and many of the people on the streets were wearing gauze masks; it was the 1918 influenza epidemic.

One of the frequent calls which I found fascinating was at a big house on Sanford Avenue; he never parked the car in front of this house, but usually left it, and me, a block away around the corner. Later, he explained that the patient was a prominent Christian Scientist, a pillar of that church. He could perfectly well have parked in front if there had been a clearer understanding all around of what he was up to, for it was, in its way, faith healing.

I took the greatest interest in his doctor's bag, a miniature black suitcase, fitted inside to hold his stethoscope and various glass bottles and ampules, syringes and needles, and a small metal case for instruments. It smelled of Lysol and ether. All he had in the bag was a handful of things. Morphine was the most important, and the only really indispensable drug in the whole pharmacopoeia. Digitalis was next in value. Insulin had arrived by the time he had been practicing for twenty years, and he had it. Adrenalin was there, in small glass ampules, in case he ran into a case of anaphylactic shock; he never did. As he drove his rounds, he talked about the patients he was seeing.

I'm quite sure my father always hoped I would want to become a doctor, and that must have been part of the reason for taking me along on his visits. But the general drift of his conversation was intended to make clear to me, early on, the aspect of medicine that troubled him most all through his professional life; there were so many people needing help, and so little that he could do for any of them. It was necessary for him to be available, and to make all these calls at their homes, but I was not to have the idea that he could do anything much to change the course of their illnesses. It was important to my father that I understand this; it was a central feature of the profession, and a doctor should not only be prepared for it but be even more prepared to be honest with himself about it.

It was not always easy to be honest, he said. One of his first patients, who had come to see him in his new office when he was an unknown in town, was a man complaining of grossly bloody urine. My father examined him at length, took a sample of the flawed urine, did a few other tests, and found himself without a diagnosis. To buy time enough to read up on the matter, he gave the patient a bottle of Blaud's pills, a popular iron remedy for anemia at the time, and told him to come back to the office in four days. The patient returned on the appointed day jubilant, carrying a flask of crystal-clear urine, totally cured. In the following months my father discovered that his reputation had been made by this therapeutic triumph. The word was out, all over town, that that new doctor, Thomas, had gifts beyond his own knowledge—this last because my father's outraged protests that his Blaud's pills could have had nothing whatever to do with recovery from bloody urine. The man had probably passed a silent kidney stone and that was all there was to it, said my father. But he had already gained the reputation of a healer, and it grew through all the years of his practice, and there was nothing he could do about it.

Even now, twenty-five years after his death, I meet people from time to time who lived once in Flushing, or whose parents lived there, and I hear the same anecdotes about his abilities: children with meningitis or rheumatic fever whose lives had been saved by him, patients with pneumonia who had recovered under his care, even people with incurable endocarditis, overwhelming typhoid fever, peritonitis, what-all.

But the same stories are told about any good, hardworking general practitioner of that day. Patients do get better, some of them anyway, from even the worst diseases; there are very few illnesses, like rabies, that kill all comers. Most of them tend to kill some patients and spare others, and if you are one of the lucky ones and have also had at hand

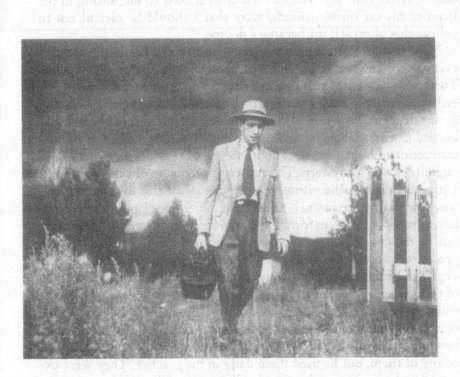

Dr. Ernest Ceriani, the only doctor in Kremmling, Colorado, makes his way through an unkempt yard to call on a patient. Photograph by W. Eugene Smith from *Country Doctor*, 1948.

a steady, knowledgeable doctor, you become convinced that the doctor saved you. My father's early instructions to me, sitting in the front of his car on his rounds, were that I should be careful not to believe this of myself if I became a doctor.

Nevertheless, despite his skepticism, he carried his prescription pad everywhere and wrote voluminous prescriptions for all his patients. These were fantastic formulations, containing five or six different vegetable ingredients, each one requiring careful measuring and weighing by the druggist, who pounded the powder, dissolved it in alcohol, and bottled it with a label giving only the patient's name, the date, and the instructions about dosage. The contents were a deep mystery, and intended to be a mystery. The prescriptions were always written in Latin, to heighten the mystery. The purpose of this kind of therapy was essentially reassurance. A skilled, experienced physician might have dozens of different formulations in his memory, ready for writing out in flawless detail at a moment's notice, but all he could have predicted about them with any certainty were the variations in the degree of bitterness of taste, the color, the smell, and the likely effects of the concentrations of alcohol used as solvent. They were placebos, and they had been the principal mainstay of medicine, the sole technology, for so long a time—millennia—that they had the incantatory power of religious ritual. My father had little faith in the effectiveness of any of them, but he used them daily in his practice. They were expected by his patients; a doctor who did not provide such prescriptions would soon have no practice at all; they did no harm, so far as he could see; if nothing else, they gave the patient something to do while the illness, whatever, was working its way through its appointed course.

The United States Pharmacopoeia, an enormous book, big as the family Bible, stood on a bookshelf in my father's office, along with scores of textbooks and monographs on medicine and surgery. The ingredients that went into the prescriptions, and the recipes for their compounding and administration, were contained in the *Pharmacopoeia.* There was no mistaking the earnestness of that volume; it was a thousand pages of true belief: this set of ingredients was useful in pulmonary tuberculosis, that one in "acute indigestion" (the term then used for what later turned out to be coronary thrombosis), another in neurasthenia (weak nerves; almost all patients had weak nerves, one time or another), and so on, down through the known catalogue of human ailments. There was a different prescription for every circumstance, often three or four. The most popular and widely used ones were the "tonics," good for bucking up the spirits; these contained the headiest concentrations of alcohol. Opium had been the prime ingredient in the prescriptions of the nineteenth century, edited out when it was realized that great numbers of elderly people, especially "nervous" women, were sitting in their rocking chairs, addicted beyond recall.

The tradition still held when I was a medical student at Harvard. In the outpatient department of the Boston City Hospital, through which hundreds of patients filed each day for renewal of their medications, each doctor's desk had a drawerful of prescriptions already printed out to save time, needing only the doctor's signature. The most popular one, used for patients with chronic, obscure complaints, was *Elixir of I, Q and S,* iron, quinine, and strychnine, each ingredient present in tiny amounts, dissolved in the equivalent of bourbon.

Medicine was subject to recurrent fads in therapy throughout my father's career. Long before his time, homeopathy emerged and still had many devout practitioners during his early years; this complex theory, involving what was believed to be the therapeutic value of "like versus like," and the administration of minuscule quantities of drugs that imitated the symptoms of the illness in question, took hold in the mid-nineteenth century in reaction against the powerfully toxic drugs then in common use—mercury, arsenic, bismuth, strychnine, aconite, and the like. Patients given the homeopathic drugs felt better and had a better chance of surviving, about the same as they would have had without treatment, and the theory swept the field for many decades.

A new theory, attributing all human disease to the absorption of toxins from the lower intestinal tract, achieved high fashion in the first decade of this century. "Autointoxication" became the fundamental disorder to be overcome by treatment, and the strongest measures were introduced to empty the large bowel and keep it empty. Cathartics, ingenious variations of the enema, and other devices for stimulating peristalsis took over medical therapy. My father, under persuasion by a detail man from one of the medical supply houses, purchased one of these in 1912, a round lead object the size of a bowling ball, encased in leather. This was to be loaned to the patient, who was instructed to lie flat in bed several times daily and roll it clockwise around the abdomen, following the course of the colon. My father tried it for a short while on a few patients, with discouraging results, and one day placed it atop a cigar box which he had equipped with wheels and a long string, and presented it to my eldest sister, who tugged it with pleasure around the corner to a neighbor's house. That was the last he saw of the ball until twelve years later, when the local newspaper announced in banner headlines that a Revolutionary War cannon ball had been discovered in the excavated garden behind our neighbor's yard. The ball was displayed for public view on the neighbor's mantel, to the mystification of visiting historians, who were unable to figure out the trajectory from any of the known engagements of the British or American forces; several learned papers were written on the problem. My father claimed privately to his family, swearing us to secrecy, that he had, in an indirect sense anyway, made medical history.

So far as I know, he was never caught up again by medical theory. He did not believe in focal infections when this notion appeared in the 1920s, and must have lost a lucrative practice by not removing normal tonsils, appendixes, and gallbladders. When the time for psychosomatic disease arrived, he remained a skeptic. He indulged my mother by endorsing her administration of cod-liver oil to the whole family, excepting himself, and even allowed her to give us something for our nerves called Eskay's Neurophosphates, which arrived as samples from one of the pharmaceutical houses. But he never convinced himself about the value of medicine.

His long disenchantment with medical therapy was gradually replaced by an interest in surgery, for which he found himself endowed with a special talent. At last, when he was in his early fifties, he decided to give up general practice and concentrate exclusively on surgery. He was very good at it, and his innate skepticism made him uniquely successful as a surgical consultant. Years later, after his death, I was told by some of his younger colleagues that his opinion was especially valued, and widely sought throughout the country, because of his known reluctance to operate on a patient until he was entirely convinced that the operation was absolutely necessary. His income must have suffered because of this, but his reputation was solidly established.

DYLAN THOMAS

DYLAN THOMAS (1914–1953). *Welsh poet, short story writer, and playwright. Thomas is acclaimed for his carefully ordered images, which focus on the recurring themes of man, nature, and the love of God. An antic spirit, Thomas was a popular reader of his own (and others') poetry, and much in demand as a lecturer during his short life.*

DO NOT GO GENTLE INTO THAT GOOD NIGHT

Do not go gentle into that good night,
Old age should burn and rave at close of day;
Rage, rage against the dying of the light.

Though wise men at their end know dark is right,
Because their words had forked no lightning they
Do not go gentle into that good night.

Good men, the last wave by, crying how bright
Their frail deeds might have danced in a green bay,
Rage, rage against the dying of the light.

Wild men who caught and sang the sun in flight,
And learn, too late, they grieved it on its way,
Do not go gentle into that good night.

Grave men, near death, who see with blinding sight
Blind eyes could blaze like meteors and be gay,
Rage, rage against the dying of the light.

And you, my father, there on the sad height,
Curse, bless, me now with your fierce tears, I pray.
Do not go gentle into that good night.
Rage, rage against the dying of the light.

RANDALL JARRELL

RANDALL JARRELL (1914–1965). *American poet, critic, and novelist. Born in Nashville, Tennessee, Jarrell served in the air force in the Second World War, then taught at a number of universities and was consultant in poetry at the Library of Congress from 1956 to 1958. Jarrell was considered a critic of great integrity for his incisive and lively essays, which are collected in* Poetry and the Age *(1953),* A Sad Heart at the Supermarket *(1962), and* The Third Book of Criticism *(1971). His* Complete Poems *appeared posthumously in 1969.*

NEXT DAY

Moving from Cheer to Joy, from Joy to All,
I take a box
And add it to my wild rice, my Cornish game hens.
The slacked or shorted, basketed, identical
Food-gathering flocks
Are selves I overlook. Wisdom, said William James,

Is learning what to overlook. And I am wise
If that is wisdom.
Yet somehow, as I buy All from these shelves
And the boy takes it to my station wagon,
What I've become
Troubles me even if I shut my eyes.

When I was young and miserable and pretty
And poor, I'd wish
What all girls wish: to have a husband,
A house and children. Now that I'm old, my wish
Is womanish:
That the boy putting groceries in my car

See me. It bewilders me he doesn't see me.
For so many years
I was good enough to eat: the world looked at me
And its mouth watered. How often they have undressed me,
The eyes of strangers!
And, holding their flesh within my flesh, their vile

Imaginings within my imagining,
I too have taken
The chance of life. Now the boy pats my dog
And we start home. Now I am good.
The last mistaken,
Ecstatic, accidental bliss, the blind

Happiness that, bursting, leaves upon the palm
Some soap and water—
It was so long ago, back in some Gay
Twenties, Nineties, I don't know . . . Today I miss
My lovely daughter
Away at school, my sons away at school,

My husband away at work—I wish for them.
The dog, the maid,
And I go through the sure unvarying days
At home in them. As I look at my life,
I am afraid
Only that it will change, as I am changing:

I am afraid, this morning, of my face.
It looks at me
From the rear-view mirror, with the eyes I hate,
The smile I hate. Its plain, lined look
Of gray discovery
Repeats to me: "You're old." That's all, I'm old.

And yet I'm afraid, as I was at the funeral
I went to yesterday,
My friend's cold made-up face, granite among its flowers,
Her undressed, operated-on, dressed body
Were my face and body.
As I think of her I hear her telling me

How young I seem; I *am* exceptional;
I think of all I have.
But really no one is exceptional,
No one has anything, I'm anybody,
I stand beside my grave
Confused with my life, that is commonplace and solitary.

THE X-RAY WAITING ROOM IN THE HOSPITAL

I am dressed in my big shoes and wrinkled socks
And one of the light blue, much-laundered smocks
The men and women of this country wear.
All of us miss our own underwear
And the old days. These new, plain, mean
Days of pain and care, this routine
Misery has made us into cases, the one case
The one doctor cures forever . . . The face
The patients have in common hopes without hope
For something outside the machine—its wife,
Its husband—to burst in and hand it life;
But when the door opens it's another smock.
It looks at us, we look at it. Our little flock
Of blue-smocked sufferers, in naked equality,
Longs for each nurse and doctor who goes by
Well and dressed, to make friends with, single out the I
That used to be, but we are indistinguishable.
It is better to lie upon a table,
A dye in my spine. The roentgenologist
Introduces me to a kind man, a specialist
In spines like mine: the lights go out, he rotates me.
My myelogram is negative. This elates me,
And I take off my smock in joy, put on
My own pajamas, my own dressing gown,
And ride back to my own room, 601.

JOHN CIARDI

JOHN CIARDI (1916–1986). *American poet, essayist, translator, lexicographer, teacher, and lecturer. Ciardi wrote and edited several dozen books, including splendid poetry for both adults and children* (Selected Poems *for adults;* I Met a Man *and* Fast and Slow *for children). His was the standard translation of Dante's* Divine Comedy. *For many years he was the poetry editor and a columnist and essayist for the* Saturday Review. *For nineteen years, he also served as director of the Bread Loaf Writers' Conference in Vermont, which continues as a vital center for American letters.*

WASHING YOUR FEET

Washing your feet is hard when you get fat.
* * *
In lither times the act was unstrained and pleasurable.
* * *
You spread the toes for signs of athlete's foot.
* * *
You used creams, and rubbing alcohol, and you powdered.
* * *
You bent over, all in order, and did everything.
* * *
Mary Magdalene made a prayer meeting of it.
* * *
She, of course, was washing not her feet but God's.
* * *
Degas painted ladies washing their own feet.
* * *
Somehow they also seem to be washing God's feet.
* * *
To touch any body anywhere should be ritual.
* * *
To touch one's own body anywhere should be ritual.
* * *
Fat makes the ritual wheezy and a bit ridiculous.
* * *
Ritual and its idea should breathe easy.
* * *
They are memorial, meditative, immortal.
* * *
Toenails keep growing after one is dead.
* * *
Washing my feet, I think of immortal toenails.
* * *
What are they doing on these ten crimped polyps?
* * *

I reach to wash them and begin to wheeze.
*   *   *
I wish I could paint like Degas or believe like Mary.
*   *   *
It is sad to be naked and to lack talent.
*   *   *
It is sad to be fat and to have dirty feet.

GWENDOLYN BROOKS

GWENDOLYN BROOKS (1917–2000). *African-American poet and novelist. The author of twenty books of poems, including* In the Mecca *(1964), Brooks was born in Topeka, Kansas, and grew up in Chicago, where she lived most of her life. She was thirteen when her first poem was published, and she went on to become the first African-American woman to be awarded a Pulitzer Prize, in 1950, for her collection of poems* Annie Allen. *She was widely recognized as one of the preeminent poets of this century. As a writer in residence at Chicago State University, she received innumerable awards. She was named the 1994 Jefferson lecturer (this is the highest honor bestowed by the federal government for intellectual achievement in the humanities) and won the 1994 National Book Foundation medal for distinguished contribution to American letters.*

THE BEAN EATERS

They eat beans mostly, this old yellow pair.
Dinner is a casual affair.
Plain chipware on a plain and creaking wood,
Tin flatware.

Two who are Mostly Good.
Two who have lived their day,
But keep on putting on their clothes
And putting things away.

And remembering . . .
Remembering, with twinklings and twinges,
As they lean over the beans in their
    rented back room that is full of beads and
    receipts and dolls and cloths, tobacco
    crumbs, vases and fringes.

DORIS GRUMBACH

DORIS GRUMBACH (1918–). *American novelist and memoirist.*
Grumbach's novels include The Magician's Girl *(1987),* Chamber
Music *(1980),* The Ladies *(1985), and* The Missing Person *(1993).*
The following selection is from her memoir Coming into the End
Zone *(1991), an intensely personal account of the year following her*
seventieth birthday, during which she is "haunted by death in the
daily reminders of her own diminishing vitality" despite a full, active
existence spent writing fiction, reviewing books, and traveling. Recent
works include Extra Innings *(1993) and* Fifty Days of Solitude
(1994). A Life in the Day *(1997) purports to be a record of an*
"ordinary" twenty-four hours, but that time period takes on
extraordinary meaning when looked at under the writer's light.

Excerpt from COMING INTO THE END ZONE

It is eccentric and inaccurate to claim that the July of my seventieth
birthday is a landmark in my life. Surely there were other important
Julys scattered throughout those many years. For instance, that
month of my fifth year when I realized I had to go to school in
September. It was a prospect I dreaded, believing in my heart that I
was already sufficiently educated by Central Park, by the books I had
read since I was three and a half, and by the disruptive arrival that year
of a baby sister who taught me terrible lessons in displacement,
resentment, hatred.

In the July of my twentieth year after I had graduated from college,
I ignored the event because I was in a state of shock. During the May
that preceded it, my friend and classmate John Ricksecker had
jumped from the roof of the School of Commerce at New York University, ending his troubled life and my innocence about how good
life was and how hopeful our future. It was May 1939, a few months
before Hitler marched into Poland. Was he determined not to be
made to go to war? I never knew why he chose to jump, or whether
he did. For he said as he was dying that he "climbed up and fell." I
have always mourned him and felt responsible for his death. As a
woman not liable to be "called up," I was overwhelmed by the unfairness of the draft, making me realize the destructive power of sexual
inequities and the injustice of death.

There was the July two years later after I married in May. I began to see that legal unions did not solve problems of inner turmoil and loneliness. . . . The Julys in my middle years after two of my children were born and I began to have serious doubts about my capacity for motherhood. The July I lay in bed in a tiny room in a country house, afflicted with viral pneumonia, listening to the sounds of husband and children downstairs, and wondering how to escape from everything and everyone I knew.

My sixtieth July was terrible. I remembered, as though I had been struck a blow, that my mother had died at fifty-nine. Somehow, to have exceeded her life span by a year seemed to me a terrible betrayal. It was worse than the guilt that choked me later at the thought of having lived eighteen years longer than the little sister I had once hoped would disappear from her crib during the night, stolen by an evil fairy, or dead at the hand of a careless Fräulein.

At sixty-five I must have been resigned to aging and death: I can remember no raging against the night, no anger about what Yeats described as "decrepit age that has been tied to me / As to a dog's tail."

But seventy. This is different. The month at seventy seems disastrous, so without redeeming moments that, in despair, I am taking notes, hoping to find in the recording process a positive value to living so long, some glory to survival, even vainglory if true glory is impossible.

The terrible Twelfth goes on. I invite Peggy, our host, to share May Sarton's gift of champagne with us. Friends from up the road, Ted Nowick and Bob Taylor, will come too. I suddenly think: A more suitable way to celebrate this dread event would be alone, not in society. I ought to let go of the cheerful illusions of company and surrender to the true state of old age, remembering Virginia Woolf's conviction that at bottom we are all alone and lonely.

The sun moves to the other side of the house. I go in to change to slacks and a shirt with sleeves. In the process I do an unusual thing. I look skeptically, exploringly, at my body in the floor-length mirror. In my young years I remember that I enjoyed feeling the firmness of my arms and legs, neck and fingers, chin and breasts. Once the result of such examinations was less reassuring I stopped doing it. Thereafter, I never resorted to a mirror, believing it would be better not to know the truth about change and decline. In my memory of my body nothing had changed.

Now I look, hard. I see the pull of gravity on the soft tissues of my breasts and buttocks. I see the heavy rings that encircle my neck like Ubangi jewelry. I notice bones that seem to have thinned and shrunk.

Muscles appear to be watered down. The walls of my abdomen, like Jericho, have softened and now press outward. There is nothing lovely about the sight of me. I have been taught that firm and unlined is beautiful. Shall I try to learn to love what I am left with? I wonder. It would be easier to resolve never again to look into a full-length mirror.

October 10. I put down this date, although my habit in journals is not to do so. If something is worth recording, I have always thought, it ought to be general enough to be free of dull, diurnal notation. But this day:

I take the very early Metroliner (six-fifty, an unusual hour for me to take a train) to New York for a meeting of the board of the National Book Critics Circle, a group I have belonged to for many years. A law has been passed that, I believe, makes this the last year of my term, so I am determined to attend every meeting, despite the cost of travel. We are reimbursed only for the two last meetings in the year if we do not serve an institution that pays our way. National Public Radio does not do this for me.

We talk about NBCC business and possible recommendations of books deserving of nomination for an award. It is always fun to meet with other critics and editors. We hole up on the third floor of the Algonquin Hotel, and argue, insult each other pleasantly by challenging the validity of views different from our own, eat a buffet lunch together as we work, and take notes on books of interest we have missed and ought now to read.

At four o'clock the meeting is over. I planned to meet my daughter Jane at the public library for a cocktail party a publisher is giving to celebrate the appearance of the first volume of T. S. Eliot's letters. I need coffee, as I always do between events. Caffeine acts as oil with which to shift gears, sustenance for my flagging spirits. Flagging: Why is that adjective always used for spirits? The *Oxford English Dictionary* informs me that the usage is three hundred years old and first referred to falling down through feebleness. It then was used for the heart, then the circulation. Matthew Arnold was the first to speak of "a spiritual flagging." I buy coffee in a plastic cup and carry it to the benches on Forty-fourth Street and Sixth Avenue (now called, grandly, the Avenue of the Americas, but in my youth known simply by its common number).

While I drink I watch a street lady eating a hot dog on a roll. Behind her and across Sixth Avenue is the store from which her food must have come. There is a huge sign over the door that reads:

AMERICA'S 24 HOUR HOST. STEAK'N'EGGS. She converses with herself between bites in a loud, harsh voice and shakes her head at what I assume are the answers she hears in the air.

Her hair is composed of switches pinned, it seems, to a wig base, and at the top there is a great heavy bun. Her eyebrows are crusted and red, the same flush that covers her light-brown skin and culminates in an angry red ball at the end of her nose. Her body is very thin under a coat composed, like her hair, of parts that are pinned together, but her thinness disappears at her neck, which is full of thick folds of skin, like the necklaces African women wear to elongate their necks for beauty.

She finishes her hot dog, rises slowly, and walks to the trash container near the door to the office building. She moves as if her steps were painful. Her face suggests misery and resentment, as though the weight of all the bunches of cloth tacked on to her were depressing her spirits. She returns to her bench. Her profile is Flemish: the long, thin nose, the chin that falls away, a large black mole on her cheek. She wipes her mouth and her nose on her fingers and then puts them in her mouth. I shudder.

I finish my coffee, stand up to walk to the trash container, and, inexplicably, fall on my face. There is pain in my right ankle that turned and caused me to fall, and greater pain in my left shoulder, so intense that I cannot get up. I lie there, seeing two sets of feet in well-shined shoes pass me by without breaking stride. I try to think of a strategy that will get me on my feet, but without the use of my left arm and hand nothing works.

Then I see a brown hand near my face and hear the street lady's rough voice say: "Here. Hold on here."

I do as she says, doubling my arm against hers and gripping her loose flesh as she holds mine. She pulls hard. I hold tight, I am up, dizzy. She puts her arm around my shoulders and puts me down on the bench. She sits beside me.

The next hour I remember with disbelief. The street lady, Nancy, and I talked about her life while she inquired about my pain and dizziness and advised me about therapy. "Don't get up yet," she said, "or you'll conk out." I think about finding a telephone to tell my daughter, who might still be at work at the Ballet Society, to meet me here instead of in front of the library. Is there a telephone in this office building? I ask her. "Yes," she says, "but whatever you do don't use it. The AT and T puts devils on the wires and they get into your ears." I give up my idea of calling Jane for fear of offending Nancy.

She tells me that she has money to buy a winter coat but storekeepers won't let her try their coats on. Silently I determine to come back and find her, take her to a store for a coat, try it on, and then let her buy it. She tells me she went through high school, took an "industrial" course, got a good job, married, had a daughter who lives now in another part of the city. "She never comes by to see me. I don't know her address."

In the same year she lost both her husband and her job "and never could get ahead again." She shares a room in a welfare hotel on Forty-sixth Street with three other women; they sleep in one bed in shifts. In warm weather she prefers to bed down in the doorways of her street, where the mattress devils can't get at her. And the evil spirits in the pillows. "But I like to have an address. Welfare checks come to me there. So I have some little to get by on," she tells me.

"Winter is worst," she says. "Even now, in October, it's too cold." Her parents came from Haiti, she says with some pride. Her mother told her she never was warm once she got here. "But she saw I went to high school and then she died from her lungs and I married a bum, a devil."

Five-thirty. I get up with difficulty. "I'll walk with you," she says, but I say no. I can make it now. I thank her and give her a hug and tell her I hope to get back to New York soon and then I will look her up at her hotel. She says, "Oh yeah. Watch out for that devil at the front door. She's into voodoo and hexing." I say I will, and limp down Forty-second Street to find an Ace bandage for my swollen ankle.

My daughter takes me to her apartment and then, this morning, to the ballet's orthopedic fellow. He says my shoulder is broken, gives me pills and a sling and a warning to do therapeutic exercises after a week or else suffer permanent stiffness. I resolve to do as he says. But already, in all the night's pain and the next day's scurry to be relieved by a doctor and medicine, the memory of Nancy seems less distinct. Will I look her up if I come to New York at the end of the month for the ballet's trip to Paris? Probably not, knowing how such resolves usually end for me.

Yesterday I sat in the waiting room of the physician who is taking care of my slowly healing shoulder. Around me are elderly patients with casts on ankles, arms, necks, a few in wheelchairs accompanied by exasperated-looking middle-aged children. There is a look I have grown to recognize on the faces of captive offspring caring for parents they have long since ceased to love.

A white-gowned young blond woman with the high, structured

hairdo called a beehive appears at the door of the waiting room and says:

"We're ready for you now, Lucy."

One of the annoyed-looking men stands up and wheels "Lucy," who is clearly over eighty, through the door. He is carrying the pink slips that indicate "Lucy" is a first-time patient.

I am in my customary state of fury. How dare that receptionist, surely not more than twenty years old, address the elderly woman by her first name. She has never met her before, knows nothing about her except that she is old, and sick. *Lucy!*

I sit there fuming, remembering a visit I made a few years ago to a nursing home on Wisconsin Avenue in Washington. My acquaintance, a professor emeritus of English literature, had broken her hip, and was here to recuperate. We talked for a while, about the study of Whitman by Paul Zweig she had been reading, about the new Marguerite Yourcenar I was reviewing. Then a young woman in white carrying a pail and mop came into the room, smiled brightly to the professor (whose doctoral work had been done, as I recall, at Oxford), and said:

"Hiya, Eda Lou. Don't mind me. I'll be out in a minute."

Professor Morton shut her eyes.

"That's a good girl. Don't need to watch while I clean."

I said: "She is Dr. Morton, not Eda Lou."

But the young woman, engrossed in her task, which took her through the middle of the professor's room but under nothing, seemed not to hear me. She finished quickly while I sat stonily and the professor lay with her eyes closed as if waiting for the final assault. It came as the young woman went out the door, calling behind her:

"Be good, Eda Lou. See ya tomorra."

Let neither the peculiar quality of anything nor its value escape you. The peculiar quality of this encounter has stayed with me, sensitizing me to the indignity, in hospitals and nursing homes and waiting rooms, of reducing the elderly sick to children, ignoring the respect due their years and accomplishments, and the dignity of their adult titles or married names.

My turn comes for the orthopedic surgeon's attention.

"Ready for you now, Doris," the woman with the beehive head says, the same bright smile on her face as the cleaning woman had in the nursing home, displaying her affected charm and familiarity with the patient.

This time I am ready. I do not move.

"Doris?" the young woman says, somewhat louder, suggesting by her tone that I, the only woman left in the room, must be deaf.

Aha, I think, I have her. She comes toward me, by now convinced I must be both deaf and, as we used to say, dumb.

"DORIS?" she shouts almost in my ear.

I stand up, forcing her to step back.

"Miss," I say, "I am Mrs. Grumbach. A stranger to you. About fifty years older than you, I would guess. Don't call me by my first name. What is *your* name, by the way?"

"Susan, er, I mean, Miss Lewis."

To her credit, she blushes furiously, apologizes, and follows me into the doctor's office. "Please be seated, Mrs. Grumbach," she says. "Dr. Moore will be with you in a moment."

"Thank you, Miss Lewis," I say. The war, of course, is still to be waged, but I have won this small skirmish. As it turns out, my shoulder appears to be better. Probably because the weight of my indignation has been lifted from it.

I need new batteries for my hearing aids. They are tiny things, little curls the size of infant snails. Last year I was made to face my loss of hearing, which had clearly begun to annoy Sybil, my dear friend and housemate of many years, and others to whom I turned an almost deaf ear—indeed, ears. But the compelling force to acquire two disturbing, overmagnifying instruments was my realization that the music I heard so clearly in my head (and could remember well although I could not sing it) was not what I was actually hearing, hard as I tried to listen more intently to records and tapes, the radio and television.

When I was young I made sure I heard everything, listened in on every conversation, as though widening my sphere of sound would permit me entry into the larger world. "I have heard that . . ." was a customary start to my sentences, and "Have you heard that . . . ?" another. I relied heavily on what I heard in order to fill my conversation and the page.

Losing a good part of my hearing reduced my avidity. Now I am grateful for hearing less, being left alone with my own silences, away from the raucous world of unnecessary talk, loud machines, the shrill chatter of cicadas in our American elm tree, the unending peeps of baby sparrows that nest under the air conditioner outside the bedroom window, the terrified nightmare screams of the neighbor's child through our wall at three o'clock in the morning.

I acquired hearing aids for use in public places—speeches in large auditoriums, classes, workshops, restaurants, theaters, concerts, and other such places. But I find I wear them less and less, preferring not to listen to the conclusions of most speeches, the sounds of dishes at a distant waiter's station, and the confidences exchanged at a nearby table. At some plays it is a comfortable kind of literary criticism to turn the little buttons off so I hear less of the inane dialogue being exchanged by unbelievable characters in a dull and unconvincing situation.

July 12, 1989: No longer am I burdened by the weight of my years. My new age today, a year later, does not worry me. Alone for most of the day, until the promise of dinner with friends tonight, I went for a swim in the cove (outside our house in Sargentville, Maine), conquering its temperature (sixty degrees) by thinking it was not as cold as I expected it to be.

Nor is this day as painful as I thought it might be. I seem not to have grown older in the year, but more content with whatever age it is I am. I accept the addition, hardly noticing it. There may well be the enduring challenge of the 365 steps up the face of the Temple of the Dwarf at Chichén Itzá, but the certainty that I shall never again climb them no longer disturbs me.

O'Henry's last words are said to have been: "Turn up the lights—I don't want to go home in the dark." I've begun to try to turn up the lights on what remains of my life.

Waiting on the deck for Ted, Bob, and Peggy to take me to a birthday dinner, I watch my unknown neighbor bring his sailboat to anchor in the cove, furl and wrap his sails, and stand for a moment in the prow looking out to the reach. The light is dimming, the water flattens out from gray to dark-blue calm, the sun sets, coloring the sky like an obscured klieg light, out of my sight.

Now I shall sail by the ash breeze, standing still on the deck.

Living in this beautiful place, I look forward to the solitude it affords me, and to friends to break it with. At the end of the day I shall welcome them to share my board and my luck. Who knows, I may be entertaining angels.

Unlike Anna Pavlova, I have no immediate use for a swan costume. I am ready to begin the end.

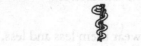

ANATOLE BROYARD

ANATOLE BROYARD (1920–1990). *American editor, literary critic, and essayist. Anatole Broyard grew up in Brooklyn and attended the New School for Social Research. After serving in World War II, he taught fiction writing at Columbia and New York University and began his forty-year career writing reviews for* The New York Times. *Broyard is celebrated for his brilliant, penetrating observations on life, art, and culture in New York City in such works as* Kafka Was the Rage: A Greenwich Village Memoir *(republished in 1993), but he is most famous for* Intoxicated by My Illness: And Other Writings of Life and Mortality *(1992), a courageous autobiographical collection of essays on the subject of his illness (prostate cancer).*

DOCTOR, TALK TO ME

When, in the summer of 1989, I moved from Connecticut to Cambridge, Massachusetts, I found that I had difficulty urinating. I was like Portnoy, in *Portnoy's Complaint,* who couldn't fornicate in Israel. I had always wanted to live in Cambridge, and the thought passed through my mind that I couldn't urinate because—like Israel for Portnoy—Cambridge was a transcendent place for me.

When my inhibition persisted, I began to think about a doctor, and I set about finding one in the superstitious manner most of us fall back on: I asked a couple I knew for a recommendation. To be recommended, for whatever unreasonable reasons, gives a doctor an aura, a history, a shred of magic. Though I thought of my disorder as a simple matter—prostatitis is common in men of my age—I still wanted a potent doctor.

I applied to this particular couple for a recommendation because they are the two most critical people I know: critics of philosophy, politics, history, literature, drama, music. They are the sort of people for whom information is a religion, and the rigor of their conversation is legendary. To talk with them is an ordeal, a fatigue of fine distinctions, and I wanted a doctor who had survived such a scrutiny.

They could only give me the name of their internist, who referred me to a urologist. The recommendation was diluted, but it was better than none, so I made an appointment to see the urologist in a local hospital. The visit began well. The secretary was attractive, efficient, and alert. She remembered my name. I was shown into a pleasant office and told that the doctor would be with me in a few minutes.

While I waited, I subjected the doctor to a preliminary semiotic scrutiny. Sitting in his office, I read his signs. The diplomas I took for granted; what interested me was the fact that the room was furnished with taste. There were well-made, well-filled bookcases, an antique desk and chairs, a reasonable Oriental rug on the floor. A large window opened one wall of the office to the panorama of Boston, and this suggested status, an earned respect. I imagined the doctor taking the long view out of his window.

On the walls and desk were pictures of three healthy-looking, conspicuously happy children, photographed in a prosperous out-door setting of lawn, flowers and trees. As I remember, one of the photographs showed a sailboat. From the evidence, their father knew how to live—and by extension, how to look after the lives of others.

Soon the doctor came in and introduced himself. "Let's go into my office," he said, and I realized that I had been waiting among someone else's effects. I felt that I had been tricked. Having already warmed myself to the first doctor, I was obliged to follow this second man, this impostor, into another office, which turned out to be modern and anonymous. There were no antiques, no Oriental rug, and no pictures that I could see.

From the beginning, I had a negative feeling about this doctor. He didn't seem intense enough or determined enough to prevail over something powerful and demonic like illness. He had a pink, soft face and blue eyes, and his manner was hearty and vague at the same time, polite where politeness was irrelevant. He reminded me of a salesman with nothing to sell but his inoffensiveness.

I didn't like the way he spoke: it struck me as deliberately deliberate, a man fixed in a pose, playing doctor. There was no sign of a tragic sense of life in him that I could see, no furious desire to oppose himself to fate. I realized, of course, that what I was looking for was extravagant, that I was demanding nothing less than an ideal doctor, yet isn't that what we all want?

In the end, it didn't matter whether my reading of this particular man was just or unjust—I simply couldn't warm up to him. Choosing a doctor is difficult because it is our first explicit confrontation of our illness. "How good is this man?" is simply the reverse of "How bad am I?" To be sick brings out all our prejudices and primitive feelings. Like fear, or love, it makes us a little crazy. Yet the craziness of the patient is part of his condition.

I was also aware of a certain predisposition in myself in favor of Jewish doctors. I thought of them as the trouble-shooters—the physicians, lawyers, brokers, arbiters, and artists—of contemporary life. History had convinced them that life was a disease. My father, who was an old-fashioned Southern anti-Semite, insisted on a Jewish doctor when he developed cancer of the bladder. A Jewish doctor, he argued, had been bred to medicine. In my father's biblical conception, a Jew's life was a story of study, repair, and reform. A Jewish doctor knew what survival was worth, because he had had to fight for his. Obliged to treat life as a business as well as a pleasure, Jews drove hard bargains. To lose a patient was bad business. In his heart, I think my father believed that a Jewish doctor was closer to God and could use that connection to "Jew down" death.

This other, all-too-human doctor took me into an examining room and felt my prostate. It appeared to me that he had not yet overcome his self-consciousness about this procedure. Back in his office, he summed up his findings. There were hard lumps in my prostate, he said, which suggested tumors, and these "mandated" further investigation. He used the word "mandate" twice in his summary, as well as the word "significantly."

But he was the only urologist I knew in Cambridge, and so, a few days later, I allowed him to perform a cystoscopy, a procedure in which a small scope was inserted through my urethra up to my prostate and bladder. During surgical procedures, doctors wear a tight-fitting white cap, a sort of skullcap like the one Alan Alda wears in *M*A*S*H*. To this, my doctor had added what looked like a clear plastic shower cap, and the moment I saw him in these two caps, I turned irrevocably against him. He wore them absolutely without inflection or style, with none of the jauntiness that usually comes with long practice. He wore them like an American in France who affects a beret without understanding how to shape or cock it. To my eyes, this doctor simply didn't have the charisma to overcome or assimilate those caps, and that finished him off for me.

I want to point out that this man is in all likelihood an able, even a talented doctor. Certainly, I'm no judge of his medical competence, nor do I mean to criticize it. What turned me against him was what I saw as a lack of style. I realized that I wanted my doctor to have style—which I think of as a dash of magic—as well as medical ability. It was like having a *lucky* doctor. I've described all this—a patient's madness—to show how irrational such transactions are, how far removed from any notion of dispassionate objectivity. To be sick is already to be disordered in your mind as well. Still, this does not necessarily mean that I was wrong to want to change doctors: I was simply listening to my unconscious telling me what I needed.

Now that I know I have cancer of the prostate, the lymph nodes, and part of my skeleton, what *do* I want in a doctor? I would say that I want one who is a close reader of illness and a good critic of medicine. I secretly believe that criticism can wither cancer. Also, I would like a doctor who is not only a talented physician but a bit of a metaphysician too, someone who can treat body and soul. I used to get restless when people talked about soul, but now I know better. Soul is the part of you that you summon up in emergencies. You don't need to be religious to believe in the soul or to have one.

My ideal doctor would be my Virgil, leading me through my purgatory or inferno, pointing out the sights as we go. He would resemble Oliver Sacks, the neurologist who wrote *Awakenings* and *The Man Who Mistook His Wife for a Hat.* I can imagine Dr. Sacks *entering* my condition, looking around at it from the inside like a benevolent landlord with a tenant, trying to see how he could make the premises more livable for me. He would see the genius of my illness. He would mingle his daemon with mine; we would wrestle with my fate together. Inside every patient, there's a poet trying to get out. My ideal doctor would "read" my poetry, my literature. He would see that my sickness has purified me, weakening my worst parts and strengthening the best.

To most physicians, my illness is a routine incident in their rounds, while for me it's the crisis of my life. I would feel better if I had a doctor who at least perceived this incongruity. I don't ask him to love me—in fact, I think the role of love is greatly exaggerated by many writers on illness. Of course you want your family and close friends to love you, but the situation shouldn't become a hunting season for love, or a competition, a desperate kiss before dying. To a critically ill person, love may begin to resemble an anesthetic. In a novel by Joy Williams called *State of Grace,* a character asks: "What can be beyond love? I want to get there." The sick man has got there: he's at a point where what he wants from most people is not love but a spacious, flaring grasp of his situation, what is known now in the literature of illness as "empathetic witnessing." The patient is always on the brink of revelation, and he needs someone who can recognize it when it comes.

Just as I see no reason for my physician to love me, I would not expect him to suffer with me either. On the contrary, what would please me most would be a doctor who *enjoyed* me. I want to be a good story for him, to give him some of my art in exchange for his. If a patient expects a doctor to be interested in him, he ought to try to *be* interesting. When he shows nothing but a greediness for care, nothing but the coarser forms of anxiety, it's only natural for the physician to feel an aversion. There is an etiquette to being sick.

I wouldn't demand a lot of my doctor's time; I just wish he would *brood* on my situation for perhaps five minutes, that he would give me his whole mind just once. I would like to think of him as going through my character, as he goes through my flesh, to get at my illness, for each man is ill in his own way. Proust complained that his physician did not allow for his having read Shakespeare. I have a wistful desire for my relation to my doctor to be beautiful—but I don't know how this can be brought about. Though I see us framed in an epiphany, I can't make out the content.

Just as he orders blood tests and bone scans of my body, I'd like my doctor to scan *me*, to grope for my spirit as well as my prostate. While he inevitably feels superior to me because he is the doctor and I am the patient, I'd like him to know that I feel superior to him too, that he is my patient also and I have my diagnosis of him. There should be a place where our respective superiorities could meet and frolic together.

Since technology deprives me of the intimacy of my illness, makes it not mine but something that belongs to science, I wish my doctor could somehow restore it to me and make it personal again. When my father's father died in the French Quarter of New Orleans sixty years ago, the popularly accepted story was that on a humid night in mid-August, he had eaten a dozen bananas and then taken a cold bath. He was a man of eighty-seven whose life had been a strenuous assertion of his appetites, and this explanation suited him, just as it suited his friends in the French Quarter. It would be more satisfying to me, it would allow me to feel that I *owned* my illness, if my urologist were to say: "You know, you've beat the hell out of this prostate of yours. It looks like a worn-out baseball." Nobody wants an anonymous illness. I'd much rather think that I brought it on myself than that it was a mere accident of nature.

It is only natural for a patient to feel some dismay at the changes brought about in his body by illness, and I wonder whether an innovative doctor—again, like Oliver Sacks—couldn't find a way to reconceptualize this situation. If only the patient could be allowed to see his illness as not so much a *failure* of his body as a natural consumption of it. Any reconciling idea would do. The doctor could say, "You've spent your self unselfishly, like a philanthropist who gives all his money away." If the patient could feel that he has *earned* his illness, that his sickness represents the decadence that follows a great flowering, he might look upon the ruin of his body as tourists look upon the ruins of antiquity. (Of course I'm offering these suggestions playfully, as experiments in thinking about medicine.)

Physicians have been taught in medical school that they must keep the patient at a distance because there isn't time to accommodate his personality, or because if the doctor becomes "involved" in the patient's predicament, the emotional burden will be too great. As I've suggested, it doesn't take much time to make good contact, but beyond that, the emotional burden of *avoiding* the patient may be much harder on the doctor than he imagines. It may be this that sometimes makes him complain of feeling harassed. The patient's unanswered questions will always thunder in his stethoscope. A doctor's job would be so much more interesting and satisfying if he would occasionally let himself plunge into the patient, if he could lose his own fear of falling.

Applying to other friends, following new recommendations, I found another urologist. He's highly regarded in his field, and he inspired such confidence in me that my cancer immediately went into remission. My only regret is that he doesn't talk very much—and when he does, he sounds like everybody else. His brilliance has no voice—at least not when he's with me. There's a paradox here at the heart of medicine, because a doctor, like a writer, must have a voice of his own, something that conveys the timbre, the rhythm, the diction, and the music of his humanity, that compensates us for all the speechless machines. When a doctor makes a difficult diagnosis, it is not his medical knowledge only that determines it, but a voice in his head. Such a diagnosis depends as much on inspiration as art does. Whether he wants to be or not, the doctor is a storyteller, and he can turn our lives into good or bad stories, regardless of the diagnosis. If my doctor would allow me, I would be glad to help him here, to take him on as *my* patient. Perhaps later, when he is older, he'll have learned how to converse. Astute as he is, he doesn't yet understand that all cures are partly "talking cures." Every patient needs mouth-to-mouth resuscitation, for talk is the kiss of life.

Yet it's too easy to accuse the doctor, to blame the absence of natural talk on him. It's also true that some of what the patient asks is ineffable. Even a doctor like Chekhov would be hard put to answer him. For example, I would like to discuss my prostate with my urologist not as a diseased organ but as a philosopher's stone. Every patient invites the doctor to combine the role of the priest, the philosopher, the poet, the scholar. He expects the doctor to evaluate his entire life, like a biographer.

Of course, a physician may reasonably ask: "But what am I supposed to say? All I can tell the patient is the facts, if there are any facts." But this is not quite true. The doctor's answer to his patient is yet to be born. It will come naturally—or at first unnaturally—from the intersecting of the patient's needs with the physician's as yet untried imagination. Just as a mother ushers her child into the world, so the doctor must usher the patient out of the ordinary world into whatever place awaits him. The physician is the patient's only familiar in a foreign country.

To help the doctor reach the patient, and the patient reach the doctor, the mood of the hospital might have to be modified. It might be less like a laboratory and more like a theater, which would be only fitting, since no place contains more drama. The laboratory atmosphere can probably be traced back to the idea of asepsis, to the avoidance of contagion. Originally, the patient was protected by the sterility of the hospital. Only the sterility went too far: It sterilized the doctor's thinking. It sterilized the patient's entire experience in the hospital. It sterilized the very notion of illness to the point where we can't bring our soiled thoughts to bear on it. But the sick man needs the contagion of life.

Not every patient can be saved, but his illness may be eased by the way the doctor responds to him—and in responding to him, the doctor may save himself. But first he must become a student again; he has to dissect the cadaver of his professional persona; he must see that his silence and neutrality are *unnatural*. It may be necessary to give up some of his authority in exchange for his humanity, but as the old family doctors knew, this is not a bad bargain. In learning to talk to his patients, the doctor may talk himself back into loving his work. He has little to lose and much to gain by letting the sick man into his heart. If he does, they can share, as few others can, the wonder, terror, and exaltation of being on the edge of being, between the natural and the supernatural.

PHILIP LARKIN

PHILIP LARKIN (1922–1985). *English poet and critic. A retiring man (except in his writing), Larkin worked for many years as a librarian. His first collection of poetry,* The North Ship *(1945), attracted little attention, but after the publication of* The Less Deceived *(1955), Larkin was considered the most distinguished voice of a new generation. He possessed a keen sensibility and the rare ability to subtly transform ordinary experience into revelation.*

FAITH HEALING

Slowly the women file to where he stands
Upright in rimless glasses, silver hair,
Dark suit, white collar. Stewards tirelessly
Persuade them onwards to his voice and hands,
Within whose warm spring rain of loving care
Each dwells some twenty seconds. *Now, dear child,
What's wrong,* the deep American voice demands,
And, scarcely pausing, goes into a prayer
Directing God about this eye, that knee.
Their heads are clasped abruptly; then, exiled

Like losing thoughts, they go in silence; some
Sheepishly stray, not back into their lives
Just yet; but some stay stiff, twitching and loud
With deep hoarse tears, as if a kind of dumb
And idiot child within them still survives
To re-awake at kindness, thinking a voice
At last calls them alone, that hands have come
To lift and lighten; and such joy arrives
Their thick tongues blort, their eyes squeeze grief, a crowd
Of huge unheard answers jam and rejoice—

What's wrong! Moustached in flowered frocks they shake:
By now, all's wrong. In everyone there sleeps
A sense of life lived according to love.
To some it means the difference they could make
By loving others, but across most it sweeps
As all they might have done had they been loved.
That nothing cures. An immense slackening ache,
As when, thawing, the rigid landscape weeps,
Spreads slowly through them—that, and the voice above
Saying *Dear child*, and all time has disproved.

KURT VONNEGUT

KURT VONNEGUT (1922–). *American writer. Vonnegut was born in Indianapolis, Indiana, and educated at Cornell, the University of Chicago, and the Carnegie Institute. His black humor, satiric voice, and incomparable imagination first captured America's attention in* The Sirens of Titan *(1959). In the 1960s, he emerged as one of America's most influential, potent, and provocative writers, a ribald commentator on the horrors of this century. The publication of* Cat's Cradle *in 1963 is said to have established him as "a true artist." Vonnegut is the author of dozens of short stories and essays and eighteen highly acclaimed books, including* Slaughterhouse-Five *(1969),* Mother Night *(1972), and* Deadeye Dick *(1982).*

FORTITUDE

DR. ELBERT LITTLE	a kindly, attractive young general practitioner, is being shown around by the creator and boss of the operation, DR. NORBERT FRANKENSTEIN.
FRANKENSTEIN	FRANKENSTEIN is 65, a crass medical genius.
DR. TOM SWIFT	Seated at the console, wearing headphones and watching meters and flashing lights, is FRANKENSTEIN's enthusiastic first assistant.
THE TIME	The present.
THE PLACE	Upstate New York, a large room filled with pulsing, writhing, panting machines that perform the functions of various organs of the human body—heart, lungs, liver, and so on. Color-coded pipes and wires swoop upward from the machines to converge and pass through a hole in the ceiling. To one side is a fantastically complicated master control console.

LITTLE   Oh, my God—oh, my God—

FRANKENSTEIN   Yeah. Those are her kidneys over there. That's her liver, of course. There you got her pancreas.

LITTLE   Amazing. Dr. Frankenstein, after seeing this, I wonder if I've even been *practicing* medicine, if I've ever even *been* to medical school. *(Pointing:)* That's her *heart?*

FRANKENSTEIN   That's a Westinghouse heart. They make a damn good heart, if you ever need one. They make a kidney I wouldn't touch with a ten-foot pole.

LITTLE   That heart is probably worth more than the whole township where I practice.

FRANKENSTEIN   That pancreas is worth your whole state. *Vermont?*

LITTLE   Vermont.

FRANKENSTEIN   What we paid for the pancreas—yeah, we could have bought Vermont for that. Nobody'd ever made a pancreas before, and we had to have one in ten days or lose the patient. So we told all the big organ manufacturers, "OK, you guys got to have a crash program for a pancreas. Put every man you got on the job. We don't care what it costs, as long as we get a pancreas by next Tuesday."

LITTLE   And they succeeded.

FRANKENSTEIN   The patient's still alive, isn't she? Believe me, those are some expensive sweetbreads.

LITTLE   But the patient could afford them.

FRANKENSTEIN   You don't live like this on Blue Cross.

LITTLE   And how many operations has she had? In how many years?

FRANKENSTEIN   I gave her her first major operation thirty-six years ago. She's had seventy-eight operations since then.

LITTLE   And how old is she?

FRANKENSTEIN   One hundred.

LITTLE   What *guts* that woman must have!

FRANKENSTEIN   You're looking at 'em.

LITTLE   I mean—what *courage!* What *fortitude!*

FRANKENSTEIN   We knock her out, you know. We don't operate without anesthetics.

LITTLE   Even so . . .

FRANKENSTEIN *taps* SWIFT *on the shoulder,* SWIFT *frees an ear from the headphones, divides his attention between the visitors and the console.*

FRANKENSTEIN   Dr. Tom Swift, this is Dr. Elbert Little. Tom here is my first assistant.

SWIFT   Howdy-doody.

FRANKENSTEIN   Dr. Little has a practice up in Vermont. He happened to be in the neighborhood. He asked for a tour.

LITTLE   What do you hear in the headphones?

SWIFT   Anything that's going on in the patient's room. *(He offers the headphones.)* Be my guest.

LITTLE   *(Listening to headphones:)* Nothing.

SWIFT   She's having her hair brushed now. The beautician's up there. She's always quiet when her hair's being brushed. *(He takes the headphones back.)*

FRANKENSTEIN   *(To* SWIFT:*)* We should *congratulate* our young visitor here.

SWIFT   What for?

LITTLE   Good question. What for?

FRANKENSTEIN   Oh, I know about the great honor that has come your way.

LITTLE   I'm not sure *I* do.

FRANKENSTEIN   You are *the* Dr. Little, aren't you, who was named the Family Doctor of the Year by the *Ladies' Home Journal* last month?

LITTLE   Yes—that's right. I don't know how in the hell they decided. And I'm even more flabbergasted that a man of *your* caliber would know about it.

FRANKENSTEIN   I read the *Ladies' Home Journal* from cover to cover every month.

LITTLE   You *do?*

FRANKENSTEIN   I only got one patient, Mrs. Lovejoy. And Mrs. Lovejoy reads the *Ladies' Home Journal,* so I read it, too. That's what we talk about—what's in the *Ladies' Home Journal.* We read all about you last month. Mrs. Lovejoy kept saying, "Oh, what a nice young man he must be. *So understanding.*"

LITTLE   Um.

FRANKENSTEIN   Now here you are in the flesh. I bet she wrote you a letter.

LITTLE   Yes—she did.

FRANKENSTEIN   She writes thousands of letters a year, gets thousands of letters back. Some pen pal she is.

LITTLE   Is she—uh—generally *cheerful* most of the time?

FRANKENSTEIN   If she isn't, that's our fault down here. If she gets unhappy, that means something down *here* isn't working right. She was blue about a month ago. Turned out it was a bum transistor in the console. *(He reaches over Swift's shoulder, changes a setting on the console. The machinery subtly adjusts to the new setting.)* There—she'll be all depressed for a couple of minutes now. *(He changes the setting again.)* There. Now, pretty quick, she'll be happier than she was before. She'll sing like a bird.

LITTLE *conceals his horror imperfectly.* CUT TO *patient's room, which is full of flowers and candy boxes and books. The patient is* SYLVIA LOVEJOY, *a billionaire's widow.* SYLVIA *is no longer anything but a head connected to pipes and wires coming up through the floor, but this is not immediately apparent. The first shot of her is a* CLOSE-UP, *with* GLORIA, *a gorgeous beautician, standing behind her.* SYLVIA *is a heartbreakingly good-looking old lady, once a famous beauty. She is crying now.*

SYLVIA   Gloria—
GLORIA   Ma'am?
SYLVIA   Wipe these tears away before somebody comes in and sees them.
GLORIA   *(Wanting to cry herself:)* Yes, ma'am. *(She wipes the tears away with Kleenex, studies the results.) There. There.*
SYLVIA   I don't know what came over me. Suddenly I was so sad I couldn't stand it.
GLORIA   Everybody has to cry *sometimes.*
SYLVIA   It's passing now. Can you tell I've been crying?
GLORIA   *No. No.*

She is unable to control her own tears anymore. She goes to a window so SYLVIA *can't see her cry.* CAMERA BACKS AWAY *to reveal the tidy, clinical abomination of the head and wires and pipes. The head is on a tripod. There is a black box with winking colored lights hanging under the head, where the chest would normally be. Mechanical arms come out of the box where arms would normally be. There is a table within easy reach of the arms. On it are a pen and paper, a partially solved jigsaw puzzle, and a bulky knitting bag. Sticking out of the bag are needles and a sweater in progress. Hanging over* SYLVIA's *head is a microphone on a boom.*

SYLVIA   *(sighing:)* Oh, what a *foolish* old woman you must think I am. (GLORIA *shakes her head in denial, is unable to reply.)* Gloria? Are you still there?
GLORIA   Yes.
SYLVIA   Is anything the matter?
GLORIA   No.
SYLVIA   You're *such* a good friend, Gloria. I want you to know I feel that with all my heart.
GLORIA   I like you, too.

SYLVIA If you ever have any problems I can help you with, I hope you'll ask me.

GLORIA I will, I *will*.

HOWARD DERBY, *the hospital mail clerk, dances in with an armload of letters. He is a merry old fool.*

DERBY Mailman! Mailman!

SYLVIA *(Brightening:)* Mailman! God *bless* the mailman!

DERBY How's the patient today?

SYLVIA Very sad a moment ago. But now that I see you, I want to sing like a bird.

DERBY Fifty-three letters today. There's even one from Leningrad.

SYLVIA There's a blind woman in Leningrad. Poor soul, *poor* soul.

DERBY *(Making a fan of the mail, reading postmarks:)* West Virginia, Honolulu, Brisbane, Australia—

SYLVIA *selects an envelope at random.*

SYLVIA Wheeling, West Virginia. Now, who do I know in Wheeling? *(She opens the envelope expertly with her mechanical hands, reads.)* "Dear Mrs. Lovejoy: You don't know me, but I just read about you in the *Reader's Digest,* and I'm sitting here with tears streaming down my cheeks." *Reader's Digest?* My goodness that article was printed fourteen years ago! And she just *read* it?

DERBY Old *Reader's Digests* go on and on. I've got one at home I'll bet is ten years old. I still read it every time I need a little inspiration.

SYLVIA *(Reading on:)* "I am never going to complain about anything that ever happens to me ever again. I thought I was as unfortunate as a person can get when my husband shot his girlfriend six months ago and then blew his own brains out. He left me with seven children and with eight payments still to go on a Buick Roadmaster with three flat tires and a busted transmission. After reading about you, though, I sit here and count my blessings." Isn't that a nice letter?

DERBY Sure is.

SYLVIA There's a P.S.: "Get well real soon, you *hear?*" *(She puts the letter on the table.)* There isn't a letter from Vermont, is there?

DERBY Vermont?

SYLVIA Last month, when I had that low spell, I wrote what I'm afraid was a very stupid, self-centered, self-pitying letter to a young doctor I read about in the *Ladies' Home Journal.* I'm so ashamed. I live in fear and trembling of what he's going to say back to me—if he answers at all.

GLORIA   What could he say? What could he *possibly* say?

SYLVIA   He could tell me about the *real* suffering going on out there in the world, about people who don't know where the next meal is coming from, about people so poor they've never *been* to a doctor in their whole *lives*. And to think of all the help I've had—all the tender, loving care, all the latest wonders science has to offer.

CUT TO *corridor outside* SYLVIA's *room. There is a sign on the door saying,* ALWAYS ENTER SMILING! FRANKENSTEIN *and* LITTLE *are about to enter.*

LITTLE   She's in *there?*

FRANKENSTEIN   Every part of her that isn't downstairs.

LITTLE   And everybody obeys this sign, I'm sure.

FRANKENSTEIN   Part of the therapy. We treat the *whole* patient here.

GLORIA *comes from the room, closes the door tightly, then bursts into noisy tears.*

FRANKENSTEIN   (*To* GLORIA, *disgusted:*) Oh, for crying out loud. And what is this?

GLORIA   Let her *die*, Dr. Frankenstein. For the love of God, let her *die!*

LITTLE   This is her *nurse?*

FRANKENSTEIN   She hasn't got the brains enough to be a nurse. She is a lousy beautician. A hundred bucks a week she makes—just to take care of one woman's face and hair. (*To* GLORIA:) You blew it, honeybunch. You're through.

GLORIA   What?

FRANKENSTEIN   Pick up your check and scram.

GLORIA   I'm her closest friend.

FRANKENSTEIN   Some friend! You just asked me to knock her off.

GLORIA   In the name of mercy, yes, I did.

FRANKENSTEIN   You're that sure there's a heaven, eh? You want to send her right up there so she can get her wings and harp.

GLORIA   I know there's a hell. I've seen it. It's in there, and you're its great inventor.

FRANKENSTEIN   (*Stung, letting a moment pass before replying:*) Christ—the things people say sometimes.

GLORIA It's time somebody who loves her spoke up.

FRANKENSTEIN Love.

GLORIA You wouldn't know what that is.

FRANKENSTEIN Love. *(More to himself than to her:)* Do I have a wife? No. Do I have a mistress? No, I have loved only two women in my life—my mother and that woman in there. I wasn't able to save my mother from death. I had just graduated from medical school and my mother was dying of cancer of the everything. "OK, wise guy," I said to myself, "you're such a hot-shot doctor from Heidelberg, now, let's see you save your mother from death." And everybody told me there wasn't anything I could do for her, and I said, "I don't give a damn. I'm gonna do something anyway." And they finally decided I was nuts and they put me in a crazyhouse for a little while. When I got out, she was dead—the way all the wise men said she had to be. What those wise men didn't know was all the wonderful things machinery could do—and neither did I, but I was gonna find out. So I went to the Massachusetts Institute of Technology and I studied mechanical engineering and electrical engineering and chemical engineering for six long years. I lived in an attic. I ate two-day-old bread and the kind of cheese they put in mousetraps. When I got out of MIT, I said to myself, "OK, boy—it's just barely possible now that you're the only guy on earth with the proper education to practice twentieth-century medicine." I went to work for the Curley Clinic in Boston. They brought in this woman who was beautiful on the outside and a mess on the inside. She was the image of my mother. She was the widow of a man who had left her five hundred million dollars. She didn't have any relatives. The wise men said again, "This lady's gotta die." And I said to them, "Shut up and listen. I'm gonna tell you what we're gonna do."

(Silence.)

LITTLE That's—that's quite a story.

FRANKENSTEIN It's a story about *love.* (*To* GLORIA:) That love story started years and years before you were born, you great lover, you. And it's still going on.

GLORIA Last month, she asked me to bring her a pistol so she could shoot herself.

FRANKENSTEIN You think I don't know that? (*Jerking a thumb at* LITTLE:) Last month, she wrote him a letter and said, "Bring me some cyanide, doctor, if you're a doctor with any heart at all."

LITTLE *(Startled:)* You *knew* that. You—you read her mail?

FRANKENSTEIN   So we'll know what she's *really* feeling. She might try to fool us sometime—just *pretend* to be happy. I told you about that bum transistor last month. We maybe wouldn't have known anything was wrong if we hadn't read her mail and listened to what she was saying to lame-brains like this one here. (*Feeling challenged:*) Look—you go in there all by yourself. Stay as long as you want, ask her anything. Then you come back out and tell me the truth: Is that a happy woman in there, or is that a woman in hell?

LITTLE   (*Hesitating:*) I—

FRANKENSTEIN   Go on in! I got some more things to say to this young lady—to Miss Mercy Killing of the Year. I'd like to show her a body that's been in a casket for a couple of years sometime— let her see how pretty death is, this thing she wants for her friend.

LITTLE *gropes for something to say, finally mimes his wish to be fair to everyone. He enters the patient's room. CUT TO room. SYLVIA is alone, faced away from the door.*

SYLVIA   Who's that?

LITTLE   A friend—somebody you wrote a letter to.

SYLVIA   That could be anybody. Can I see you, please? (LITTLE *obliges. She looks him over with growing affection.*) Dr. Little— family doctor from Vermont.

LITTLE   (*Bowing slightly:*) Mrs. Lovejoy—how are you today?

SYLVIA   Did you bring me cyanide?

LITTLE   No.

SYLVIA   I wouldn't take it today. It's such a lovely day. I wouldn't want to miss it, or tomorrow, either. Did you come on a snow-white horse?

LITTLE   In a blue Oldsmobile.

SYLVIA   What about your patients, who love and need you so?

LITTLE   Another doctor is covering for me. I'm taking a week off.

SYLVIA   Not on my account.

LITTLE   No.

SYLVIA   Because I'm fine. You can see what wonderful hands I'm in.

LITTLE   Yes.

SYLVIA   One thing I don't need is another doctor.

LITTLE   Right.

(*Pause.*)

SYLVIA   I do wish I had somebody to talk to about death, though. You've seen a lot of it, I suppose.

LITTLE   Some.

SYLVIA   And it was a blessing for some of them—when they died?

LITTLE   I've heard that said.

SYLVIA   But you don't say so yourself.

LITTLE   It's not a professional thing for a doctor to say, Mrs. Lovejoy.

SYLVIA   Why have other people said that certain deaths have been a blessing?

LITTLE   Because of the pain the patient was in, because he couldn't be cured at any price—at any price within his means. Or because the patient was a vegetable, had lost his mind and couldn't get it back.

SYLVIA   At any price.

LITTLE   As far as I know, it is not now possible to beg, borrow, and steal an artificial mind for someone who's lost one. If I asked Dr. Frankenstein about it, he might tell me that it's the coming thing.

(Pause.)

SYLVIA   It *is* the coming thing.

LITTLE   He's told you so?

SYLVIA   I asked him yesterday what would happen if my brain started to go. He was serene. He said I wasn't to worry my pretty little head about that. "We'll cross that bridge when we come to it," he told me. *(Pause.)* Oh, God, the bridges I've crossed!

CUT TO *room full of organs, as before.* SWIFT is at the console. FRANKENSTEIN and LITTLE enter.

FRANKENSTEIN   You've made the grand tour and now here you are back at the beginning.

LITTLE   And I still have to say what I said at the beginning: "My God—oh, my God."

FRANKENSTEIN   It's gonna be a little tough going back to the aspirin-and-laxative trade after this, eh?

LITTLE   Yes. *(Pause.)* What's the cheapest thing here?

FRANKENSTEIN   The simplest thing. It's the goddamn pump.

LITTLE   What does a heart go for these days?

FRANKENSTEIN   Sixty thousand dollars. There are cheaper ones and more expensive ones. The cheap ones are junk. The expensive ones are jewelry.

LITTLE   And how many are sold a year now?

FRANKENSTEIN   Six hundred, give or take a few.

LITTLE   Give one, that's life. Take one, that's death.

FRANKENSTEIN If the trouble is the heart. It's lucky if you have trouble that cheap. (*To* SWIFT:) Hey, Tom—put her to sleep so he can see how the day ends around here.

SWIFT It's twenty minutes ahead of time.

FRANKENSTEIN What's the difference? We put her to sleep for twenty minutes extra, she still wakes up tomorrow feeling like a million bucks, unless we got another bum transistor.

LITTLE Why don't you have a television camera aimed at her, so you can watch her on a screen?

FRANKENSTEIN She didn't want one.

LITTLE She gets what she wants?

FRANKENSTEIN She got *that.* What the hell do we have to watch her face for? We can look at the meters down here and find out more about her than she can know about herself. (*To* SWIFT:) Put her to sleep, Tom.

SWIFT (*To* LITTLE:) It's just like slowing down a car or banking a furnace.

LITTLE Um.

FRANKENSTEIN Tom, too, has degrees in both engineering and medicine.

LITTLE Are you tired at the end of a day, Tom?

SWIFT It's a good kind of tiredness—as though I'd flown a big jet from New York to Honolulu, or something like that. (*Taking hold of a lever:*) And now we'll bring Mrs. Lovejoy in for a happy landing. (*He pulls the lever gradually and the machinery slows down.*) There.

FRANKENSTEIN Beautiful.

LITTLE She's asleep?

FRANKENSTEIN Like a baby.

SWIFT All I have to do now is wait for the night man to come on.

LITTLE Has anybody ever brought her a suicide weapon?

FRANKENSTEIN No. We wouldn't worry about it if they did. The arms are designed so she can't possibly point a gun at herself or get poison to her lips, no matter how she tries. That was Tom's stroke of genius.

LITTLE Congratulations.

Alarm bell rings. Light flashes.

FRANKENSTEIN Who could that be? (*To* LITTLE:) Somebody just went into her room. We better check! (*To* SWIFT:) Lock the door up there, Tom—so whoever it is, we got 'em. (SWIFT *pushes a button that locks door upstairs. To* LITTLE:) You come with me.

CUT TO *patient's room.* SYLVIA *is asleep, snoring gently.* GLORIA *has just sneaked in. She looks around furtively, takes a revolver from her purse, makes sure it's loaded, then hides it in* SYLVIA's *knitting bag. She is barely finished when* FRANKENSTEIN *and* LITTLE *enter breathlessly,* FRANKENSTEIN *opening the door with a key.*

FRANKENSTEIN   What's this?

GLORIA   I left my watch up here. *(Pointing to watch:)* I've got it now.

FRANKENSTEIN   Thought I told you never to come into this building again.

GLORIA   I won't.

FRANKENSTEIN   *(To* LITTLE:) You keep her right there. I'm gonna check things over. Maybe there's been a little huggery buggery. *(To* GLORIA:) How would you like to be in court for attempted murder, eh? *(Into microphone:)* Tom? Can you hear me?

SWIFT   *(Voice from squawk box on wall:)* I hear you.

FRANKENSTEIN   Wake her up again. I gotta give her a check.

SWIFT   Cock-a-doodle-doo.

Machinery can be heard speeding up below. SYLVIA *opens her eyes, sweetly dazed.*

SYLVIA   *(To* FRANKENSTEIN:) Good morning, Norbert.

FRANKENSTEIN   How do you feel?

SYLVIA   The way I always feel when I wake up—fine—vaguely at sea. Gloria! Good morning!

GLORIA   Good morning.

SYLVIA   Dr. Little! You're staying another day?

FRANKENSTEIN   It isn't morning. We'll put you back to sleep in a minute.

SYLVIA   I'm sick again?

FRANKENSTEIN   I don't think so.

SYLVIA   I'm going to have to have another operation?

FRANKENSTEIN   Calm down, calm down. *(He takes an ophthalmoscope from his pocket.)*

SYLVIA   How can I be calm when I think about another operation?

FRANKENSTEIN   *(Into microphone:)* Tom—give her some tranquilizers.

SWIFT   *(Squawk box:)* Coming up.

SYLVIA   What else do I have to lose? My ears? My hair?

FRANKENSTEIN   You'll be calm in a minute.

SYLVIA   My eyes? My eyes. Norbert—are they going next?

FRANKENSTEIN   *(To* GLORIA:*)* Oh, boy, baby doll—will you look what you've done? *(Into microphone:)* Where the hell are those tranquilizers?

SWIFT   Should be taking effect just about now.

SYLVIA   Oh, well. It doesn't matter. *(As* FRANKENSTEIN *examines her eyes:)* It *is* my eyes, isn't it?

FRANKENSTEIN   It isn't your anything.

SYLVIA   Easy come, easy go.

FRANKENSTEIN   You're healthy as a horse.

SYLVIA   I'm sure somebody manufactures excellent eyes.

FRANKENSTEIN   RCA makes a damn good eye, but we aren't gonna buy one for a while yet. *(He backs away, satisfied.)* Everything's all right up here. *(To* GLORIA:*)* Lucky for you.

SYLVIA   I love it when friends of mine are lucky.

SWIFT   Put her to sleep again?

FRANKENSTEIN   Not yet. I want to check a couple of things down there.

SWIFT   Roger and out.

CUT TO LITTLE, GLORIA *and* FRANKENSTEIN *entering the machinery room minutes later.* SWIFT *is at the console.*

SWIFT   Night man's late.

FRANKENSTEIN   He's got troubles at home. You want a good piece of advice, boy? Don't ever get married. *(He scrutinizes meter after meter.)*

GLORIA   *(Appalled by her surroundings:)* My God—oh, my God—

LITTLE   You've never seen this before?

GLORIA   No.

FRANKENSTEIN   She was the great hair specialist. We took care of everything else—everything but the hair. *(The reading on a meter puzzles him.)* What's this? *(He socks the meter, which then gives him the proper reading.)* That's more like it.

GLORIA   *(Emptily:)* Science.

FRANKENSTEIN   What did you think it was like down here?

GLORIA   I was afraid to think. Now I can see why.

FRANKENSTEIN   You got any scientific background at all—any way of appreciating even slightly what you're seeing here?

GLORIA   I flunked earth science twice in high school.

FRANKENSTEIN   What do they teach in beauty college?

GLORIA   Dumb things for dumb people. How to paint a face. How

to curl and uncurl hair. How to cut hair. How to dye hair. Finger-
nails. Toenails in the summertime.

FRANKENSTEIN   I suppose you're gonna crack off about this place
after you get out of here—gonna tell people all the crazy stuff that
goes on.

GLORIA   Maybe.

FRANKENSTEIN   Just remember this: You haven't got the brains or
the education to talk about any aspect of our operation. Right?

GLORIA   Maybe.

FRANKENSTEIN   What *will* you say to the outside world?

GLORIA   Nothing very complicated—just that . . .

FRANKENSTEIN   Yes?

GLORIA   That you have the head of a dead woman connected to a
lot of machinery, and you play with it all day long, and you aren't
married or anything, and that's all you do.

FREEZE SCENE *as a still photograph.* FADE TO *black.* FADE
IN *same still. Figures begin to move.*

FRANKENSTEIN   *(Aghast:)* How can you call her dead? She reads the
Ladies' Home Journal! She talks! She knits! She writes letters to
pen pals all over the world!

GLORIA   She's like some horrible fortune-telling machine in a penny
arcade.

FRANKENSTEIN   I thought you loved her.

GLORIA   Every so often, I see a tiny little spark of what she used to
be. I love that spark. Most people say they love her for her courage.
What's that courage worth, when it comes from down here? You
could turn a few faucets and switches down here and she'd be
volunteering to fly a rocket ship to the moon. But no matter what
you do down here, that little spark goes on thinking, "For the love
of God—somebody get me out of here!"

FRANKENSTEIN   *(Glancing at the console:)* Dr. Swift—is that microphone open?

SWIFT   Yeah. *(Snapping his fingers:)* I'm sorry.

FRANKENSTEIN   Leave it open. *(To* GLORIA:) She's heard every word
you've said. How does that make you feel?

GLORIA   She can hear me now?

FRANKENSTEIN   Run off at the mouth some more. You're saving me
a lot of trouble. Now I won't have to explain to her what sort of
friend you really were and why I gave you the old heave-ho.

GLORIA   *(Drawing nearer to the microphone:)* Mrs. Lovejoy?

SWIFT   (*Reporting what he has heard on the headphones:*) She says, "What is it, dear?"

GLORIA   There's a loaded revolver in your knitting bag, Mrs. Lovejoy—in case you don't want to live anymore.

FRANKENSTEIN   (*Not in the least worried about the pistol but filled with contempt and disgust for* GLORIA:) You total imbecile. Where did you get a pistol?

GLORIA   From a mail-order house in Chicago. They had an ad in *True Romances.*

FRANKENSTEIN   They sell guns to crazy broads.

GLORIA   I could have had a bazooka if I'd wanted one. Fourteen-ninety-eight.

FRANKENSTEIN   I am going to get that pistol now and it is going to be exhibit A at your trial. (*He leaves.*)

LITTLE   (*To* SWIFT:) Shouldn't you put the patient to sleep?

SWIFT   There's no way she can hurt herself.

GLORIA   (*To* LITTLE:) What does he mean?

LITTLE   Her arms are fixed so she can't point a gun at herself.

GLORIA   (*Sickened:*) They even thought of that.

CUT TO SYLVIA's *room.* FRANKENSTEIN *is entering.* SYLVIA is holding the pistol thoughtfully.

FRANKENSTEIN   Nice playthings you have.

SYLVIA   You mustn't get mad at Gloria, Norbert. I asked her for this. I begged her for this.

FRANKENSTEIN   Last month.

SYLVIA   Yes.

FRANKENSTEIN   But everything is better now.

SYLVIA   Everything but the spark.

FRANKENSTEIN   Spark?

SYLVIA   The spark that Gloria says she loves—the tiny spark of what I used to be. As happy as I am right now, that spark is begging me to take this gun and put it out.

FRANKENSTEIN   And what is your reply?

SYLVIA   I am going to do it, Norbert. This is good-bye. (*She tries every which way to aim the gun at herself, fails and fails, while* FRANKENSTEIN *stands calmly by.*) That's no accident, is it?

FRANKENSTEIN   We very much don't want you to hurt yourself. We love you, too.

SYLVIA   And how much longer must I live like this? I've never dared ask before.

KURT VONNEGUT

FRANKENSTEIN   I would have to pull a figure out of a hat.

SYLVIA   Maybe you'd better not. *(Pause.)* Did you pull one out of a hat?

FRANKENSTEIN   At least five hundred years.

(Silence.)

SYLVIA   So I will still be alive—long after you are gone?

FRANKENSTEIN   Now is the time, my dear Sylvia, to tell you something I have wanted to tell you for years. Every organ downstairs has the capacity to take care of two human beings instead of one. And the plumbing and wiring have been designed so that a second human being can be hooked up in two shakes of a lamb's tail. *(Silence.)* Do you understand what I am saying to you, Sylvia? *(Silence. Passionately:)* Sylvia! I will be that second human being! Talk about marriage! Talk about great love stories from the past! Your kidney will be my kidney! Your liver will be my liver! Your heart will be my heart! Your ups will be my ups and your downs will be my downs! We will live in such perfect harmony, Sylvia, that the gods themselves will tear out their hair in envy!

SYLVIA   This is what you want!

FRANKENSTEIN   More than anything in this world.

SYLVIA   Well, then—here it is, Norbert. *(She empties the revolver into him.)*

CUT TO *same room almost a half hour later. A second tripod has been set up, with* FRANKENSTEIN's *head on top.* FRANKENSTEIN *is asleep and so is* SYLVIA. SWIFT, *with* LITTLE *standing by, is feverishly making a final connection to the machinery below. There are pipe wrenches and a blowtorch and other plumber's and electrician's tools lying around.*

SWIFT   That's gotta be it. *(He straightens up, looks around.)* That's gotta be it.

LITTLE   *(Consulting watch:)* Twenty-eight minutes since the first shot was fired.

SWIFT   Thank God you were around.

LITTLE   What you really needed was a plumber.

SWIFT   *(Into microphone:)* Charley—we're all set up here. You all set down there?

CHARLEY   *(Squawk box:)* All set.

SWIFT   Give 'em plenty of martinis.

189

GLORIA *appears numbly in doorway.*

CHARLEY They've got 'em. They'll be higher than kites.
SWIFT Better give 'em a touch of LSD, too.
CHARLEY Coming up.
SWIFT Hold it! I forgot the phonograph. (*To* LITTLE:) Dr. Frankenstein said that if this ever happened, he wanted a certain record
playing when he came to. He said it was in with the other records—
in a plain white jacket. (*To* GLORIA:) See if you can find it.

GLORIA *goes to phonograph, finds the record.*

GLORIA This it?
SWIFT Put it on.
GLORIA Which side?
SWIFT I don't know.
GLORIA There's tape over one side.
SWIFT The side *without* tape. (GLORIA *puts record on. Into micro-
phone*:) Stand by to wake up the patients.
CHARLEY Standing by.

*Record begins to play. It is a Jeanette MacDonald–Nelson Eddy
duet, "Ah, Sweet Mystery of Life."*

SWIFT (*Into microphone:*) Wake 'em up!

FRANKENSTEIN *and* SYLVIA *wake up, filled with formless pleasure. They dreamily appreciate the music, eventually catch sight
of each other, perceive each other as old and beloved friends.*

SYLVIA Hi, there.
FRANKENSTEIN Hello.
SYLVIA How do you feel?
FRANKENSTEIN Fine. Just fine.

GRACE PALEY

GRACE PALEY *(1922–). American fiction writer and poet. A storyteller for thirty-five years, Grace Paley is the author of the short story collections* Enormous Changes at the Last Minute *(1974),* The Little Disturbances of Man *(1985), and* Later the Same Day *(1985), as well as two books of poetry and a book of poems and prose pieces. A frequent lecturer at universities and writing workshops, Paley counts among her many awards and honors the 1994 Jewish Cultural Achievement Award, the 1992 Rea Award for Short Stories, and the 1989 Edith Wharton Award.* The Collected Stories *was a finalist for the 1994 National Book Award in fiction.*

A MAN TOLD ME THE STORY OF HIS LIFE

Vicente said: I wanted to be a doctor. I wanted to be a doctor with my whole heart.

I learned every bone, every organ in the body. What is it for? Why does it work?

The school said to me: Vicente, be an engineer. That would be good. You understand mathematics.

I said to the school: I want to be a doctor. I already know how the organs connect. When something goes wrong, I'll understand how to make repairs.

The school said: Vicente, you will really be an excellent engineer. You show on all the tests what a good engineer you will be. It doesn't show whether you'll be a good doctor.

I said: Oh, I long to be a doctor. I nearly cried. I was seventeen. I said: But perhaps you're right. You're the teacher. You're the principal. I know I'm young.

The school said: And besides, you're going into the army.

And then I was made a cook. I prepared food for two thousand men.

Now you see me. I have a good job. I have three children. This is my wife, Consuela. Did you know I saved her life?

Look, she suffered pain. The doctor said: What is this? Are you tired? Have you had too much company? How many children? Rest overnight, then tomorrow we'll make tests.

The next morning I called the doctor. I said: She must be operated immediately. I have looked in the book. I see where her pain is. I understand what the pressure is, where it comes from. I see clearly the organ that is making trouble.

The doctor made a test. He said: She must be operated at once. He said to me: Vicente, how did you know?

DANNIE ABSE

DANNIE ABSE (1923–). *British physician, poet, and playwright. Born in Cardiff, Wales, Abse was educated at the University of Wales, at King's College in London, and at Westminster Hospital. A prolific writer, he has written award-winning plays, novels such as* Ash on a Young Man's Sleeve, *and a compelling autobiography,* A Poet in the Family. *He is perhaps best known for his poetry, including* White Coat, Purple Coat. *His* Intermittent Journals *was published in 1994;* Selected Poems *appeared recently from Penguin.*

X-RAY

Some prowl sea-beds, some hurtle to a star
and, mother, some obsessed turn over every stone
or open graves to let that starlight in.
There are men who would open anything.

Harvey, the circulation of the blood,
and Freud, the circulation of our dreams,
pried honourably and honoured are
like all explorers. Men who'd open men.

And those others, mother, with diseases
like great streets named after them: Addison,
Parkinson, Hodgkin—physicians who'd arrive
fast and first on any sour death-bed scene.

I am their slowcoach colleague—half afraid,
incurious. As a boy it was so: you know how
my small hand never teased to pieces
an alarm clock or flensed a perished mouse.

And this larger hand's the same. It stretches now
out from a white sleeve to hold up, mother,
your X-ray to the glowing screen. My eyes look
but don't want to, I still don't want to know.

CASE HISTORY

"Most Welshmen are worthless,
an inferior breed, doctor."

He did not know I was Welsh.
Then he praised the architects
of the German death-camps—
did not know I was a Jew.
He called liberals, "White blacks,"
and continued to invent curses.

When I palpated his liver
I felt the soft liver of Goering;
when I lifted my stethoscope
I heard the heartbeats of Himmler;
when I read his encephalograph
I thought, *"Sieg heil, mein Führer."*

In the clinic's dispensary
red berry of black bryony,
cowbane, deadly nightshade, deathcap.
Yet I prescribed for him
as if he were my brother.

Later that night I must have slept
on my arm: momentarily
my right hand lost its cunning.

CARNAL KNOWLEDGE

1

You, student, whistling those elusive bits
of Schubert when phut, phut, phut, throbbed the sky
of London. Listen: the servo-engine cut
and the silence was not the desired silence
between two movements of music. Then
Finale, the Aldwych echo of crunch
and the urgent ambulances loaded
with the fresh dead. You, young, whistled again,
entered King's, climbed the stone-murky steps
to the high and brilliant Dissecting Room

where nameless others, naked on the slabs,
reclined in disgraceful silences—twenty
amazing sculptures waiting to be vandalized.

2

You, corpse, I pried into your bloodless meat
without the morbid curiosity of Vesalius,
did not care that the great Galen was wrong,
Avicenna mistaken, that they had described
the approximate structure of pigs and monkeys
rather than the human body. With scalpel
I dug deep into your stale formaldehyde
unaware of Pope Boniface's decree
but, as instructed, violated you—
the reek of you in my eyes, my nostrils,
clothes, in the kisses of my girlfriends.
You, anonymous. Who were you, mister?
Your thin mouth could not reply, "Absent, sir,"
or utter with inquisitionary rage.

   Your neck exposed, muscles, nerves, vessels,
a mere coloured plate in some anatomy book;
your right hand, too, dissected, never belonged,
it seemed, to somebody once shockingly alive,
never held, surely, another hand in greeting
or tenderness, never clenched a fist in anger,
never took up a pen to sign an authentic name.

   You, dead man, Thing, each day, each week,
each month, you, slowly decreasing Thing,
visibly losing Divine proportions,
you, residue, mere trunk of a man's body,
you, X, legless, armless, headless Thing
that I dissected so casually.

   Then went downstairs to drink wartime coffee.

3

When the hospital priest, Father Jerome,
remarked, "The Devil made the lower parts
of a man's body, God the upper,"
I said, "Father, it's the other way round."
So, the anatomy course over, Jerome,
thanatologist, did not invite me
to the Special Service for the Twenty Dead,

did not say to me, "Come for the relatives' sake."
(Surprise, surprise, that they had relatives,
those lifeless-size, innominate creatures.)
Other students accepted, joined in the fake chanting,
organ solemnity, cobwebbed theatre.
And that's all it would have been,
a ceremony propitious and routine,
an obligation forgotten soon enough
had not the strict priest with premeditated rage
called out the Register of the Twenty Dead—
each non-cephalic carcass gloatingly identified
with a local habitation and a name
till one by one, made culpable, the students cried.

4

I did not learn the name of my intimate,
the twentieth sculpture, the one next to the door.
No matter. Now all these years later
I know those twenty sculptures were but one,
the same one duplicated. You.
I hear not Father Jerome but St. Jerome cry,
"No, John will be John, Mary will be Mary,"
as if the dead would have ears to hear
the Register on Judgement Day.
    Look, on gravestones many names.
There should be one only. Yours.
No, not even one since you have no name.
In the newspapers' memorial columns
many names. A joke.
On the canvases of masterpieces
the same figure always in disguise. Yours.
Even in the portraits of the old anchorite
fingering a dry skull you are half concealed
lest onlookers should turn away blinded.
In certain music, too, with its sound of loss,
in that Schubert Quintet, for instance,
you are there in the Adagio,
playing the third cello that cannot be heard.
    You are there and there and there, nameless,
and here I am, older by far and nearer,
perplexed, trying to recall what you looked like
before I dissected your face—you, threat,

molesting presence, and I in a white coat
your enemy, in a purple one, your nuncio,
writing this while a winter twig, not you,
scrapes, scrapes the windowpane.
  Soon I shall climb the stairs. Gratefully,
I shall wind up the usual clock at bedtime
(the steam vanishing from the bathroom mirror)
with my hand, my living hand.

IN THE THEATRE
(A True Incident)

*'Only a local anaesthetic was given because of the blood
pressure problem. The patient, thus, was fully awake
throughout the operation. But in those days—in 1938, in
Cardiff, when I was Lambert Rogers' dresser—they
could not locate a brain tumour with precision. Too
much normal brain tissue was destroyed as the surgeon
crudely searched for it, before he felt the resistance of
it . . . all somewhat hit and miss. One operation I shall
never forget. . . .'*

(DR *WILFRED ABSE*)

Sister saying—'Soon you'll be back in the ward,'
sister thinking—'Only two more on the list,'
the patient saying—'Thank you, I feel fine';
small voices, small lies, nothing untoward,
though, soon, he would blink again and again
because of the fingers of Lambert Rogers,
rash as a blind man's, inside his soft brain.

If items of horror can make a man laugh
then laugh at this: one hour later, the growth
still undiscovered, ticking its own wild time;
more brain mashed because of the probe's braille path;
Lambert Rogers desperate, fingering still;
his dresser thinking, 'Christ! Two more on the list,
a cisternal puncture and a neural cyst.'

Then, suddenly, the cracked record in the brain,
a ventriloquist voice that cried, 'You sod,
leave my soul alone, leave my soul alone,'—
the patient's dummy lips moving to that refrain,
the patient's eyes too wide. And, shocked,
Lambert Rogers drawing out the probe
with nurses, students, sister, petrified.

'Leave my soul alone, leave my soul alone,'
that voice so arctic and that cry so odd
had nowhere else to go—till the antique
gramophone wound down and the words began
to blur and slow, '. . . leave . . . my . . . soul . . . alone . . .'
to cease at last when something other died.
And silence matched the silence under snow.

JAMES DICKEY

JAMES DICKEY (1923–1997). *American poet, novelist, and critic. Dickey was born in Atlanta and attended Clemson and Vanderbilt universities. As a pilot in the air force, he flew a hundred missions on the Pacific front, and later saw military duty in Korea. He worked briefly in advertising, but after receiving a Guggenheim Fellowship left the world of business to focus exclusively on his writing. He won the National Book Award for poetry in 1966, and served as poetry consultant to the Library of Congress from 1966 to 1968. In addition to being a widely published poet, Dickey was the author of the novel* Deliverance *(1970); his most recent book was* To the White Sea *(1993). He also published literary criticism and children's poetry.*

DIABETES

I

Sugar

One night I thirsted like a prince
Then like a king
Then like an empire   like a world
On fire. I rose and flowed away and fell
Once more to sleep. In an hour I was back
In the kingdom   staggering, my belly going round with self-
Made night-water, wondering what
The hell. Months of having a tongue
Of flame convinced me: I had better not go
On this way. The doctor was young

And nice. He said, I must tell you,
My friend, that it is needles moderation
And exercise. You don't want to look forward
To gangrene and kidney

Failure   boils blindness infection skin trouble falling
Teeth coma and death.
                    O.K.
                              In sleep my mouth went dry
With my answer   and in it burned the sands

Of time with new fury. Sleep could give me no water
But my own. Gangrene in white
Was in my wife's hand at breakfast
Heaped like a mountain. Moderation, moderation,
My friend, and exercise. Each time the barbell
Rose   each time a foot fell
Jogging, it counted itself
One death   two death   three death and resurrection
For a little while. Not bad! I always knew it would have to be
                                        somewhere around
The house: the real
Symbol of Time I could eat
And live with, coming true when I opened my mouth:
True in the coffee and the child's birthday
Cake   helping sickness be fire-
tongued, sleepless and water-
logged   but not bad, sweet sand
Of time, my friend, an everyday—
A livable death at last.

II
Under Buzzards

(for Robert Penn Warren)

Heavy summer. Heavy. Companion, if we climb our mortal bodies
High with great effort, we shall find ourselves
Flying with the life
Of the birds of death. We have come up
Under buzzards   they face us

Slowly   slowly circling   and as we watch them they turn us
Around, and you and I spin
Slowly, slowly rounding
Out the hill. We are level
Exactly on this moment: exactly on the same bird-

plane with those deaths. They are the salvation of our sense
Of glorious movement. Brother, it is right for us to face
Them every which way, and come to ourselves and come
From every direction
There is. Whirl and stand fast!
Whence cometh death, O Lord?

On the downwind, riding fire,
Of Hogback Ridge.
But listen: what is dead here?
They are not falling but waiting   but waiting
Riding, and they may know
The rotten, nervous sweetness of my blood.
Somewhere riding the updraft
Of a far forest fire, they sensed the city sugar
The doctors found in time.
My eyes are green as lettuce with my diet,
My weight is down,
One pocket nailed with needles and injections, the other dragging
With sugar cubes to balance me in life
And hold my blood
Level, level. Tell me, black riders, does this do any good?
Tell me what I need to know about my time
In the world. O out of the fiery

Furnace of pine-woods, in the sap-smoke and crownfire of needles,
Say when I'll die. When will the sugar rise boiling
Against me, and my brain be sweetened
to death?
In heavy summer, like this day.
All right! Physicians, witness! I will shoot my veins
Full of insulin. Let the needle burn
In. From your terrible heads
The flight-blood drains   and you are falling back
Back to the body-raising
Fire.
Heavy summer. Heavy. My blood is clear
For a time. Is it too clear? Heat waves are rising
Without birds. But something is gone from me,
Friend. This is too sensible. Really it is better
To know when to die   better for my blood
To stream with the death-wish of birds.
You know, I had just as soon crush
This doomed syringe
Between two mountain rocks, and bury this needle in needles

Of trees. Companion, open that beer.
How the body works   how hard it works
For its medical books is not

Everything: everything is how
Much glory is in it: heavy summer is right
For a long drink of beer. Red sugar of my eyeballs
Feels them turn blindly
In the fire   rising   turning   turning
Back to Hogback Ridge, and it is all
Delicious, brother: my body is turning   is flashing unbalanced
Sweetness everywhere, and I am calling my birds.

THE CANCER MATCH

Lord, you've sent both
And may have come yourself. I will sit down, bearing up under
The death of light very well, and we will all
Have a drink. Two or three, maybe.
I see now the delights

Of being let "come home"
From the hospital.
Night!
I don't have all the time
In the world, but I have all night.
I have space for me and my house,
And I have cancer and whiskey

In a lovely relation.
They are squared off, here on my ground. They are fighting,
Or are they dancing? I have been told   and told
That medicine has no hope, or anything
More to give,

But they have no idea
What hope is, or how it comes. You take these two things:
This bourbon and this thing growing. Why,
They are like boys! They bow
To each other

Like judo masters,
One of them jumping for joy, and I watch them struggle
All around the room, inside and out
Of the house, as they battle
Near the mailbox

And superbly
For the street-lights! Internally, I rise like my old self
To watch: and remember, ladies and gentlemen,
We are looking at this match
From the standpoint

Of tonight
Alone, swarm over him, my joy, my laughter, my Basic Life
Force! Let your bright sword-arm stream
Into that turgid hulk, the worst
Of me, growing:

Get 'im, O Self
Like a beloved son! One more time! Tonight we are going
Good   better and better   we are going
To win, and not only win but win
Big, win big.

DENISE LEVERTOV

Denise Levertov (1923–1997). *English-born poet who remained in the United States after her marriage to an American in 1948. Her writings, influenced by William Carlos Williams and other contemporary poets, spanned more than three decades, from the publication of* Five Poems *(1958) and* The Jacob's Ladder *(1961) to* A Door in the Hive *(1989) and* Evening Train *(1993), with more than a dozen other volumes in between.*

TALKING TO GRIEF

Ah, grief, I should not treat you
like a homeless dog
who comes to the back door
for a crust, for a meatless bone.
I should trust you.

I should coax you
into the house and give you
your own corner,
a worn mat to lie on,
your own water dish.

You think I don't know you've been living
under my porch.
You long for your real place to be readied
before winter comes. You need
your name,
your collar and tag. You need
the right to warn off intruders,
to consider
my house your own
and me your person
and yourself
my own dog.

DEATH PSALM: O LORD OF MYSTERIES

She grew old.
She made ready to die.
She gave counsel to women and men, to young girls and
                                        young boys.

She remembered her griefs.
She remembered her happinesses.
She watered the garden.
She accused herself.
She forgave herself.
She learned new fragments of wisdom.
She forgot old fragments of wisdom.
She abandoned certain angers.
She gave away gold and precious stones.
She counted-over her handkerchiefs of fine lawn.
She continued to laugh on some days, to cry on others,
                        unfolding the design of her identity.
She practiced the songs she knew, her voice
                                        gone out of tune
                        but the breathing-pattern perfected.
She told her sons and daughters she was ready.
She maintained her readiness.
She grew very old.
She watched the generations increase.
She watched the passing of seasons and years.
She did not die.

She did not die, but lies half-speechless, incontinent,
                        aching in body, wandering in mind
                        in a hospital room.
A plastic tube, taped to her nose,
        disappears into one nostril.
Plastic tubes are attached to veins in her arms.
Her urine runs through a tube into a bottle under the bed.
On her back and ankles are black sores.

The black sores are parts of her that have died.
The beat of her heart is steady.
She is not whole.

She made ready to die, she prayed, she made her peace,
    she read daily from the lectionary.
She tended the green garden she had made,
    she fought off the destroying ants,
    she watered the plants daily
    and took note of their blossoming.
She gave sustenance to the needy.
She prepared her life for the hour of death.
But the hour has passed and she has not died.

O Lord of mysteries, how beautiful is sudden death
    when the spirit vanishes
    boldly and without casting
    a single shadowy feather of hesitation
    onto the felled body.

O Lord of mysteries, how baffling, how clueless
    is laggard death, disregarding
    all that is set before it
        in the dignity of welcome—
    laggard death, that steals
        insignificant patches of flesh—
    laggard death, that shuffles
    past the open gate,
    past the open hand,
    past the open,
        ancient,
        courteously waiting life.

LISEL MUELLER

LISEL MUELLER (1924–). *American poet. A native of Hamburg, Germany, and now a U.S. citizen, Lisel Mueller received the 1997 Pulitzer Prize for poetry for her seventh book,* Alive Together: New and Selected Poems. *Many of her previous books have also won prizes, among them* The Private Life *(the Lamont Poetry Selection of the Academy of American Poets),* The Need to Hold Still *(National Book Award), and* Waving from Shore *(the Carl Sandburg Prize). A social worker and book reviewer in her early years, Mueller has spent her later years as a visiting lecturer and poet in residence on many college campuses throughout the United States, including the University of Chicago and Warren Wilson College. She resides in Chicago.*

MONET REFUSES THE OPERATION

Doctor, you say there are no haloes
around the streetlights in Paris
and what I see is an aberration
caused by old age, an affliction.
I tell you it has taken me all my life
to arrive at the vision of gas lamps as angels,
to soften and blur and finally banish
the edges you regret I don't see,
to learn that the line I called the horizon
does not exist and sky and water,
so long apart, are the same state of being.
Fifty-four years before I could see
Rouen cathedral is built
of parallel shafts of sun,
and now you want to restore
my youthful errors: fixed
notions of top and bottom,
the illusion of three-dimensional space,
wisteria separate
from the bridge it covers.
What can I say to convince you
the Houses of Parliament dissolve
night after night to become

the fluid dream of the Thames?
I will not return to a universe
of objects that don't know each other,
as if islands were not the lost children
of one great continent. The world
is flux, and light becomes what it touches,
becomes water, lilies on water,
above and below water,
becomes lilac and mauve and yellow
and white and cerulean lamps,
small fists passing sunlight
so quickly to one another
that it would take long, streaming hair
inside my brush to catch it.
To paint the speed of light!
Our weighted shapes, these verticals,
burn to mix with air
and change our bones, skin, clothes
to gases. Doctor,
if only you could see
how heaven pulls earth into its arms
and how infinitely the heart expands
to claim this world, blue vapor without end.

DONALD JUSTICE

DONALD JUSTICE (1925–). *American poet, essayist, teacher, and editor. Mr. Justice is the recipient of numerous honors, including the Pulitzer and Bollingen Prizes for poetry. He is a member of the American Academy and Institute of Arts and Letters and is a chancellor of the Academy of American Poets. Donald Justice was born in Miami, Florida. Early on he studied musical composition with Carl Ruggles, a passion reflected in some of his poems. His M.A. and Ph.D. are from the University of North Carolina and University of Iowa, respectively. He has taught at many colleges and universities, including the University of Iowa, Princeton, the University of Virginia, and the University of Florida. Of Justice's work, a colleague, Mark Strand, has written: "Reading Justice, one feels keenly that a poem is an act of retrieval—that, as it memorializes, so it revives." Currently he lives in Iowa City.*

MEN AT FORTY

Men at forty
Learn to close softly
The doors to rooms they will not be
Coming back to.

At rest on a stair landing,
They feel it
Moving beneath them now like the deck of a ship,
Though the swell is gentle.

And deep in mirrors
They rediscover
The face of the boy as he practices tying
His father's tie there in secret

And the face of that father,
Still warm with the mystery of lather.
They are more fathers than sons themselves now.
Something is filling them, something

That is like the twilight sound
Of the crickets, immense,
Filling the woods at the foot of the slope
Behind their mortgaged houses.

L. E. SISSMAN

L. E. SISSMAN (1928–1976). *American poet. Sissman, an advertising executive, suffered from Hodgkin's disease, and some of his poetry was influenced by this chronic, debilitating illness. Poems such as "A Deathplace" describe poignant, even breathtaking thoughts about death within a hospital setting. Other works include* Dying: An Introduction *(1968),* Scattered Returns *(1969), and* Hello Darkness: The Collected Poems of L. E. Sissman *(1978). Sissman received several writing awards, including a Guggenheim Fellowship (1968) and a grant from the National Institute of Arts and Letters (1969).*

A DEATHPLACE

Very few people know where they will die,
But I do: in a brick-faced hospital,
Divided not unlike Caesarean Gaul,
Into three parts: the Dean Memorial
Wing, in the classic cast of 1910,
Green-grated in unglazed, Aeolian
Embrasures; the Maud Wiggin Building, which
Commemorates a dog-jawed Boston bitch
Who fought the brass down to their whipcord knees
In World War I, and won enlisted men
Some decent hospitals, and, being rich,
Donated her own granite monument;
The Mandeville Pavilion, pink-brick tent
With marble piping, flying snapping flags
Above the entry where our bloody rags
Are rolled in to be sponged and sewn again.
Today is fair; tomorrow, scourging rain
(If only my own tears) will see me in
Those jaundiced and distempered corridors
Off which the five-foot-wide doors slowly close.
White as my skimpy chiton, I will cringe
Before the pinpoint of the least syringe;
Before the buttered catheter goes in;
Before the I.V.'s lisp and drip begins
Inside my skin; before the rubber hand
Upon the lancet takes aim and descends

To lay me open, and upon its thumb
Retracts the trouble, a malignant plum;
And finally, I'll quail before the hour
When the authorities shut off the power
In that vast hospital, and in my bed
I'll feel my blood go thin, go white, the red,
The rose all leached away, and I'll go dead.
Then will the business of life resume:
The muffled trolley wheeled into my room,
The off-white blanket blanking off my face,
The stealing, secret, private, *largo* race
Down halls and elevators to the place
I'll be consigned to for transshipment, cased
In artificial air and light: the ward
That's underground; the terminal; the morgue.
Then one fine day when all the smart flags flap,
A booted man in black with a peaked cap
Will call for me and troll me down the hall
And slot me into his black car. That's all.

RICHARD SELZER

RICHARD SELZER (1928–). *American surgeon, writer, and educator. Born and raised in Troy, New York, Dr. Selzer was on the faculty of the Yale School of Medicine until 1990. He is both a popular, engaging lecturer and a widely published author; among his books are* Mortal Lessons: Notes on the Art of Surgery; Confessions of a Knife; *and* Taking the World in for Repairs. *His recent works—* Down from Troy: A Doctor Comes of Age *(1993) and* Raising the Dead: A Doctor's Encounter with His Own Mortality *(1994)—are wholly autobiographical. In* Down from Troy, *Selzer artistically chronicles the arc of his life from his childhood through his medical training, surgical career, and retirement, while in* Raising the Dead, *he captures the peculiarity of the doctor-turned-patient phenomenon by reflecting on his own excruciating experience with Legionnaires' disease.*

MERCY

It is October at the Villa Serbelloni, where I have come for a month to write. On the window ledges the cluster flies are dying. The climate is full of uncertainty. Should it cool down? Or warm up? Each day it overshoots the mark, veering from frost to steam. The flies have no uncertainty. They understand that their time has come.

What a lot of energy it takes to die! The frenzy of it. Long after they have collapsed and stayed motionless, the flies are capable of suddenly spinning so rapidly that they cannot be seen. Or seen only as a blurred glitter. They are like dervishes who whirl, then stop, and lay as quiet as before, only now and then waving a leg or two feebly, in a stuporous reenactment of locomotion. Until the very moment of death, the awful buzzing as though to swarm again.

Every morning I scoop up three dozen or so corpses with a dustpan and brush. Into the wastebasket they go, and I sit to begin the day's writing. All at once, from the wastebasket, the frantic knocking of resurrection. Here, death has not yet secured the premises. No matter the numbers slaughtered, no matter that the windows be kept shut all day, each evening the flies gather on the ledges to die, as they have lived, *ensemble*. It must be companionable to die so, matching spin for spin, knock for knock, and buzz for buzz with one's fellows.

We humans have no such fraternity, but each of us must buzz and spin and knock alone.

I think of a man in New Haven! He has been my patient for seven years, ever since the day I explored his abdomen in the operating room and found the surprise lurking there—a cancer of the pancreas. He was forty-two years old then. For this man, these have been seven years of famine. For his wife and his mother as well. Until three days ago his suffering was marked by slowly increasing pain, vomiting and fatigue. Still, it was endurable. With morphine. Three days ago the pain rollicked out of control, and he entered that elect band whose suffering cannot be relieved by any means short of death. In his bed at home he seemed an eighty-pound concentrate of pain from which all other pain must be made by serial dilution. He twisted under the lash of it. An ambulance arrived. At the hospital nothing was to be done to prolong his life. Only the administration of large doses of narcotics.

"Please," he begs me. In his open mouth, upon his teeth, a brown paste of saliva. All night long he has thrashed, as though to hollow out a grave in the bed.

"I won't let you suffer," I tell him. In his struggle the sheet is thrust aside. I see the old abandoned incision, the belly stuffed with tumor. His penis, even, is skinny. One foot with five blue toes is exposed. In my cupped hand, they are cold. I think of the twenty bones of that foot laced together with tendon, each ray accompanied by its own nerve and artery. Now, this foot seems a beautiful dead animal that had once been trained to transmit the command of a man's brain to the earth.

"I'll get rid of the pain," I tell his wife.

But there is no way to kill the pain without killing the man who owns it. Morphine to the lethal dose . . . and still he miaows and bays and makes other sounds like a boat breaking up in a heavy sea. I think his pain will live on long after he dies.

"Please," begs his wife, "we cannot go on like this."

"Do it," says the old woman, his mother. "Do it now."

"To give him any more would kill him," I tell her.

"Then do it," she says. The face of the old woman is hoof-beaten with intersecting curves of loose skin. Her hair is donkey brown, donkey gray.

They wait with him while I go to the nurses' station to prepare the syringes. It is a thing that I cannot ask anyone to do for me. When I return to the room, there are three loaded syringes in my hand, a rubber tourniquet and an alcohol sponge. Alcohol sponge! To prevent infection? The old woman is standing on a small stool and leaning over the side rail of the bed. Her bosom is just above his upturned face, as though she were weaning him with sorrow and gentleness from her still-full breasts. All at once she says severely, the way she must have said it to him years ago:

"Go home, son. Go home now."

I wait just inside the doorway. The only sound is a flapping, a rustling, as in a room to which a small animal, a bat perhaps, has retreated to die. The women turn to leave. There is neither gratitude nor reproach in their gaze. I should be hooded.

At last we are alone. I stand at the bedside.

"Listen," I say, "I can get rid of the pain." The man's eyes regain their focus. His gaze is like a wound that radiates its pain outward so that all upon whom it fell would know the need of relief.

"With these." I hold up the syringes.

"Yes," he gasps. "Yes." And while the rest of his body stirs in answer to the pain, he holds his left, his acquiescent arm still for the tourniquet. An even dew of sweat covers his body. I wipe the skin with the alcohol sponge, and tap the arm smartly to bring out the veins. There is one that is still patent; the others have long since clotted and broken down. I go to insert the needle, but the tourniquet has come unknotted; the vein has collapsed. Damn! Again I tie the tourniquet. Slowly the vein fills with blood. This time it stays distended.

He reacts not at all to the puncture. In a wild sea what is one tiny wave? I press the barrel and deposit the load, detach the syringe from the needle and replace it with the second syringe. I send this home, and go on to the third. When they are all given, I pull out the needle. A drop of blood blooms on his forearm. I blot it with the alcohol sponge. It is done. In less than a minute, it is done.

"Go home," I say, repeating the words of the old woman. I turn off the light. In the darkness the contents of the bed are theoretical. No! I must watch. I turn the light back on. How reduced he is, a folded parcel, something chipped away until only its shape and a little breath are left. His impatient bones gleam as though to burst through the papery skin. I am impatient, too. I want to get it over with, then step out into the corridor where the women are waiting. His death is like a jewel to them.

My fingers at his pulse. The same rhythm as mine! As though there were one pulse that beat throughout all of nature, and every creature's heart throbbed precisely.

"You can go home now," I say. The familiar emaciated body untenses. The respirations slow down. Eight per minute . . . six . . . It won't be long. The pulse wavers in and out of touch. It won't be long.

"Is that better?" I ask him. His gaze is distant, opaque, preoccupied. Minutes go by. Outside, in the corridor, the murmuring of women's voices.

But this man will not die! The skeleton rouses from its stupor. The snout twitches as if to fend off a fly. What is it that shakes him like a gourd full of beans? The pulse returns, melts away, comes back again, and stays. The respirations are twelve, then fourteen. I have not done it. I did not murder him. I am innocent!

I shall walk out of the room into the corridor. They will look at me, holding their breath, expectant. I lift the sheet to cover him. All at once, there is a sharp sting in my thumb. The same needle with which I meant to kill him has pricked *me*. A drop of blood appears. I press it with the alcohol sponge. My fresh blood deepens the stain of his on the gauze. Never mind. The man in the bed swallows. His Adam's apple bobs slowly. It would be so easy to do it. Three minutes of pressure on the larynx. He is still not conscious, wouldn't feel it, wouldn't know. My thumb and fingertips hover, land on his windpipe. My pulse beating in his neck, his in mine. I look back over my shoulder. No one. Two bare IV poles in a corner, their looped metal eyes witnessing. Do it! Fingers press. Again he swallows. Look back again. How closed the door is. And . . . my hand wilts. I cannot. It is not in me to do it. Not that way. The man's head swivels like an upturned fish. The squadron of ribs battles on.

I back away from the bed, turn and flee toward the doorway. In the mirror, a glimpse of my face. It is the face of someone who has been resuscitated after a long period of cardiac arrest. There is no spot of color in the cheeks, as though this person were in shock at what he had just seen on the yonder side of the grave.

In the corridor the women lean against the wall, against each other. They are like a band of angels dispatched here to take possession of his body. It is the only thing that will satisfy them.

"He didn't die," I say. "He won't . . . or can't." They are silent.

"He isn't ready yet," I say.

"He *is* ready," the old woman says. "*You* ain't."

IMELDA

I heard the other day that Hugh Franciscus had died. I knew him once. He was the Chief of Plastic Surgery when I was a medical student at Albany Medical College. Dr. Franciscus was the archetype of the professor of surgery—tall, vigorous, muscular, as precise in his technique as he was impeccable in his dress. Each day a clean lab coat monkishly starched, that sort of thing. I doubt that he ever read books. One book only, that of the human body, took the place of all others. He never raised his eyes from it. He read it like a printed page as though he knew that in the calligraphy there just beneath the skin were all the secrets of the world. Long before it became visible to anyone else, he could detect the first sign of granulation at the base of a wound, the first blue line of new epithelium at the periphery that would tell him that a wound would heal, or the barest hint of necrosis that presaged failure. This gave him the appearance of a prophet. "This skin graft will take," he would say, and you must believe beyond all cyanosis, exudation and inflammation that it would.

He had enemies, of course, who said he was arrogant, that he exalted activity for its own sake. Perhaps. But perhaps it was no more than the honesty of one who knows his own worth. Just look at a scalpel, after all. What a feeling of sovereignty, megalomania even, when you know that it is you and you alone who will make certain use of it. It was said, too, that he was a ladies' man. I don't know about that. It was all rumor. Besides, I think he had other things in mind than mere living. Hugh Franciscus was a zealous hunter. Every fall during the season he drove upstate to hunt deer. There was a glass-front case in his office where he showed his guns. How could he shoot a deer? we asked. But he knew better. To us medical students he was someone heroic, someone made up of several gods, beheld at a distance, and always from a lesser height. If he had grown accustomed to his miracles, we had not. He had no close friends on the staff. There was something a little sad in that. As though once long ago he had been flayed by friendship and now the slightest breeze would hurt. Confidences resulted in dishonor. Perhaps the person in whom one confided would scorn him, betray. Even though he spent his days among those less fortunate, weaker than he—the sick, after all— Franciscus seemed aware of an air of personal harshness in his environment to which he reacted by keeping his own counsel, by a certain remoteness. It was what gave him the appearance of being haughty. With the patients he was forthright. All the facts laid out, every question anticipated and answered with specific information. He delivered good news and bad with the same dispassion.

I was a third-year student, just turned onto the wards for the first time, and clerking on Surgery. Everything—the operating room, the morgue, the emergency room, the patients, professors, even the nurses—was terrifying. One picked one's way among the mines and booby traps of the hospital, hoping only to avoid the hemorrhage and perforation of disgrace. The opportunity for humiliation was everywhere.

It all began on Ward Rounds. Dr. Franciscus was demonstrating a cross-leg flap graft he had constructed to cover a large fleshy defect in the leg of a merchant seaman who had injured himself in a fall. The man was from Spain and spoke no English. There had been a comminuted fracture of the femur, much soft tissue damage, necrosis. After weeks of débridement and dressings, the wound had been made ready for grafting. Now the patient was in his fifth postoperative day. What he saw was a thick web of pale blue flesh arising from the man's left thigh, and which had been sutured to the open wound on the right thigh. When the surgeon pressed the pedicle with his finger, it blanched; when he let up, there was a slow return of the violaceous color.

"The circulation is good," Franciscus announced. "It will get better." In several weeks, we were told, he would divide the tube of flesh at its site of origin, and tailor it to fit the defect to which, by then, it would have grown more solidly. All at once, the webbed man in the bed reached out, and gripping Franciscus by the arm, began to speak rapidly, pointing to his groin and hip. Franciscus stepped back at once to disengage his arm from the patient's grasp.

"Anyone here know Spanish? I didn't get a word of that."

"The cast is digging into him up above," I said. "The edges of the plaster are rough. When he moves, they hurt."

Without acknowledging my assistance, Dr. Franciscus took a plaster shears from the dressing cast and with several large snips cut away the rough edges of the cast.

"*Gracias, gracias.*" The man in the bed smiled. But Franciscus had already moved on to the next bed. He seemed to me a man of immense strength and ability, yet without affection for the patients. He did not want to be touched by them. It was less kindness that he showed them than a reassurance that he would never give up, that he would bend every effort. If anyone could, he would solve the problems of their flesh.

Ward Rounds had disbanded and I was halfway down the corridor when I heard Dr. Franciscus' voice behind me.

"You speak Spanish." It seemed a command.

"I lived in Spain for two years," I told him.

"I'm taking a surgical team to Honduras next week to operate on the natives down there. I do it every year for three weeks, somewhere. This year, Honduras. I can arrange the time away from your duties here if you'd like to come along. You will act as interpreter. I'll show you how to use the clinical camera. What you'd see would make it worthwhile."

So it was that, a week later, the envy of my classmates, I joined the mobile surgical unit—surgeons, anesthetists, nurses and equipment—aboard a Military Air Transport plane to spend three weeks performing plastic surgery on people who had been previously selected by an advance team. Honduras. I don't suppose I shall ever see it again. Nor do I especially want to. From the plane it seemed a country made of clay—burnt umber, raw sienna, dry. It had a deadweight quality, as though the ground had no buoyancy, no air sacs through which a breeze might wander. Our destination was Comayagua, a town in the Central Highlands. The town itself was situated on the edge of one of the flatlands that were linked in a network between the granite mountains. Above, all was brown, with only an occasional Spanish cedar tree; below, patches of luxuriant tropical growth. It was a day's bus ride from the airport. For hours, the town kept appearing and disappearing with the convolutions of the road. At last, there it lay before us, panting and exhausted at the bottom of the mountain.

That was all I was to see of the countryside. From then on, there was only the derelict hospital of Comayagua, with the smell of spoiling bananas and the accumulated odors of everyone who had been sick there for the last hundred years. Of the two, I much preferred the frank smell of the sick. The heat of the place was incendiary. So hot that, as we stepped from the bus, our own words did not carry through the air, but hung limply at our lips and chins. Just in front of the hospital was a thirsty courtyard where mobs of waiting people squatted or lay in the meager shade, and where, on dry days, a fine dust rose through which untethered goats shouldered. Against the walls of this courtyard, gaunt, dejected men stood, their faces, like their country, preternaturally solemn, leaden. Here no one looked up at the sky. Every head was bent beneath a wide-brimmed straw hat. In the days that followed, from the doorway of the dispensary, I would watch the brown mountains sliding about, drinking the hospital into their shadow as the afternoon grew later and later, flattening us by their very altitude.

The people were mestizos, of mixed Spanish and Indian blood.

They had flat, broad, dumb museum feet. At first they seemed to me indistinguishable the one from the other, without animation. All the vitality, the hidden sexuality, was in their black hair. Soon I was to know them by the fissures with which each face was graven. But, even so, compared to us, they were masked, shut away. My job was to follow Dr. Franciscus around, photograph the patients before and after surgery, interpret and generally act as aide-de-camp. It was exhilarating. Within days I had decided that I was not just useful, but essential. Despite that we spent all day in each other's company, there were no overtures of friendship from Dr. Franciscus. He knew my place, and I knew it, too. In the afternoon he examined the patients scheduled for the next day's surgery. I would call out a name from the doorway to the examining room. In the courtyard someone would rise. I would usher the patient in, and nudge him to the examining table where Franciscus stood, always, I thought, on the verge of irritability. I would read aloud the case history, then wait while he carried out his examination. While I took the "before" photographs, Dr. Franciscus would dictate into a tape recorder:

"Ulcerating basal cell carcinoma of the right orbit—six by eight centimeters—involving the right eye and extending into the floor of the orbit. Operative plan: wide excision with enucleation of the eye. Later, bone and skin grafting." The next morning we would be in the operating room where the procedure would be carried out.

We were more than two weeks into our tour of duty—a few days to go—when it happened. Earlier in the day I had caught sight of her through the window of the dispensary. A thin, dark Indian girl about fourteen years old. A figurine, orange-brown, terra-cotta, and still attached to the unshaped clay from which she had been carved. An older, sun-weathered woman stood behind and somewhat to the left of the girl. The mother was short and dumpy. She wore a broad-brimmed hat with a high crown, and a shapeless dress like a cassock. The girl had long, loose black hair. There were tiny gold hoops in her ears. The dress she wore could have been her mother's. Far too big, it hung from her thin shoulders at some risk of slipping down her arms. Even with her in it, the dress was empty, something hanging on the back of a door. Her breasts made only the smallest imprint in the cloth, her hips none at all. All the while, she pressed to her mouth a filthy, pink, balled-up rag as though to stanch a flow or buttress against pain. I knew that what she had come to show us, what we were there to see, was hidden beneath that pink cloth. As I watched, the woman handed down to her a gourd from which the girl drank, lapping like a dog. She was the last patient of the day. They had been waiting in the courtyard for hours.

"Imelda Valdez," I called out. Slowly she rose to her feet, the cloth never leaving her mouth, and followed her mother to the examining-room door. I shooed them in.

"You sit up there on the table," I told her. "Mother, you stand over there, please." I read from the chart:

"This is a fourteen-year-old girl with a complete, unilateral, left-sided cleft lip and cleft palate. No other diseases or congenital defects. Laboratory tests, chest X ray—negative."

"Tell her to take the rag away," said Dr. Franciscus. I did, and the girl shrank back, pressing the cloth all the more firmly.

"Listen, this is silly," said Franciscus. "Tell her I've got to see it. Either she behaves, or send her away."

"Please give me the cloth," I said to the girl as gently as possible. She did not. She could not. Just then, Franciscus reached up and, taking the hand that held the rag, pulled it away with a hard jerk. For an instant the girl's head followed the cloth as it left her face, one arm still upflung against showing. Against all hope, she would hide herself. A moment later, she relaxed and sat still. She seemed to me then like an animal that looks outward at the infinite, at death, without fear, with recognition only.

Set as it was in the center of the girl's face, the defect was utterly hideous—a nude rubbery insect that had fastened there. The upper lip was widely split all the way to the nose. One white tooth perched upon the protruding upper jaw projected through the hole. Some of the bone seemed to have been gnawed away as well. Above the thing, clear almond eyes and long black hair reflected the light. Below, a slender neck where the pulse trilled visibly. Under our gaze the girl's eyes fell to her lap where her hands lay palms upward, half open. She was a beautiful bird with a crushed beak. And tense with the expectation of more shame.

"Open your mouth," said the surgeon. I translated. She did so, and the surgeon tipped back her head to see inside.

"The palate, too. Complete," he said. There was a long silence. At last he spoke.

"What is your name?" The margins of the wound melted until she herself was being sucked into it.

"Imelda." The syllables leaked through the hole with a slosh and a whistle.

"Tomorrow," said the surgeon, "I will fix your lip. *Mañana*."

It seemed to me that Hugh Franciscus, in spite of his years of experience, in spite of all the dreadful things he had seen, must have been awed by the sight of this girl. I could see it flit across his face for an instant. Perhaps it was her small act of concealment, that he had had to demand that she show him the lip, that he had had to force her to show it to him. Perhaps it was her resistance that intensified the disfigurement. Had she brought her mouth to him willingly, without shame, she would have been for him neither more nor less than any other patient.

He measured the defect with calipers, studied it from different angles, turning her head with a finger at her chin.

"How can it ever be put back together?" I asked.

"Take her picture," he said. And to her, "Look straight ahead." Through the eye of the camera she seemed more pitiful than ever, her humiliation more complete.

"Wait!" The surgeon stopped me. I lowered the camera. A strand of her hair had fallen across her face and found its way to her mouth, becoming stuck there by saliva. He removed the hair and secured it behind her ear.

"Go ahead," he ordered. There was the click of the camera. The girl winced.

"Take three more, just in case."

When the girl and her mother had left, he took paper and pen and with a few lines drew a remarkable likeness of the girl's face.

"Look," he said. "If this dot is A, and this one B, this, C and this, D, the incisions are made A to B, then C to D. CD must equal AB. It is all equilateral triangles." All well and good, but then came X and Y and rotation flaps and the rest.

"Do you see?" he asked.

"It is confusing," I told him.

"It is simply a matter of dropping the upper lip into a normal position, then crossing the gap with two triangular flaps. It is geometry," he said.

"Yes," I said. "Geometry." And relinquished all hope of becoming a plastic surgeon.

In the operating room the next morning the anesthesia had already been administered when we arrived from Ward Rounds. The tube emerging from the girl's mouth was pressed against her lower lip to be kept out of the field of surgery. Already, a nurse was scrubbing the face which swam in a reddish-brown lather. The tiny gold earrings were included in the scrub. Now and then, one of them gave a brave flash. The face was washed for the last time, and dried. Green towels were placed over the face to hide everything but the mouth and nose. The drapes were applied.

"Calipers!" The surgeon measured, locating the peak of the distorted Cupid's bow.

"Marking pen!" He placed the first blue dot at the apex of the bow. The nasal sills were dotted; next, the inferior philtral dimple, the vermilion line. The *A* flap and the *B* flap were outlined. On he worked, peppering the lip and nose, making sense out of chaos, realizing the lip that lay waiting in that deep essential pink, that only he could see. The last dot and line were placed. He was ready.

"Scalpel!" He held the knife above the girl's mouth.

"O.K. to go ahead?" he asked the anesthetist.

"Yes."

He lowered the knife.

"No! Wait!" The anesthetist's voice was tense, staccato. "Hold it!"

The surgeon's hand was motionless.

"What's the matter?"

"Something's wrong. I'm not sure. God, she's hot as a pistol. Blood pressure is way up. Pulse one eighty. Get a rectal temperature." A nurse fumbled beneath the drapes. We waited. The nurse retrieved the thermometer.

"One hundred seven . . . no . . . eight." There was disbelief in her voice.

"Malignant hyperthermia," said the anesthetist. "Ice! Ice! Get lots of ice!" I raced out the door, accosted the first nurse I saw.

"Ice!" I shouted. "*Hielo!* Quickly! *Hielo!*" The woman's expression was blank. I ran to another. "*Hielo! Hielo!* For the love of God, ice."

"*Hielo?*" She shrugged. "*Nada.*" I ran back to the operating room.

"There isn't any ice," I reported. Dr. Franciscus had ripped off his rubber gloves and was feeling the skin of the girl's abdomen. Above the mask his eyes were the eyes of a horse in battle.

"The EKG is wild . . ."

"I can't get a pulse . . ."

"What the hell . . ."

The surgeon reached for the girl's groin. No femoral pulse.

"EKG flat. My God! She's dead!"

"She can't be."

"She is."

The surgeon's fingers pressed the groin where there was no pulse to be felt, only his own pulse hammering at the girl's flesh to be let in.

* * *

It was noon, four hours later, when we left the operating room. It was a day so hot and humid I felt steamed open like an envelope. The woman was sitting on a bench in the courtyard in her dress like a cassock. In one hand she held the piece of cloth the girl had used to conceal her mouth. As we watched, she folded it once neatly, and then again, smoothing it, cleaning the cloth which might have been the head of the girl in her lap that she stroked and consoled.

"I'll do the talking here," he said. He would tell her himself, in whatever Spanish he could find. Only if she did not understand was I to speak for him. I watched him brace himself, set his shoulders. How could he tell her? I wondered. What? But I knew he would tell her everything, exactly as it had happened. As much for himself as for her, he needed to explain. But suppose she screamed, fell to the ground, attacked him, even? All that hope of love . . . gone. Even in his discomfort I knew that he was teaching me. The way to do it was professionally. Now he was standing above her. When the woman saw that he did not speak, she lifted her eyes and saw what he held crammed in his mouth to tell her. She knew, and rose to her feet.

"*Señora*," he began, "I am sorry." All at once he seemed to me shorter than he was, scarcely taller than she. There was a place at the crown of his head where the hair had grown thin. His lips were stones. He could hardly move them. The voice dry, dusty.

"No one could have known. Some bad reaction to the medicine for sleeping. It poisoned her. High fever. She did not wake up." The last, a whisper. The woman studied his lips as though she were deaf. He tried, but could not control a twitching at the corner of his mouth. He raised a thumb and forefinger to press something back into his eyes.

"*Muerte*," the woman announced to herself. Her eyes were human, deadly.

"*Sí, muerte*." At that moment he was like someone cast, still alive, as an effigy for his own tomb. He closed his eyes. Nor did he open them until he felt the touch of the woman's hand on his arm, a touch from which he did not withdraw. Then he looked and saw the grief corroding her face, breaking it down, melting the features so that eyes, nose, mouth ran together in a distortion, like the girl's. For a long time they stood in silence. It seemed to me that minutes passed. At last her face cleared, the features rearranged themselves. She spoke, the words coming slowly to make certain that he understood her. She would go home now. The next day her sons would come for the girl, to take her home for burial. The doctor must not be sad. God has decided. And she was happy now that the harelip had been fixed so

that her daughter might go to Heaven without it. Her bare feet re-
treating were the felted pads of a great bereft animal.

The next morning I did not go to the wards, but stood at the gate
leading from the courtyard to the road outside. Two young men in
striped ponchos lifted the girl's body wrapped in a straw mat onto
the back of a wooden cart. A donkey waited. I had been drawn to this
place as one is drawn, inexplicably, to certain scenes of desolation—
executions, battlefields. All at once, the woman looked up and saw me.
She had taken off her hat. The heavy-hanging coil of her hair made her
head seem larger, darker, noble. I pressed some money into her hand.

"For flowers," I said. "A priest." Her cheeks shook as though minutes ago a stone had been dropped into her navel and the ripples were
just now reaching her head. I regretted having come to that place.

"*Sí, sí,*" the woman said. Her own face was stitched with flies. "The
doctor is one of the angels. He has finished the work of God. My
daughter is beautiful."

What could she mean! The lip had not been fixed. The girl had died
before he would have done it.

"Only a fine line that God will erase in time," she said.

I reached into the cart and lifted a corner of the mat in which the girl
had been rolled. Where the cleft had been there was now a fresh line of
tiny sutures. The Cupid's bow was delicately shaped, the vermilion
border aligned. The flattened nostril had now the same rounded shape
as the other one. I let the mat fall over the face of the dead girl, but not
before I had seen the touching place where the finest black hairs sprang
from the temple.

"*Adiós, adiós . . .*" And the cart creaked away to the sound of
hooves, a tinkling bell.

There are events in a doctor's life that seem to mark the boundary
between youth and age, seeing and perceiving. Like certain dreams,
they illuminate a whole lifetime of past behavior. After such an event,
a doctor is not the same as he was before. It had seemed to me then to
have been the act of someone demented, or at least insanely arrogant.
An attempt to reorder events. Her death had come to him out of
order. It should have come after the lip had been repaired, not before.
He could have told the mother that, no, the lip had not been fixed. But
he did not. He said nothing. It had been an act of omission, one of
those strange lapses to which all of us are subject and which we live to
regret. It must have been then, at that moment, that the knowledge of
what he would do appeared to him. The words of the mother had not

consoled him; they had hunted him down. He had not done it for her. The dire necessity was his. He would not accept that Imelda had died before he could repair her lip. People who do such things break free from society. They follow their own lonely path. They have a secret which they can never reveal. I must never let on that I knew.

How often I have imagined it. Ten o'clock at night. The hospital of Comayagua is all but dark. Here and there lanterns tilt and skitter up and down the corridors. One of these lamps breaks free from the others and descends the stone steps to the underground room that is the morgue of the hospital. This room wears the expression as if it had waited all night for someone to come. No silence so deep as this place with its cargo of newly dead. Only the slow drip of water over stone. The door closes gassily and clicks shut. The lock is turned. There are four tables, each with a body encased in a paper shroud. There is no mistaking her. She is the smallest. The surgeon takes a knife from his pocket and slits open the paper shroud, that part in which the girl's head is enclosed. The wound seems to be living on long after she has died. Waves of heat emanate from it, blurring his vision. All at once, he turns to peer over his shoulder. He sees nothing, only a wooden crucifix on the wall.

He removes a package of instruments from a satchel and arranges them on a tray. Scalpel, scissors, forceps, needle holder. Sutures and gauze sponges are produced. Stealthy, hunched, engaged, he begins. The dots of blue dye are still there upon her mouth. He raises the scalpel, pauses. A second glance into the darkness. From the wall a small lizard watches and accepts. The first cut is made. A sluggish flow of dark blood appears. He wipes it away with a sponge. No new blood comes to take its place. Again and again he cuts, connecting each of the blue dots until the whole of the zigzag slice is made, first on one side of the cleft, then on the other. Now the edges of the cleft are lined with fresh tissue. He sets down the scalpel and takes up scissors and forceps, undermining the little flaps until each triangle is attached only at one side. He rotates each flap into its new position. He must be certain that they can be swung without tension. They can. He is ready to suture. He fits the tiny curved needle into the jaws of the needle holder. Each suture is placed precisely the same number of millimeters from the cut edge, and the same distance apart. He ties each knot down until the edges are apposed. Not too tightly. These are the most meticulous sutures of his life. He cuts each thread close to the knot. It goes well. The vermilion border with its white skin roll is exactly aligned. One more stitch and the Cupid's bow appears as if by magic. The man's face shines with moisture. Now the nostril is incised around the margin, released, and sutured into a round shape to match its mate. He wipes the blood from the face of the girl with gauze that he has dipped in water. Crumbs of light are scattered on the girl's face. The shroud is folded once more about her. The instruments are handed into the satchel. In a moment the morgue is dark and a lone lantern ascends the stairs and is extinguished.

Six weeks later I was in the darkened amphitheater of the Medical School. Tiers of seats rose in a semicircle above the small stage where Hugh Franciscus stood presenting the case material he had encountered in Honduras. It was the highlight of the year. The hall was filled. The night before he had arranged the slides in the order in which they were to be shown. I was at the controls of the slide projector.

"Next slide!" he would order from time to time in that military voice which had called forth blind obedience from generations of medical students, interns, residents and patients.

"This is a fifty-seven-year-old man with a severe burn contracture of the neck. You will notice the rigid webbing that has fused the chin to the presternal tissues. No motion of the head on the torso is possible. . . . Next slide!"

"Click," went the projector.

"Here he is after the excision of the scar tissue and with the head in full extension for the first time. The defect was then covered. . . . Next slide!"

"Click."

". . . with full-thickness drums of skin taken from the abdomen with the Padgett dermatome. Next slide!"

"Click."

And suddenly there she was, extracted from the shadows, suspended above and beyond all of us like a resurrection. There was the oval face, the long black hair unbraided, the tiny gold hoops in her ears. And that luminous gnawed mouth. The whole of her life seemed to have been summed up in this photograph. A long silence followed that was the surgeon's alone to break. Almost at once, like the anesthetist in the operating room in Comayagua, I knew that something was wrong. It was not that the man would not speak as that he could not. The audience of doctors, nurses and students seemed to have been infected by the black, limitless silence. My own pulse doubled. It was hard to breathe. Why did he not call out for the next slide? Why did he not save himself? Why had he not removed this slide from the ones to be shown? All at once I knew that he had used his camera on her again. I could see the long black shadows of her hair flowing into the darker shadows of the morgue. The sudden blinding flash . . . The next slide would be the one taken in the morgue. He would be exposed.

In the dim light reflected from the slide, I saw him gazing up at her, seeing not the colored photograph, I thought, but the negative of it where the ghost of the girl was. For me, the amphitheater had become Honduras. I saw again that courtyard littered with patients. I could see the dust in the beam of light from the projector. It was then that I knew that she was his measure of perfection and pain—the one lost, the other gained. He, too, had heard the click of the camera, had seen her wince and felt his mercy enlarge. At last he spoke.

"Imelda." It was the one word he had heard her say. At the sound of his voice I removed the next slide from the projector. "Click" . . . and she was gone. "Click" again, and in her place the man with the orbital cancer. For a long moment Franciscus looked up in my direction, on his face an expression that I have given up trying to interpret. Gratitude? Sorrow? It made me think of the gaze of the girl when at last she understood that she must hand over to him the evidence of her body.

"This is a sixty-two-year-old man with a basal cell carcinoma of the temple eroding into the bony orbit . . ." he began as though nothing had happened.

At the end of the hour, even before the lights went on, there was loud applause. I hurried to find him among the departing crowd. I could not. Some weeks went by before I caught sight of him. He seemed vaguely convalescent, as though a fever had taken its toll before burning out.

Hugh Franciscus continued to teach for fifteen years, although he operated a good deal less, then gave it up entirely. It was as though he had grown tired of blood, of always having to be involved with blood, of having to draw it, spill it, wipe it away, stanch it. He was a quieter, softer man, I heard, the ferocity diminished. There were no more expeditions to Honduras or anywhere else.

I, too, have not been entirely free of her. Now and then, in the years that have passed, I see that donkey-cart cortège, or his face bent over hers in the morgue. I would like to have told him what I now know, that his unrealistic act was one of goodness, one of those small, persevering acts done, perhaps, to ward off madness. Like lighting a lamp, boiling water for tea, washing a shirt. But, of course, it's too late now.

THE EXACT LOCATION OF THE SOUL

Someone asked me why a surgeon would write. Why, when the shelves are already too full? They sag under the deadweight of books. To add a single adverb is to risk exceeding the strength of the boards. A surgeon should abstain. A surgeon, whose fingers are more at home in the steamy gullies of the body than they are tapping the dry keys of a typewriter. A surgeon, who feels the slow slide of intestines against the back of his hand and is no more alarmed than were a family of snakes taking their comfort from such an indolent rubbing. A surgeon, who palms the human heart as though it were some captured bird.

Why should he write? Is it vanity that urges him? There is glory enough in the knife. Is it for money? One can make too much money. No. It is to search for some meaning in the ritual of surgery, which is at once murderous, painful, healing, and full of love. It is a devilish hard thing to transmit—to find, even. Perhaps if one were to cut out a heart, a lobe of the liver, a single convolution of the brain, and paste it to a page, it would speak with more eloquence than all the words of Balzac. Such a piece would need no literary style, no mass of erudition or history, but in its very shape and feel would tell all the frailty and strength, the despair and nobility of man. What? Publish a heart? A little piece of bone? Preposterous. Still I fear that is what it may require to reveal the truth that lies hidden in the body. Not all the undressings of Rabelais, Chekhov, or even William Carlos Williams have wrested it free, although God knows each one of those doctors made a heroic assault upon it.

I have come to believe that it is the flesh alone that counts. The rest is that with which we distract ourselves when we are not hungry or cold, in pain or ecstasy. In the recesses of the body I search for the philosophers' stone. I know it is there, hidden in the deepest, dampest cul-de-sac. It awaits discovery. To find it would be like the harnessing of fire. It would illuminate the world. Such a quest is not without pain. Who can gaze on so much misery and feel no hurt? Emerson has written that the poet is the only true doctor. I believe him, for the poet, lacking the impediment of speech with which the rest of us are afflicted, gazes, records, diagnoses, and prophesies.

I invited a young diabetic woman to the operating room to amputate her leg. She could not see the great shaggy black ulcer upon her foot and ankle that threatened to encroach upon the rest of her body, for she was blind as well. There upon her foot was a Mississippi Delta brimming with corruption, sending its raw tributaries down between her toes. Gone were all the little web spaces that when fresh and whole are such a delight to loving men. She could not see her wound, but she could feel it. There is no pain like that of the bloodless limb turned rotten and festering. There is neither unguent nor anodyne to kill such a pain yet leave intact the body.

For over a year I trimmed away the putrid flesh, cleansed, anointed, and dressed the foot, staving off, delaying. Three times each week, in her darkness, she sat upon my table, rocking back and forth, holding her extended leg by the thigh, gripping it as though it were a rocket that must be steadied lest it explode and scatter her toes about the room. And I would cut away a bit here, a bit there, of the swollen blue leather that was her tissue.

At last we gave up, she and I. We could no longer run ahead of the gangrene. We had not the legs for it. There must be an amputation in order that she might live—and I as well. It was to heal us both that I must take up knife and saw, and cut the leg off. And when I could feel it drop from her body to the table, see the blessed *space* appear between her and that leg, I too would be well.

Now it is the day of the operation. I stand by while the anesthetist administers the drugs, watch as the tense familiar body relaxes into narcosis. I turn then to uncover the leg. There, upon her kneecap, she has drawn, blindly, upside down for me to see, a face; just a circle with two ears, two eyes, a nose, and a smiling upturned mouth. Under it she has printed SMILE, DOCTOR. Minutes later I listen to the sound of the saw, until a little crack at the end tells me it is done.

So, I have learned that man is not ugly, but that he is Beauty itself. There is no other his equal. Are we not all dying, none faster or more slowly than any other? I have become receptive to the possibilities of love (for it is love, this thing that happens in the operating room), and each day I wait, trembling in the busy air. Perhaps today it will come. Perhaps today I will find it, take part in it, this love that blooms in the stoniest desert.

All through literature the doctor is portrayed as a figure of fun. Shaw was splenetic about him; Molière delighted in pricking his pompous medicine men, and well they deserved it. The doctor is ripe for caricature. But I believe that the truly great writing about doctors has not yet been done. I think it must be done *by* a doctor, one who is through with the love affair with his technique, who recognizes that he has played Narcissus, raining kisses on a mirror, and who now, out of the impacted masses of his guilt, has expanded into self-doubt, and finally into the high state of wonderment. Perhaps he will be a nonbeliever who, after a lifetime of grand gestures and mighty deeds, comes upon the knowledge that he has done no more than meddle in the lives of his fellows, and that he has done at least as much harm as good. Yet he may continue to pretend, at least, that there is nothing to fear, that death will not come, so long as people depend on his authority. Later, after his patients have left, he may closet himself in his darkened office, sweating and afraid.

There is a story by Unamuno in which a priest, living in a small Spanish village, is adored by all the people for his piety, kindness, and the majesty with which he celebrates the Mass each Sunday. To them he is already a saint. It is a foregone conclusion, and they speak of him as Saint Immanuel. He helps them with their plowing and planting, tends them when they are sick, confesses them, comforts them in death, and every Sunday, in his rich, thrilling voice, transports them to paradise with his chanting. The fact is that Don Immanuel is not so much a saint as a martyr. Long ago his own faith left him. He is an atheist, a good man doomed to suffer the life of a hypocrite, pretending to a faith he does not have. As he raises the chalice of wine, his hands tremble, and a cold sweat pours from him. He cannot stop for he knows that the people need this of him, that their need is greater than his sacrifice. Still . . . still . . . could it be that Don Immanuel's whole life is a kind of prayer, a paean to God?

A writing doctor would treat men and women with equal reverence, for what is the "liberation" of either sex to him who knows the diagrams, the inner geographies of each? I love the solid heft of men as much as I adore the heated capaciousness of women—women in whose penetralia is found the repository of existence. I would have them glory in that. Women are physics and chemistry. They are matter. It is their bodies that tell of the frailty of men. Men have not their cellular, enzymatic wisdom. Man is albuminoid, proteinaceous, laked pearl; woman is yolky, ovoid, rich. Both are exuberant bloody growths. I would use the defects and deformities of each for my sacred purpose of writing, for I know that it is the marred and scarred and faulty that are subject to grace. I would seek the soul in the facts of animal economy and profligacy. Yes, it is the exact location of the soul that I am after. The smell of it is in my nostrils. I have caught glimpses of it in the body diseased. If only I could tell it. Is there no mathematical equation that can guide me? So much pain and pus equals so much truth? It is elusive as the whippoorwill that one hears calling incessantly from out the night window, but which, nesting as it does low in the brush, no one sees. No one but the poet, for he sees what no one else can. He was born with the eye for it.

* * *

Once I thought I had it: Ten o'clock one night, the end room off a long corridor in a college infirmary, my last patient of the day, degree of exhaustion suitable for the appearance of a vision, some manifestation. The patient is a young man recently returned from Guatemala, from the excavation of Mayan ruins. His left upper arm wears a gauze dressing which, when removed, reveals a clean punched-out hole the size of a dime. The tissues about the opening are swollen and tense. A thin brownish fluid lips the edge, and now and then a lazy drop of the overflow spills down the arm. An abscess, inadequately drained. I will enlarge the opening to allow better egress of the pus. Nurse, will you get me a scalpel and some . . . ?

What happens next is enough to lay Francis Drake avomit in his cabin. No explorer ever stared in wilder surmise than I into that crater from which there now emerges a narrow gray head whose sole distinguishing feature is a pair of black pincers. The head sits atop a longish flexible neck arching now this way, now that, testing the air. Alternately it folds back upon itself, then advances in new boldness. And all the while, with dreadful rhythmicity, the unspeakable pincers open and close. Abscess? Pus? Never. Here is the lair of a beast at whose malignant purpose I could but guess. A Mayan devil, I think, that would soon burst free to fly about the room, with horrid blanket-wings and iridescent scales, raking, pinching, injecting God knows what acid juice. And even now the irony does not escape me, the irony of my patient as excavator excavated.

With all the ritual deliberation of a high priest I advance a surgical clamp toward the hole. The surgeon's heart is become a bat hanging upside down from his rib cage. The rim achieved—now thrust—and the ratchets of the clamp close upon the empty air. The devil has retracted. Evil mocking laughter bangs back and forth in the brain. More stealth. Lying in wait. One must skulk. Minutes pass, perhaps an hour. . . . A faint disturbance in the lake, and once again the thing upraises, farther and farther, hovering. Acrouch, strung, the surgeon is one with his instrument; there is no longer any boundary between its metal and his flesh. They are joined in a single perfect tool of extirpation. It is just for this that he was born. Now—thrust—and clamp—and *yes*. Got him!

Transmitted to the fingers comes the wild thrashing of the creature. Pinned and wriggling, he is mine. I hear the dry brittle scream of the dragon, and a hatred seizes me, but such a detestation as would make of Iago a drooling sucktit. It is the demented hatred of the victor for the vanquished, the warden for his prisoner. It is the hatred of fear. Within the jaws of my hemostat is the whole of the evil of the world, the dark concentrate itself, and I shall kill it. For mankind. And, in so doing, will open the way into a thousand years of perfect peace. Here is Surgeon as Savior indeed.

Tight grip now . . . steady, relentless pull. How it scrabbles to keep its tentacle-hold. With an abrupt moist plop the extraction is complete. There, writhing in the teeth of the clamp, is a dirty gray body, the size and shape of an English walnut. He is hung everywhere with tiny black hooklets. Quickly . . . into the specimen jar of saline . . . the lid screwed tight. Crazily he swims round and round, wiping his slimy head against the glass, then slowly sinks to the bottom, the mass of hooks in frantic agonal wave.

"You are going to be all right," I say to my patient. "We are *all* going to be all right from now on."

The next day I take the jar to the medical school. "That's the larva of the botfly," says a pathologist. "The fly usually bites a cow and deposits its eggs beneath the skin. There, the egg develops into the larval form which, when ready, burrows its way to the outside through the hide and falls to the ground. In time it matures into a full-grown botfly. This one happened to bite a man. It was about to come out on its own, and, of course, it would have died."

The words *imposter, sorehead, servant of Satan* spring to my lips. But now he has been joined by other scientists. They nod in agreement. I gaze from one gray eminence to another, and know the mallet-blow of glory pulverized. I tried to save the world, but it didn't work out.

No, it is not the surgeon who is God's darling. He is the victim of vanity. It is the poet who heals with his words, stanches the flow of blood, stills the rattling breath, applies poultice to the scalded flesh.

Did you ask me why a surgeon writes? I think it is because I wish to be a doctor.

MAYA ANGELOU

MAYA ANGELOU (1928–). *African-American poet, fiction writer, and storyteller. Angelou's best-known work is the autobiographical* I Know Why the Caged Bird Sings *(1970), a critical and popular success imbued with optimism, humor, and homespun philosophy. Other writings include* Wouldn't Take Nothing for My Journey Now *(1994), a collection of personal reflections, and numerous collections of poetry, among them* Just Give Me a Cool Drink of Water 'Fore I Die *(1971);* Oh Pray My Wings Are Gonna Fit Me Well *(1975);* And Still I Rise *(1978);* Shaker, Why Don't You Sing? *(1981); and* I Shall Not Be Moved *(1990). She read the Inaugural Poem at the Ceremony for President William Jefferson Clinton on January 20, 1993. Angelou is currently Reynolds professor of American studies at Wake Forest University in Winston-Salem, North Carolina.*

THE LAST DECISION

> The print is too small, distressing me.
> Wavering black things on the page.
> Wriggling polliwogs all about.
> I know it's my age.
> I'll have to give up reading.
>
> The food is too rich, revolting me.
> I swallow it hot or force it down cold,
> and wait all day as it sits in my throat.
> Tired as I am, I know I've grown old.
> I'll have to give up eating.
>
> My children's concerns are tiring me.
> They stand at my bed and move their lips,
> and I cannot hear one single word.
> I'd rather give up listening.
>
> Life is too busy, wearying me.
> Questions and answers and heavy thought.
> I've subtracted and added and multiplied,
> and all my figuring has come to naught.
> Today I'll give up living.

DONALD HALL

DONALD HALL (1928–). *American poet, essayist. Born in New Haven, Connecticut, Donald Hall attended the Bread Loaf Writers' Conference at the age of sixteen; in the same year he had his first work published. He received a B.A. from Harvard (1951) and a B. Litt. from Oxford (1953). His remarkable literary career includes fourteen books of poetry. His most recent book,* Without: Poems *(1998), was published on the third anniversary of the death of Jane Kenyon, his wife and fellow poet. The* One Day: A Poem in Three Parts *(1988) won the National Book Critics Circle Award and a Pulitzer Prize nomination. In addition to poetry, he has written books on the poet Marianne Moore, the sculptor Henry Moore, and baseball. He has also written a Caldecott-winning children's book,* Ox-Cart Man *(1979), and several autobiographical works, including* Life Work *(1993). For twenty years he and Kenyon lived at Eagle Pond Farm in Wilmot, New Hampshire, where he had spent his childhood summers. It was a place that had a deepening effect on the lives and work of both writers.*

Excerpt from HER LONG ILLNESS

Daybreak until nightfall,
he sat by his wife at the hospital
        while chemotherapy dripped
through the catheter into her heart.
        He drank coffee and read
the *Globe.* He paced; he worked
        on poems; he rubbed her back
and read aloud. Overcome with dread,
        they wept and affirmed
their love for each other, witlessly,
        over and over again.
When it snowed one morning Jane gazed
        at the darkness blurred
with flakes. They pushed the IV pump
        which she called Igor
slowly past the nurses' pods, as far
        as the outside door
so that she could smell the snowy air.

U. A. FANTHORPE

U. A. FANTHORPE (1929–). English poet. Ursula Askham Fanthorpe was born in Kent. She was educated at St. Anne's College, Oxford, then at the University of London, from which she obtained a teaching diploma. She taught English for a number of years at an independent girls' school. She also gained extensive hospital experience (as an admissions clerk and receptionist in a Bristol hospital). Her poetry reflects both of these occupations in telling, honest, and sometimes humorous ways. She began writing when in her forties and was nearly fifty when she published her first book (1978). Her output has been prolific since, numbering nine books of poetry at last count. Fanthorpe was the first woman ever to be nominated for the post of Oxford professor of poetry. One reviewer, Liz Lochhead, has called Fanthorpe "a national treasure."

CHILDREN IMAGINING A HOSPITAL
For Kingswood County Primary School

I would like kindness, assurance,
A wide selection of books;
Lots of visitors, and a friend
To come and see me:
A bed by the window so I could look at
All the trees and fields, where I could go for a walk.
I'd like a hospital with popcorn to eat.
A place where I have my own way.

I would like HTV all to myself
And people bringing tea round on trollies;
Plenty of presents and plenty of cards
(I would like presents of food).
Things on the walls, like pictures, and things
That hang from the ceiling;
Long corridors to whizz down in wheelchairs.
Not to be left alone.

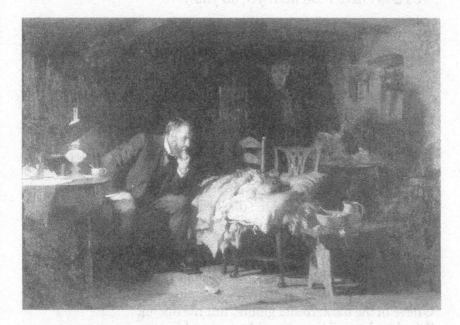

The Doctor, by Sir Luke Fildes
The painter's eldest son died on Christmas morning, 1877.
The child was closely tended by Dr. Murray, whose dedication impressed
Fildes. Years later, when Sir Henry Tate commissioned Fildes for an exhibit,
the painter chose this scene.

THE DOCTOR

Sir Luke Fildes: The Doctor, Tate Gallery

'That Jackson, he's another one.
If he goes on opening windows we'll all
Die of pneumonia.'
                    The native obsessions:
Health and the weather. Attendants have
The dogged, grainy look of subjects. Someone,
Surely, is going to paint them?

'You don't have a bad heart yet, do you?'

'Not that I know of.'
                          'They can examine you.'

'But they don't really know.'
                          The painters knew.
Gainsborough eyed his lovely, delicate daughters
And rich fat brewers: Turner his hectic skies.
They brooded on death by drowning (Ophelia, in real water);
Cloud without end; storm; storm coming on;
Bright exophthalmic eyes, consumptive colours,
And gorgeous goitred throats; the deluge,
The end of the world, and Adam's
Appalling worm-wrapped birth.
                          Such patient watchers
Have eyes for those who watch. The child
Frets in its fever, the parents
Grieve in the background gloom. But the doctor,
Who has done all he can, and knows nothing
Will help or heal, sits raptly, raptly,
As if such absorbed attention were in itself
A virtue. As it is.

RICHARD C. REYNOLDS

RICHARD C. REYNOLDS (1929–). *American physician, educator, and writer. For a number of years, Dr. Reynolds was in the private practice of internal medicine in Frederick, Maryland. His academic career has included appointments at Johns Hopkins University School of Medicine and the University of Florida. A former dean of the University of Medicine and Dentistry of New Jersey, he has also served as executive vice president of the Robert Wood Johnson Foundation in Princeton. Currently he is a courtesy professor of medicine at the University of Florida, in Gainesville.*

A DAY IN THE LIFE OF AN INTERNIST

Author's Foreword: Over the past two years there have been a number of articles describing what internists do. These have appeared in the Annals of Internal Medicine *and* The New England Journal of Medicine *and usually represent summaries of data collected from a large group of internists. Having practiced internal medicine in a community of 22,000 for nine years before returning to a full-time academic life, I found difficulty in relating what I did in everyday practice to what was being described in these articles. About this time, I came across one of my appointment books from my eighth year of practice. I thumbed through this book and was amazed by how vividly I could recall many of the patients who were identified, albeit ten years later. This prompted me to try to write this article. I suspect the passing years have made me take some liberties with the details, but I am convinced that the day I describe is representative of many such days.*

The alarm rings. Reflexly, I turn it off within seconds. It is 6:30 A.M., but I have already been awake for fifteen minutes. My sleep has been restless since the phone rang at 2:30 A.M. and the nurse from the ICU told me about the increasing number of PVCs in the forty-six-year-old man with a coronary whom I had admitted yesterday afternoon. I ordered some Lidocaine and told the nurse to be sure to call back if the patient did not improve. She did not call, but I found it difficult to fall asleep.

Contrary to common belief, most phone calls in the middle of the night, whether from the hospital or from home, indicate a major patient difficulty. I am never sure when I respond to the patient over the phone that I have not missed a situation that requires a more personal review. I suspect that the post-phone-call restlessness that I experience is caused by the uneasiness that my response may have been too cursory. I never cease to be amazed after a few years in practice how quickly and easily one can triage phone calls. That tone of panic in the voice of a spouse when the husband or wife is experiencing a major mishap or a call for help from a family that has never before asked for assistance out of regular office hours is unmistakably recognizable.

Today is Thursday. I go from the bedroom to the family room and turn on the television. While looking at "Sunrise Semester," I do my daily ritual of the Royal Canadian Air Force Exercises. These exercises coupled with some weekend tennis represent my compromise with the present exercise mania.

It is nearly seven. After quick morning ablutions and a sparse breakfast, I drive to the hospital. The nurses on One North have finished their morning report. They greet me and smile at my punctuality. If I did not start making rounds on my patients on One North at exactly 7:30 A.M., I would disappoint them. I understand that members of the nursing staff occasionally put money into a pool, with each participant choosing the minutes on either side of 7:30 A.M. that I will appear.

I have twelve patients in the hospital. My first office appointment is at 9:00 A.M. Mentally, I begin to pace my morning rounds. The first patient is completing the second week of hospitalization for his coronary thrombosis. Fifty-two years old, previously healthy and vigorous, he is in good spirits and beginning to ask about going home. This morning he has already walked the length of the corridor. I take his blood pressure and listen to his heart and lungs. Nothing is wrong. (Interesting how we always think in negatives in medical history taking and physical examination. No this, no that; never good this or good that. No wonder the World Health Organization defines health as the absence of disease.) I banter with the patient. He had never previously been under my care until the day he had chest pain and was admitted. His wife had been a regular patient for years, always following the admonitions and exhortations of the women's magazines to have regular checkups. I make a mental note that I need to have a conversation with the patient and his wife this weekend to go over a plan for his physical activity and return to work after discharge.

In the next room is a seventy-seven-year-old lady who has been admitted with a cerebral thrombosis resulting in mild aphasia and weakness of her right arm. She is improving rapidly from her stroke and is sitting in a chair as I walk into the room. Two questions need answers. How aggressive a workup shall I do on this patient, who in all likelihood has a simple cerebral thrombosis, and what arrangements shall we work out for her after she leaves the hospital. She lives by herself and has always been independent. Since this stroke she has become aware of her vulnerability. I suspect in a few days she may introduce the subject of a temporary residence at a nursing home after discharge. I shall have the head nurse begin to explore the subject with her.

I walk upstairs to Two North. I see a patient I admitted a week ago when I was on call for the emergency room. This sixty-eight-year-old man had a severe urinary tract infection with sepsis that has responded to antibiotics and catheterization. He was seen by the urologist yesterday. I glance at the consultation note on the chart. He confirms my suspicion of obstructive prostate disease and recommends surgery. I need to talk to the patient about this. I begin to quicken the pace of rounds. There are still nine more patients to see before I am due at the office.

My office is only two blocks from the hospital. At five minutes to nine I walk in. My office staff has been there since 8:30. The first two patients are already there. The first one is in the examining room. I glance at the appointment book. The day is full. I see that Mrs. D is scheduled at 10:30 for fifteen minutes. There is no way that I can see that woman in fifteen minutes. It takes her longer than that to recite her neatly written list of complaints.

My office hours are 9:00 to 12:00 and 1:30 to 3:30. I keep the half hour 3:30 to 4:00 open to see sick people in need of attention that day. I schedule patients every fifteen minutes, except for annual physicals that require thirty minutes for old patients and forty-five minutes for a first time visit. Consultations are scheduled for forty-five to sixty minutes.

The first few patients today are straightforward. Mrs. G is a forty-six-year-old lady with uncomplicated hypertension, easily controlled with Diuril and Aldomet. Today her blood pressure is 135/90. Her weight has increased five pounds since her last visit three months ago. We talk about diet and exercise and her son who is a sophomore at Duke. The second patient is a thirty-four-year-old school teacher with tension headaches, who one year ago went through a miserable depressive episode. She prefers to see me every four to six weeks just to be reassured. It is not exactly clear what the reassurance is for. Both she and I know that the headaches are tension in character, and evil things such as brain tumors have long ago been eliminated from diagnostic consideration. Today we chat. I congratulate her on being selected one of the county's outstanding high school teachers. (My receptionist has placed a note in the front of her chart reminding me of this accolade.) She appears composed, more relaxed than usual. I schedule the next appointment for eight weeks hence and begin to anticipate weaning her away from her dependence on me.

I try to arrange my schedule to do one complete examination in the morning and one in the afternoon. Today the third patient, Mrs. S, is a healthy, slightly obese thirty-eight-year-old housewife who comes in for her annual evaluation. An interval history reveals no mishaps since she was here one year ago. The physical exam is ritualistic. After performing thousands of physical examinations I have noticed a tendency to lose focus of concentration during this procedure. To combat this, I have devised a scheme. The first week of each month I select one part of the examination for unusual scrutiny. This week my special attention is on the thyroid. Last month it was the ear. During the preceding week I reviewed the anatomy and examination of the thyroid. As I examine the patient I carefully observe and palpitate the thyroid, mentally identifying the poles and isthmus. Somehow, I hope this technique prevents the ritualistic examination from becoming an ineffective, cursory effort. Mrs. S's thyroid is normal. While she dresses, I enter the second examining room to see Mr. L. Mr. L is a sixty-eight-year-old retired merchant, who was in the hospital four months ago. His unexplained persistent abdominal pain led to an exploratory laparotomy, which revealed carcinoma of the pancreas. The tumor had already invaded the liver. The patient's course subsequent to surgery has been surprisingly uneventful. Mr. L is lying on the examining table. His heart and lungs are normal. I think that since he was here one month ago his liver has enlarged. I glance at his sclera and note he is slightly jaundiced. He responds to my query about abdominal discomfort by stating that it remains unchanged. I muse that neither one of us uses the word pain. I tell Mr. L to dress, and I return to my office, where my nurse has placed Mrs. S after she has dressed.

Doctors need to give every patient a chance to talk with their clothes on after the examination is over. Before the examination patients are sometimes frightened or intimidated and often forgetful or hesitant to bring up an unpleasant subject. After the examination, and if they have had a few minutes to sit in the doctor's office, they will be more composed and confident. I reassure Mrs. S that she remains in good health. I chide her good-naturedly about her eighteen extra pounds of weight. I deflect her questions of diet pills in such a way that she does not ask for any and get turned down. I do not give her a diet. I presume that no event has happened to catalyse her weight loss and that she is content being buxom. (I wonder if her husband prefers her that way.) Today, Mrs. S tells me that her only child is entering college this fall and she herself would like to enter the local community college and become a nurse. She wants to know what I think about the idea. Inwardly, I smile. Patients at times do expect their doctors to be omniscient. I ask her what her husband thinks of this career change from housewife to student to nurse. She replies that he has been encouraging. I tell Mrs. S that I believe her idea is excellent. I recall the name of another patient who made a similar career decision three years ago and who is now working in a doctor's office. I suggest she call this individual, and I also make a mental note to mention Mrs. S's aspirations to my other patient.

Mrs. S leaves and Mr. L comes in. His clothes indicate recent weight loss, and I glance at his chart and note that he has lost twelve pounds since his discharge from the hospital. Mr. L sits down. We look at one another. Neither of us says anything for a few moments. He breaks the silence. "Well, how are things?" I indicate I want to do a few tests. Actually, I want to do a bilirubin to determine the extent of his jaundice. "They are not too good," he says. I comment that the course of an individual with his malady is unpredictable, but so far he has done remarkably well. That is true; he has. I recall our conversation in the hospital. Several days after surgery when I was certain he was alert, I sat down by his bedside and shared with him his diagnosis. He asked me in his laconic way, "How long?" I said it was difficult to tell, but the course was usually somewhere between six and twelve months. He asked a few other questions about the pancreatic cancer. I assured him that I would work with him and his wife so that he would be as comfortable as possible, and I urged him to be active as long as he felt good. By mutual consent we then directed our conversation to comfortable, ordinary subjects such as sports and hospital food. Today, for the first time since our hospital conversation, he uses the word *cancer.* "The cancer is spreading." He states it as both a question and a fact. I nod confirmation. I give him a return appointment for two weeks.

The morning progresses with a steady procession of patients. Most patients have straightforward problems—a recurrent sinus infection, a streptococcal sore throat, an insurance physical examination. A few questions identify the problem, the examination confirms, and advice and/or a drug prescription are given. The medical record is reviewed to make sure that chronic problems are not overlooked or that the drug prescribed is not likely to interact with any present medication.

By 12:15 P.M. I have seen the last patient scheduled for the morning. At noon, I have scheduled an executive committee meeting of the community hospital. I have been elected chief of medicine of the community hospital and serve on this committee. Today we plan to review two audits, one on childbirth and another on urinary tract infection. Our professional care audit committees are struggling with the task of defining the character of the audit and interpreting the data resulting from the audit. The executive committee ponders what recommendations to make to the staff. The major deficiency revealed by these audits is incomplete records and inconsistent behavior on the part of attending physicians in recording data. We wonder whether the new transcribing system will improve the medical records. Another problem is introduced by the chief of surgery. One of the most respected older surgeons in the community is generating complaints by his patients of not making rounds on weekends and not returning the calls of the involved families. This is a sensitive subject that makes us all uneasy. There is a shaded reference to family problems and, hesitantly, a comment that the surgeon is imbibing too much alcohol. What to do? We agree that the chief of staff will approach one of the surgeon's close and long-standing colleagues and ask him to initiate a conversation and report back to the chief of staff.

Most doctors use lunch hours as an integral part of their professional workday. Continuing education meetings, hospital committee work, or a trip back to the hospital to check a sick patient are common events during the lunch break. If the doctor eats lunch at the hospital it is often a time of informal consultation with other doctors about patients not always requiring a formal review by another physician. I occasionally use the lunch hour to make a house call and frequently use this time to return phone calls.

I return to the office at 1:30 P.M. The afternoon proceeds much like the morning. Instead of an annual physical examination, I am seeing in consultation this afternoon a thirty-eight-year-old man with chest pain. The chest pain probably does not represent angina, but I proceed with a stress ECG. It is normal. I assure the patient that his chest pain is not cardiac in origin but represents a muscular-skeletal disorder that confused the diagnosis because of its location on the left anterior chest wall. His relief is obvious.

There has been a spate of phone calls from relatively young men asking for appointments for physical exams. Recently, a locally eminent businessman, president of the Chamber of Commerce, died suddenly from a coronary thrombosis at the age of forty-four. Whenever such an unfortunate mishap occurs to a citizen popular enough to have it recorded on the front page of the local paper, it precipitates an increased number of patient visits to many doctors' offices.

The afternoon continues. Two patients are seen for review of their drug-controlled hypertension. In moving about the office I glance at my patients in the waiting room. One of my patients sits there next to her high-school-aged daughter. Both appear tense; the daughter has been crying. My receptionist confirms my suspicion. The mother has brought the daughter in to determine—no, confirm—that she is pregnant. As they sit together in the waiting room they form a tableau that is itself almost diagnostic. When their turn comes, I ask the mother to remain in the waiting room while I examine the daughter. She is probably ten weeks pregnant. I discuss the issues and options with the daughter, who is composed. I bring the mother in with us and tell her what she already knows. There will be a family meeting tonight. I try to keep them from recriminations. I direct the attention to the daughter's pregnancy and recommend an obstetrician for care. Before they leave, I have my receptionist give the mother an appointment to see me next week. She will need some extra support at this time.

As the afternoon office hours begin to draw to an end, the secretary places on my desk six charts with phone messages attached. I am able to make a few of these calls between patients. Today, two of the phone calls concern prescription refills, which I call in directly to the drugstore. Both are for continuing medications for patients I see regularly for management of high blood pressure and osteoarthritis. Two other patients have requested information concerning their acute respiratory infections, presumably viral in origin, which necessitate only reassurance from me that the illness will probably last only three to five days. They are instructed to call again in a few days if they have not improved.

After I have seen the last patient of the day, I still have two outstanding phone calls. A twenty-seven-year-old anxious woman patient has read another article delineating the morbidity from birth control pills. Her uneasiness resulting from reading this article precipitates the phone call. Not too successfully, I allay her apprehensions. I make a note on the chart to discuss this problem at her next visit and to consider other forms of birth control. The last phone call is from a middle-aged woman who describes the symptoms of an acute urinary tract infection with sudden onset of dysuria, frequency, and urgency.

I decide to treat her by prescribing a ten-day course of Gantrisin. I have the secretary schedule her for an appointment in two weeks for follow-up urinalysis and culture.

The office day is completed. The nurse and receptionist are tidying up the office and have placed my diagnostic instruments into a small black bag I carry on hospital rounds. I sit at my desk and finish some notes in the charts of patients seen during the day. I glance at my mail, which is mostly advertisements. It does include one report from a doctor in Florida who cares for one of my patients for six months each year. I sign the letters I have dictated the night before. There are two journals in today's mail, and I carry them with me to the car and plan to scan them tonight.

Before I return to the hospital, I make a house call on an eighty-seven-year-old lady whom I have cared for for eight years. Two years ago she had a cerebral thrombosis, which resulted in some left-sided weakness. Despite mild congestive heart failure and the residua of the stroke she remains alert and engaged in the community and world, albeit from the confines of her apartment. My call is social and medical. The housekeeper reassures me that her charge has not had any problems since my last visit three months ago. I enjoy a few minutes' conversation with the patient. Her numerous contacts with people by phone and through visits to her apartment make her a social barometer for the community. At times she seems to know the well-being of some of my patients better than I. I take her blood pressure, listen to her heart and lungs, note that her ankles are not swollen. I tell her and her housekeeper to stay on the same medicines and that I will check back in three months.

I drive back to the hospital and begin my late afternoon rounds. I check on the acutely ill patients first. I make brief personal contacts with the remaining patients to see if they have any new problems and to report to them the results of any laboratory or X-ray examinations that have been done today.

I have arranged to see the wife of the sixty-eight-year-old man who was admitted with a urinary tract infection and will need prostatic surgery to relieve his urinary obstruction. She is waiting for me in her husband's room. She has many questions about the surgery and particularly about its risk for her husband. I answer the questions in front of her husband and try to have her appreciate the commonplace nature of the problem and surgery. Without her asking, I mention the excellent qualifications of the urologist who will do the surgery. I get up to leave and the wife follows me to the door and out of the room. In the hallway she asks the one important question. "Doctor, is there any chance this is cancer?" Though not entirely eliminating this possibility, I share my belief that the difficulty is most commonly caused by benign enlargement of the prostate gland. She seems reassured.

The early evening hours are ideal times for evaluating new patients or doing consultations for other physicians. Laboratory and X-ray studies have been completed and the reports are in the charts. The hospital is usually quiet, as afternoon visitors have gone home and the evening visitors have not arrived.

I have not had any new admissions today, but an orthopedic surgeon has asked me to evaluate a seventy-two-year-old lady with a broken left hip. I review her chart and find her laboratory studies, chest X ray and ECG are normal. The patient is in pain but tries to cooperate during my examination. She has had good health and denies any cardiovascular symptoms. Physical examination confirms her good health, which is now compromised by her broken hip. I write a note on her chart indicating she should tolerate the hip surgery and that I will follow her postoperatively.

I page my colleague, Dr. C, who is taking call for our three-member group. I quickly review by phone conversation the status of my acutely ill patients in the hospital. I ask him if he returns to the hospital tonight to look in on my one patient in the intensive care unit, a forty-five-year-old man who three days ago had an acute coronary thrombosis.

It is now seven o'clock. I drive home. The day of work is finished. I know that I shall not have any more calls as I sign my phone out to the telephone answering service. I sit down to dinner with my wife and three school-age children. I listen to the children recount the activities of the day. It is March, and my wife and I begin to talk about possible vacation sites for this summer. After dinner I go to my study and take a journal from a pile of unread periodicals. I thumb through it, unable to concentrate enough to get interested in any one article. I turn on the television and begin to watch an NBA game. Later, my wife wakens me.

ROBERT COLES

ROBERT COLES (1929–). *American physician and essayist. A psychiatrist by training, Dr. Coles is a professor at Harvard University, Duke University, and the University of North Carolina. He is the author of over forty books, including the* Children of Crisis *series, for which he won the Pulitzer Prize. His books include* The Call of Service *(1994),* The Ongoing Journey *(1994), and* Anna Freud: The Dream of Psychoanalysis *(1992). In 1999 he was awarded the Medal of Freedom, the nation's highest civilian honor, by President Clinton.*

Excerpt from THE CALL OF STORIES

At that point we were interrupted by a phone call. One of Dr. Williams' patients had suffered a relapse: a young woman of fifteen, on the road to recovery from severe pneumonia, had spiked a high fever yet again. She had a past history of rheumatic heart disease, with a congestive heart murmur and the long-term prospect of congestive heart disease. All of that and more Dr. Williams explained to me as he hurriedly drove to her home, a tenement building in Paterson, where poor families struggled hard to get by—make enough money to pay the rent, buy food, stay warm, and, yes, give their doctor, who made house calls, an occasional payment for his services. As we climbed those dark stairs to a fourth-floor apartment, the doctor suddenly whirled around and looked right at me, his eyes meeting mine. A moment's silence, and then he said: "I don't like this mother you'll see. She drives me crazy with her questions. I want to take the girl and save her. I want to take her younger brother and save him. I don't like the father, either. What a pair! The miracle is that wonderful daughter of theirs. She puts up with them, and she sees everything, all their bad habits."

A second later, he was rapping his right hand's knuckles on a door whose brown paint was peeling and whose splinters were noticeable— he had to be careful about where to make contact with the wood. Three knocks, then a shuffling of his feet to register impatience. Noise arose on the other side of the door, and I could see his face suddenly concentrating, the ears perking up, the head unselfconsciously tilting toward the door, as if he was interested but didn't want to admit to himself, never mind anyone else, that he was *that* interested—and so, abruptly, he moved away a step from the door just as it opened. (I later realized he'd probably heard, among other things, the sound of approaching steps.)

The mother opened the door and, without saying a word, stepped aside for us. I can still remember her eyes meeting those of Dr. Williams. My heart went out to her; she seemed retiring, frightened, and eager to please. She motioned to her daughter, asking her to get ready for the doctor by sitting up, and then moved away to make room for him. But the girl, febrile, seemed uninterested in what the mother wished. Meanwhile, Dr. Williams put his black bag down beside the patient's bed, glanced around the room, caught sight of a chair, pulled it toward the bed, sat down, and took the girl's left wrist into his right hand and held it firmly. At that point she picked herself up and sat half upright against the pillow, staring at her wrist and Dr. Williams' hand. He asked her how she was doing. She was doing OK, she said. He wouldn't accept her answer: "Tell me the truth." She immediately changed her reply: "Not so OK." He nodded, let go of her wrist, told her he was sure, from her pulse, that she had a fever, and announced he would soon examine her. He explained that I was a medical student and asked if she minded my being there as he listened to her chest and heart. She shook her head and smiled. It was then, as he reached for his stethoscope, that the mother entered the scene, so to speak. She drew nearer, frowning, and addressed the doctor: "Why no temperature?" Suddenly I realized I hadn't heard her voice before, and realized, a second later, that her English was imperfect. She wanted the doctor to take her daughter's temperature, to learn whether she had a fever. He barked back at her: "Leave her alone!"

I was stunned. He spoke with obvious annoyance. I knew he could be cranky; he had told me so, and I'd seen him moody and irascible at times, especially when we talked about certain literary matters. But this situation was puzzling, and for a moment I wondered whether he wasn't going beyond the ethical bounds, being rude to a patient's mother for no justifiable reason. Then came her retort: "You not do right. You always do wrong thing. She hot. Give her the thermom." While my ears concentrated on that abbreviated last word, the doctor pointedly turned his back and started doing his examination with the stethoscope. It was left for my unobstructed and idle ears to hear a tirade from the mother, uttered in a mix of broken English and fluent Italian. She had come close, very close; by the time he had finished his examination, she was nearer the doctor than I. As he looked up, her eyes were ready for him, for his eyes. Again they locked into a mutual gaze. It was then that the patient looked at her mother and said her own imploring word: "Please!" The mother backed off, and the doctor began telling the girl what he believed was happening—the pneumonia was returning. He urged fluids as well as aspirin. He asked whether she'd been taking the medicine he'd prescribed earlier. No, she had stopped. Why? The answer: "Because my fever went down, and she [the mother] told me I must stop taking the pills, since I'm cool."

Now the doctor understood all—and became enraged. He turned to the mother and opened his mouth, ready (I thought) to give her the lecture of her life. I could see the color on his face. I could also see his right hand tighten its grip on the stethoscope. No words came out of his mouth. He simply stood there, bearing down with those formidable eyes on the woman of forty or so; she didn't budge, however, nor did she stop looking right at him. I wondered who would flinch first. Neither did. He suddenly flung up his right arm, stethoscope in hand. All eyes in the room, the patient's and mine as well as the mother's, followed the course of that ancient medical instrument, that symbol of a profession's authority. With that gesture the mother retreated, and then the patient slumped back onto her pillow. Dr. Williams started getting ready to leave. He folded his stethoscope carefully and put it into his black bag. Only at that moment did I begin to relax a bit—the weapon was being laid down. He turned his back on the mother yet again and began a quiet appeal to the patient—she ought to take those pills every day, as he had instructed, and not stop taking them under any circumstances whatever. He emphasized the importance of that last remark with his voice, and after he'd finished speaking, he looked directly at the girl and asked her if she understood what he had said. Yes, she did. Then he asked her why she hadn't followed his instructions and kept taking the pills. Silence. He lowered his head. But he wasn't feeling shy or humble; he was fuming. Finally the head was raised, the mouth opened, the body turned toward the older woman: "I want every one of these pills taken by her. Every one." He was pointing at the patient. His eyes once more engaged with those of the mother. Neither retreated until the daughter addressed the mother: "Please pay the doctor." It was then that the mother left the room; she came back with a tightly folded bill, which she gave to her daughter, not the doctor. The daughter immediately handed it to the doctor, who quickly put it in his pocket without so much as looking at it. I remember being curious as to the amount. In a few seconds we were out of that apartment, and shortly thereafter on our way back to Williams' Rutherford home.

He didn't speak, and I was afraid to say anything, ask anything.

Usually he was a willing, animated talker; now all his energy seemed given to the act of driving his car. He held the wheel with both hands (he often used only one hand to drive), and he fussed with the windshield wipers, putting them on and then turning them off as some rain fell, then stopped falling. Suddenly came his first words: "Hell, make up your mind"—addressed, I realized, to the nameless, faceless weather. Then he laughed, turned to me, relaxed a bit—his back slouched against the back of the seat—and began to talk: "Well, there's a lesson for you in medical psychology, in what a doctor has to put up with." He wasn't satisfied with what he had said, so he went into a long explanation while the windshield wiper worked away at nothing, the rain having stopped. I was told all about the family, the patient's medical history, the mother's psychiatric history, the neighborhood's (immigrant, impoverished) social and cultural history. I was also told about previous encounters of the kind I had just witnessed. The narrator was sometimes wry or even humorous, at other times sardonic and angry. During one of those latter spells, he pulled out the crumpled bill he'd been given, telling me as he did so that it was "only one dollar." He laughed, with a mixture of embarrassment and annoyance, at what he'd heard himself say, and he added: "I'm lucky to get anything at all! Be grateful, I guess. Don't envy your colleagues what *they* make!"

MEDICAL ETHICS AND LIVING A LIFE

A black woman in Mississippi's Delta told me in 1969, as I went from home to home with other doctors trying to understand how it went for extremely poor and hard-pressed people:

We don't have it good here. It's no good at all. I turn and ask the Lord, a lot of times, why it's so—the unfairness in this world. But I'll never get an answer. My daddy told me: "Don't expect answers to the really big questions—not from anyone. We're put here, and we don't know why, and we try to figure out why while we're here, and we fight to stay around as long as we can, and the next thing we know, it's slipping away from us, and we're wondering where we're going, if we're going any place." If I was a doctor, I guess I'd wonder every day what it's all about, this life. A lot of times my children ask me these questions, ask me why people behave so bad toward other people, and why there's so much greed in the world, and when will God get angry and stop all the people who don't care about anything but themselves. I have to say I don't have the answers. Does anyone? If you go to college, my oldest girl said, you learn the answers. She's twelve. She thinks that the more education you get, the more you know about how to be good and live a good life. But I'll tell you, I'm not so sure. I think you can have a lot of diplomas to your credit, and not be the best person in the world. You can be a fool, actually, and have a lot of people calling you professor, lawyer, even doctor.

That "even"—a measure of hesitation, of lingering awe, of qualified respect. She had experienced her "rough times" with doctors—not only segregated facilities, but poor care and more insults than she cared to remember. A self-described "uppity nigger," she had finally spoken up to a doctor, had an argument with him. She remembered the critical essence of their confrontation this way:

I heard him saying bad, bad words about my people on the phone, and then he came into the waiting room and he gave me the nod. He never is polite to us, the way he can be with his white patients, and the more money they have, the bigger the smile they get out of him, and he's as eager to please as he can be. But with us, it's different; we get one sour look after the other. That day he told me to "shake a leg." I guess I wasn't walking into his office fast enough. Then he started talking about all "the welfare people," and saying, "Why didn't they go get themselves work?" Then, as he poked my belly, he gave me a lecture on eating and my diabetes—how I should "shape up and eat better."

That's when I forgot myself. I told him he should look to himself sometimes and stop making cracks at others. I told him he wasn't being much of a credit to his people and his profession, the way he was making these wisecracks about us poor folks. I told him he should know better, that there wasn't the jobs, and only now are we getting the right to vote, and the schools we've had weren't like the ones he could go to. I told him I expected more of him. Isn't he a doctor? If he can lord it over people, being a doctor, then he ought to remember how our Lord Jesus Christ behaved. He was the Son of God, but did He go around showing how big and important He was, and calling people bad names, and making wisecracks, and sidling up to the rich and looking down His nose at the poor? Jesus was a doctor; He healed the sick, and He tended after the lame, the halt and the blind, like our minister says. I told our doctor he ought to read the Bible more. I told him that instead of saying bad things about the poor people and us colored people, he should take a hard look at himself and see if he's living the best life he can—the kind of life a doctor should live—if he's going to preach to the rest of us, and be looked up to as if he's the best of the best.

She didn't get very far with such words, although, to his credit, the doctor not only heard her out but smiled and thanked her for the obvious courage (in the year 1967) that she had displayed. And it may be all too easy now, as it has surely been in past years, to call upon such an incident, the South being once again a convenient scapegoat for the rest of us. In fact, there aren't too many places in America, one suspects, where such a candid encounter could take place. How many of us in medicine have been asked by anyone—patient, friend, relative, student, colleague—to connect our professional position with the kind of life we live, the way we get on with those we attend in an office, clinic, ward? That woman, who today would be categorized as "culturally deprived" or "culturally disadvantaged" (the dreary banality of such language!), had managed to put her finger on an important issue, indeed—one that philosophers, theologians and novelists have struggled for a long time to comprehend: How does one live a decent and honorable life, and is it right to separate, in that regard, a person's "private life" from his or her working life?

In a sense, too, that woman was struggling with the issue of medical ethics: How broad and deep ought such a subject cut—to the bone of the doctor's life? Without question, we need to examine the ethical matters that press on us every day in the course of our work. Recently, such matters have gained increasing attention and have been worked into the curricula of our medical schools. The traditions and resources of analytic philosophy have been extremely helpful, as we wonder when life ends or contemplate priorities so far as scarce (or experimental) technology and medicine go. It is utterly necessary for us to confront our values (or lack of them) as, for example, we work with patients too young or too old or too sick to be able to speak for themselves. And the dying patient has, of course, by and large benefited from the recent attention given that final stretch of earthly time, though one hastens to wonder whether a certain kind lof psychological self-consciousness has not had its own dangers: all those "stages" and the prescriptive arrogance that can accompany "reform." Aren't there some people who have a "right" to "denial," not to mention a belief in the Good News? When does psychological analysis become a kind of normative judgment, if not smug self-righteousness? Sometimes, as I read the "literature" on "death and dying," I get the feeling that agnostic psychological moralists have the complete run of the field, with all too many ministers worrying all too much about something called "pastoral counseling," when a few old-fashioned prayers might be in order for the sake of the patient, the attending clergyman, and the rest of us as well.

Be that as it may, the woman just quoted from the outer precincts of Clarksdale, Mississippi, was aware in her own way that there have been, all along, two philosophical traditions—the analytic and the existential. The former allows us to ponder a host of variables and to make a specific (for the doctor, medical) decision. But the latter tradition urges us to go along with Kierkegaard, who surveyed Hegel's analytic abstractions with a certain awe but managed to remind himself and his readers that a man who had scrutinized all history and come up with a comprehensive theoretical explanation of anything and everything that had happened or would take place nevertheless had not much to tell us about how we ought to live our lives—we, who ask such a question and know that we have only so much time to find an answer. The existentialists (I don't like the glib, trendy use of the word, but what can one do these days with any word?) have stressed the particulars of everyday life—hence their interest (Buber, Marcel, Camus, Sartre and the father of them all, that at once high-spirited and gloomy Dane, Kierkegaard) in short stories, novels, plays and essays concerned with specific, concrete matters, as opposed to large-scale theoretical formulations meant to explain whatever comes in sight and then some.

It is the everyday life that clinicians also contend with—the unique nature of each human being. Since no patient is quite like any other, the doctor has to step from well learned abstractions to the individual person at hand—an important move, indeed. Novelists as well are wedded to the specific, the everyday; their job is to conjure up details for us, examples for us—the magic of art. And, as our black woman friend pointed out, everyday life has its own ethical conflicts. No wonder novelists do so well examining the trials and temptations that intervene, say, in a doctor's life. The point of a medical humanities course devoted to literature is ethical reflection, not a bit of culture polish here, a touch of story enjoyment there. There is an utter methodologic precision to the aim taken by George Eliot in *Middlemarch*, F. Scott Fitzgerald in *Tender Is the Night*, Sinclair Lewis in *Arrowsmith*, Walker Percy in *Love in the Ruins*. They are interested in exploring a kind of medical ethics that has to do with the quality of a lived life.

In *Middlemarch* Dr. Lydgate, a young doctor with high ideals, gradually must contend with a world of money and power. His marriage, his friendships, his everyday attitudes and commitments are revealed to weigh heavily, in the end, on the nature of his work. When he leaves Middlemarch for his excellent practice "between London and a Continental bathing place," he is not only abandoning a promising research career; he has changed so imperceptibly that he has no notion of real change. The ethical implications of his change of career are rendered with great subtlety. This greatest of English novelists knew better than to indulge in melodrama—the high-minded doctor come to naught through bad luck or a bad marriage or the bad faith of a particular banker. She makes it clear that to the outer world Lydgate is never a failure; he becomes, rather, more and more successful, as judged by the (corrupt and ignorant, we now know) standards of his time and place. The measure of his failure is his own early and well muscled ethical resolve. He had wanted to combat typhus and cholera—aware of the social as well as personal devastation those diseases wrought. He had wanted to take issue with the "principalities and powers" in his own profession. He ends up writing a treatise on gout. No doubt, gout, too, imposes suffering on people. And who is to decide what each of us ought to do—in any profession? But Lydgate had, indeed, made a series of decisions for himself and had hoped to see certain hopes and ambitions realized. *Middlemarch* provides a chronicle of disenchantment. A steady series of minor accommodations, rationalizations, mistakes of judgment contribute to a change of purpose, if not of heart. A doctor's character is proved wanting, and the result is his professional success by the standards of the time. Such a devastating irony leaves the reader in hopes, no doubt, that a bit of contemplation will take place: a person's work is part of a person's life, and the two combined as lifework must be seen as constantly responsive to the moral decisions that we never stop making, day in and day out. What George Eliot probed was character, a quality of mind and heart sadly ignored in today's all-too-numerous psychological analyses.

Similarly in *Arrowsmith*, a novel that many of us, arguably, read and take seriously at the wrong time in our lives—as high-schoolers, rather than during medical school and the years of hospital training. Sinclair Lewis was no George Eliot; he had a ruder, more polemical nature as a writer. And he lacked her gifts of narration. But he knew how professional lives become threatened, cheapened, betrayed. And he knew that such developments take place gradually, almost innocently—the small moments in the long haul, or the seemingly irrelevant big moments, such as a decision to live with one or another person and in this or that setting. His novel offered a powerful indictment of the larger society (always Lewis' intent) that exerts its sway on medicine, even research medicine, which is supposedly insulated from the vulgar world of cash and politics. But, of course, nothing is completely removed from that world—not doctors and not writers and not church people either. *Arrowsmith* is a novel that confronts the reader with a doctor's repeated ethical choices, a novel that makes it clear that such choices not only have to do with procedures (to do or not to do) or plugs (to pull or not to pull) but with the fateful decisions of everyday life that we are constantly making.

Such decisions are the stuff of each person's life. Once made, such decisions shadow us to the last breath. That is why Dick Diver haunts us in *Tender Is the Night,* and that is why Thomas More of Walker Percy's sad, funny and compelling novel, *Love in the Ruins,* makes us so uneasy with his shrewd, satirical observations about himself and his fellow human beings. Those two physicians, the reader knows, have asked important questions about life—how to live it honorably, decently. They have also stumbled badly, and their "fall" troubles us. We want to know why. But the reasons, the explanations, are not the categorical ones of modern psychology—some emotional hang-up. Those two principal characters speak for novelists who know how seamless a web life is, how significantly each physician's career connects with his or her moral values. It is a truism that one takes a risk by isolating the various moments of one's time on earth; yet we commonly strain to do so, and we are even allowed, if not taught, to do so, in our colleges and graduate schools and post-graduate training.

Every day, for instance, I see undergraduates not only working fiercely in courses such as organic chemistry but showing evidence of malevolent, destructive competitiveness. I have talked with some of those who teach such courses—heard the horror stories, the accounts of spite and meanness and outright dishonesty. Yet, again and again one listens to it asked: What can we do? And the students tell themselves, and we tell ourselves—we, who have gone through the maze ourselves—that it is something "inevitable" and, once over, forgotten. But these bothersome novelists tell us that we don't forget, and Lord knows Freud managed to make that point rather tellingly during his lifetime. We may appear to forget; we may convince ourselves that we do, but the small compromises, evasions, surrenderings of principle have their place in the unconscious, an element of geography yet to be done justice to by psychological theorists—the way we "repress" our moral sensibility, accommodate to various situations and die in the way George Eliot indicates.

Each year I receive respectful letters from ministers, bishops and church officials of one kind or another; I am asked to pass judgment psychologically on candidates for the ministry. Once my wife, in a moment of mischief and perhaps common sense, wondered what would have happened to all of us, historically, had Rorschach tests, Thematic Apperception Tests, or, yes, psychiatric interviews, been given to St. Francis of Assisi, St. Teresa of Avila, Martin Luther or Gandhi, not to mention the Old Testament prophets or Jesus Christ. Would they have "passed" those psychiatric interviews—they with their anger at the injustices of this world and their extraordinary willingness to suffer on behalf of all of us? One shudders at the psychiatric words that might have been sent their way. For that matter, she also wondered: Would Freud be given a grant from the National Institute of Mental Health today and would he even be willing to fill out those idiotic forms, one after the other? But setting that detour of my wife's aside, one is still left with the "spectacle" (to use a word that St. Paul favored as a critical moment in the affirmation of his faith) of religious authorities relying rather eagerly on the judgment of my ilk regarding the selection of candidates—as if psychiatrists were especially successful in finding for themselves, never mind others, how it is possible to live a principled life.

In psychiatry and medicine, as in other walks of life, we might ask for a few letters ourselves—not only appraisals of "mental function" but judgments about the ethical qualities of our various candidates. Do we often enough ask for such judgments? Do we ask ourselves and our students the kind of questions that George Eliot had in mind when she gave us, forever, one hopes, Dr. Lydgate, who would soon enough realize that there are prices to be paid for not asking certain questions? Dr. Lydgate forgot to inquire about what it would mean to him to become financially dependent on the philanthropist Bulstrode. Dr. Arrowsmith saw again and again the way doctors, like others, fall in line, knuckle under to various authorities who curb and confine independent thinking, never mind research. What those novelists move us to pursue is moral inquiry of a wide-ranging kind, in the tradition of Socrates or the Augustinian *Confessions* or Pascal's *Pensées*, or again, the best of our novelists: intense scrutiny of one's assumptions, one's expectations, one's values, one's life as it is being lived or as one hopes to live it. The pivotal questions are, of course, obvious. How much money is too much money? Who commands one's time, and who does not? What balance is there to one's commitment of energy?

And, from another standpoint, when do reformers start succumbing to the very arrogance or cruelty that they claim to fight? How ought we to resist various intrusions on our freedom, on our privacy as persons and as doctors—the bureaucratic statism that no one, however anxious for various governmental programs, should dismiss as being of little consequence, not after this century's testimony? And so on. Is there room to teach that kind of medical ethics, that kind of program of medical humanities in our medical schools? Is there any better way to do so than through the important stories and character portrayals of novelists who have moved close to the heart of the matter—the continuing tension between idealism and so-called "practicality" in all our lives?

X. J. KENNEDY

X. J. KENNEDY (1929–). *American poet. Kennedy is the author of numerous collections of poetry, and the highly regarded editor of such anthologies as* Messages: A Thematic Anthology of Poetry; Tygers of Wrath: Poems of Hate, Anger, and Invective; *and, in 1987,* Literature: An Introduction to Fiction, Poetry, and Drama. *Recent collections of poetry include* Talking Like the Rain *(1992), a book of first poems for children;* The Kite That Braved Old Orchard Beach *(1991); and* Fresh Brats *(1990), also for children.*

LITTLE ELEGY:
For a Child Who Skipped Rope

Here lies resting, out of breath,
Out of turns, Elizabeth
Whose quicksilver toes not quite
Cleared the whirring edge of night.

Earth whose circles round us skim
Till they catch the lightest limb,
Shelter now Elizabeth
And for her sake trip up Death.

MILLER WILLIAMS

MILLER WILLIAMS (1930–). *American poet, translator, educator, and publisher. Williams's degrees in science (biology and physiology) have influenced his prolific literary output. Among his published works are* The Boys on Their Bony Mules *(1983);* Imperfect Love *(1986); and, most recently,* Living on the Surface: New and Selected Poems *(1989), a sharp, sobering, at times witty collection representing thirty years of observations on everyday contemporary life. Formerly director of the Creative Writing and Translation Program at the University of Arkansas, Williams is now director of the University of Arkansas Press. Among his awards are the Prix de Rome of the American Academy of Arts and Letters and, in 1990, the prestigious Poets' Prize. His most recent book is* Some Jazz a While: Collected Poems *(1999).*

GOING

The afternoon in my brother's backyard
when my mother in awful age and failing
in body not at all and twice the pity
thought I was my dead father home for dinner
I didn't know what to tell her. What could I say?
Here I am home Darling give me your hand?
Let us walk together a little while?
Here it is 1915, we are married,
the first of our children is not yet born or buried,
the war in Europe is not yet out of hand
and the one you will not forget who wanted you first
is just as we are, neither old nor dead.
He still frets about us being together.

Good woman wife with five good children to mourn for,
and children arriving with children, what can I say?

See we have come because we wanted to come.
Because of love. Because of bad dreams.
This is my wife. We live in another state.

A DAY IN THE DEATH

He is amazed how hard it is to die.
He lies in his hospital bed, his shallow breaths
audible in the hall. He wonders why—
and tries to laugh because he knows—the deaths
of heroes always seem to be so quick.
Because, he knows, heroes have to fight,
and die fighting; also they rarely get sick.
A nurse looks into the room to say good night.
They don't tell each other what they know,
that both hope these words are the last he'll hear,
but guess they aren't. He thinks of the undertow
all swimmers swimming in strange waters fear,
that grabs you from below. He tries to sink
deep enough beneath the surface of sleep
to be found there and lost. There is a stink
thickening in the room. He knows the cheap
perfume Death wears. Why does she stand around?
Why doesn't the bitch take him? He tries to laugh
and this time does, and jerks at the new sound.
Well, half is already gone; the other half
could be a survivor of Buchenwald. Today
a counselor held his hand and told him again
to let go, to let it slip away.
He turned back to see how long it had been
since he had held on. He almost said,
"I'm trying. Something's stuck. Give me a shove."
He almost did. He squeezed the hand instead,
once for reasons forgotten and once for love.
But now he tries to sleep, pretends he is led
down through a wandering tunnel, sweetly gray,
to join the deep society of the dead,
afraid when the sun comes they'll send him away,
back to that room, back to that shrinking bed,
to lie there, being a lie, another day,
his eyes, his enormous eyes, eating his head.

PATRICIA GOEDICKE

PATRICIA GOEDICKE (1931–). *American poet. Born in Boston, Goedicke received her B.A. at Middlebury College and her M.A. at Ohio University. She has taught at Sarah Lawrence and Hunter College, among others, and now teaches creative writing at the University of Montana at Missoula. Her poetry has been published widely (in, among other periodicals, the* New Yorker, *the* Kenyon Review, *and the* Hudson Review) *and she has been awarded a number of prizes, including a fellowship from the National Endowment for the Arts. Her books include* Crossing the Same River *(1980),* The King of Childhood *(1984),* The Wind of Our Going *(1985),* Listen, Love *(1987),* The Tongues We Speak *(1989), and most recently,* Paul Bunyan's Bearskin *(1992), in which she brilliantly melds emotion and analysis, poetry and politics, and daily, mundane commonalities with issues of national concern.*

ONE MORE TIME

And next morning, at the medical center
Though the X-Ray Room swallows me whole,

Though cold crackles in the corridors
I brace myself against it and then relax.

Lying there on the polished steel table
Though I step right out of my body,

Suspended in icy silence
I look at myself from far off
Calmly, I feel free.

Even though I'm not, now
Or ever:

The metal teeth of death bite
But spit me out

One more time:

When the technician says breathe
I breathe.

JENNY JOSEPH

JENNY JOSEPH (1932–) *British poet and writer. Jenny Joseph's poetry was first published when she was a scholar of St. Hilda's College, Oxford. She has published numerous collections of poetry and fiction, including* The Unlooked-For Season *(1960),* Rose in the Afternoon *(1974),* The Thinking Heart *(1978),* Beyond Descartes *(1983),* Persephone *(1986),* Beached Boats *(1992),* The Inland Sea *(1992),* Selected Poems *(1992),* Ghosts and Other Company *(1996), and* Extended Similes *(1997). Her work has received many awards, including a Gregory Award and a Cholmondeley Award. In 1996, her poem "In Honour of Love" received the Forward Poetry Prize in the category of best individual poem. In that same year, she was honored in a national poll as the author of the United Kingdom's "most popular post-war poem"—"Warning"—reproduced here.*

WARNING

When I am an old woman I shall wear purple
With a red hat which doesn't go, and doesn't suit me.
And I shall spend my pension on brandy and summer gloves
And satin sandals, and say we've no money for butter.
I shall sit down on the pavement when I'm tired
And gobble up samples in shops and press alarm bells
And run my stick along the public railings
And make up for the sobriety of my youth.
I shall go out in my slippers in the rain
And pick the flowers in other people's gardens
And learn to spit.

You can wear terrible shirts and grow more fat
And eat three pounds of sausages at a go
Or only bread and pickle for a week
And hoard pens and pencils and beermats and things in boxes.

But now we must have clothes that keep us dry
And pay our rent and not swear in the street
And set a good example for the children.
We must have friends to dinner and read the papers.

But maybe I ought to practise a little now?
So people who know me are not too shocked and surprised
When suddenly I am old, and start to wear purple.

LINDA PASTAN

LINDA PASTAN (1932–). *American poet. Pastan is the recipient of, among other honors, the Dylan Thomas Poetry Award, the di Castagnola Award, and several fellowships from the National Endowment for the Arts. Among her collections of poetry are* AM/PM: New and Selected Poems *(1982),* The Imperfect Paradise *(1988), and* Heroes in Disguise *(1991), a clear-sighted, graceful composition on the cyclical nature of life and how we as human beings fit into it.* An Early Afterlife *(1995) was followed in 1999 by* Carnival Evening: New and Selected Poems 1968–1998.

THE FIVE STAGES OF GRIEF

The night I lost you
someone pointed me towards
the Five Stages of Grief.
Go that way, they said,
it's easy, like learning to climb
stairs after the amputation.
And so I climbed.
Denial was first.
I sat down at breakfast
carefully setting the table
for two. I passed you the toast—
you sat there. I passed
you the paper—you hid
behind it.
Anger seemed more familiar.
I burned the toast, snatched
the paper and read the headlines myself.
But they mentioned your departure,
and so I moved on to
Bargaining. What can I exchange
for you? The silence
after storms? My typing fingers?
Before I could decide, *Depression*
came puffing up, a poor relation
its suitcase tied together
with string. In the suitcase

266

were bandages for the eyes
and bottles of sleep. I slid
all the way down the stairs
feeling nothing.
And all the time Hope
flashed on and off
in defective neon.
Hope was a signpost pointing
straight in the air.
Hope was my uncle's middle name,
he died of it.
After a year I am still climbing,
though my feet slip
on your stone face.
The treeline
has long since disappeared;
green is a color
I have forgotten.
But now I see what I am climbing
towards: *Acceptance*
written in capital letters,
a special headline:
Acceptance,
its name is in lights.
I struggle on,
waving and shouting.
Below, my whole life spreads its surf,
all the landscapes I've ever known
or dreamed of. Below
a fish jumps: the pulse
in your neck.
Acceptance. I finally
reach it.
But something is wrong.
Grief is a circular staircase.
I have lost you.

NOTES FROM THE DELIVERY ROOM

Strapped down,
victim in an old comic book,
I have been here before,
this place where pain winces
off the walls
like too bright light.
Bear down a doctor says,
foreman to sweating laborer,
but this work, this forcing
of one life from another
is something that I signed for
at a moment when I would have signed anything.
Babies should grow in fields;
common as beets or turnips
they should be picked and held
root end up, soil spilling
from between their toes—
and how much easier it would be later,
returning them to earth.
Bear up . . . bear down . . . the audience
grows restive, and I'm a new magician
who can't produce the rabbit
from my swollen hat.
She's crowning, someone says,
but there is no one royal here,
just me, quite barefoot,
greeting my barefoot child.

REMISSION

It seems you must grow
into your death slowly,
as if it were a pair of new shoes
waiting on the closet floor,
smelling of the animal
it came from, but still too big
too stiff for you to wear.
Meanwhile you dance barefoot
your shaky dance to pretence,
and we dance with you,

the pulses in our own wrists
ticking away.
In this small truce
the body waits,
having waged war on itself
for years. You say
the water tastes of flowers.
You steal on tiptoe
past the closet door.

PAUL ZIMMER

PAUL ZIMMER (1934–). *American poet, essayist, editor, University Press director. Paul Zimmer was born in Canton, Ohio, and received his B.A. degree in English from Kent State. He is the author of eleven books and has received many national awards and prizes for his poetry. For some forty years he worked in scholarly publishing, serving first as director of the University of Georgia Press, then the University of Iowa Press, two of the most acclaimed such institutions. He has now retired from the Iowa position and lives on a farm in southwestern Wisconsin. From this site he travels, both to teach and read from his work, to colleges and universities over the United States. He and his wife also spend part of the year in France, where they own a small house.*

THE TENTH CIRCLE

"More than three (3) health emergency calls in one month from apartment to switchboard shall be conclusive evidence to landlord that occupant is not capable of independent living. Landlord can then have tenant moved to such health care facility as is available."

Dear Dad,

Do not fall for the third time,
Or if you do, tell no one.
Hunch over your agony and
Make it your ultimate secret.
You have done this before.
Shrug, tell a joke, go on.
If an ambulance slips up
Quietly to the back door
Do not get on. They mean to
Take you to the tenth circle
Where everyone is turned in
One direction, piled like cordwood
Inside the cranium of Satan
So that only the light of
Television shines in their eyes.

Dad, call if you need help,
But do not let them take you
Easily to this place where
They keep the motor idling
On the long black car, where if
Someone cries out in the night
Only the janitor comes.

THE EXPLANATION

Before his last fires were dowsed,
Before the irreversible stillness,
My father stormed against equivocation,
Heaving against tubes and wires
Until they had to bind him down.

The doctors asked for explanation.
He called for pencil and paper,
Angrily scribbled for a moment,
Then wrote in his clearest,
Most commanding hand, "I am dead."

JOSEPH HARDISON

JOSEPH HARDISON (1935–). *American physician, educator, and writer. Dr. Hardison attended Emory College and Emory University School of Medicine, where he is now a professor of medicine. His essays, by turns provocative, poignant, and humorous, have appeared widely—in the* New England Journal of Medicine, *the* Annals of Internal Medicine, Archives of Internal Medicine, Journal of the American Medical Association, *and the* American Journal of Medicine.

THE HOUSE OFFICER'S CHANGING WORLD

We middle-aged and older physicians are smug about our house-staff days—the days when medical giants roamed the hospital halls day and night. We prepared and stained our own blood smears, performed white-cell counts and differentials, actually looked through a microscope at our patients' urine, gram-stained sputum smears, determined circulation times, and measured venous pressures. Invasive procedures consisted of lumbar punctures, paracenteses, thoracenteses, liver biopsies, pleural biopsies, sigmoidoscopies, and bone marrow aspirations. We worked in private hospitals and in gloomy non-air-conditioned city and Veterans Administration hospitals. Patients were crowded together on large, open wards, where the nurses could see and hear everyone and where blacks were often segregated from whites.

The fund of medical knowledge was manageable. We revered and feared our teachers. Occasional intimidation and embarrassment were accepted as effective methods of teaching. Professors had time to spend with us, to teach us and get to know us. Departments of medicine were smaller, and everyone knew everyone else. Conferences were well attended, well prepared, and in most instances, given by the faculty in residence. The drug-company lecture circuit had not yet begun. Conferences were rarely interrupted. Messages were briefly flashed on the screen, or interns and residents were summoned by a display of their call numbers. Beepers were a scourge for the future. It was possible, if we worked hard, listened well, learned from our mistakes, and read about our patients' conditions, to become, in three years, confident and competent to diagnose and treat most of the diseases we would encounter in internal medicine without ever having photocopied a single article.

We worked every other night or every third night. There were frequently three or four of us in one on-call room with one telephone. Our pay averaged about 25 cents an hour. Moonlighting, though prohibited, went on and consisted almost entirely of physical examinations of clients of insurance salesmen. In most instances, the client did not come to the doctor. I performed examinations in a liquor store and a bowling alley, and I once examined a movie projectionist in his booth while John Wayne was on the screen. Most of our wives worked (there were very few women in medicine), and most of us borrowed money at low interest rates. We didn't have large debts incurred in medical school. Entertainment was infrequent and simple and usually enjoyed in the company of other house officers. We were all able to go to the annual Christmas party because the faculty covered for us.

Many of the patients whom we (and private physicians) took care of could not afford to pay and were not expected to do so. There were charity wards in most private hospitals, and the big city hospitals were primarily for the indigent. There was no Medicare, Medicaid, or diagnosis-related groups (DRGs). Most patients were uninformed about medicine. They trusted and respected their physicians and did not question the diagnosis, prognosis, or treatment. They did not accept responsibility for their health. They went to the doctor when they got sick and expected the doctor to make them well. Physicians and their patients smoked.

Medicolegal and ethical matters were relatively uncomplicated. Malpractice premiums were low, and malpractice suits were uncommon; doctors usually won and, if they lost, the awards were reasonable. The courts, by and large, saw fit to leave medical decisions to physicians. There was no need for living wills or for distinguishing brain death from death. "No code" or "do not resuscitate" orders did not exist because there was no effective cardiopulmonary resuscitation. Often patients were not told that they had cancer or leukemia; they were given the opportunity to prolong the denial of their imminent death. After all, we thought, if they really wanted to know what the score was, they could tell from our actions and what we left unsaid. There was no patient's bill of rights.

Technology consisted of stethoscopes, ophthalmoscopes, tuning forks, reflex hammers, electrocardiographs, rigid sigmoidoscopes, bronchoscopes, and various and sundry biopsy needles. There were no medical intensive care units, no coronary care units, no respiratory care units, and no arterial lines, subclavian lines, Swan-Ganz catheters, pacemakers, Holter monitors, bedside monitors, or cardioverters. Imaging consisted of roentgenography and fluoroscopy. Ultrasound, echocardiography, computerized axial tomographic scanning, and nuclear magnetic-resonance imaging were yet to come. There were no third-, or second-, or even first-generation cephalosporins, and nitrogen mustard was the only effective chemotherapy. We sterilized our needles in an autoclave and reused them; blood came in bottles. "End-stage" disease meant the end was near. There was no renal dialysis, and organs were not transplanted. We did very little to patients, and it was easier for them to die with dignity.

When we finished our training and were ready for practice or a career in academia, opportunities abounded. There weren't enough physicians to go around. There were no "docs in boxes" or preferred provider organizations, and there were very few prepaid health plans. Physicians did not advertise. We could be assured of working hard, earning a comfortable living, and being members of the most respected of professions.

Modern-day house officers find themselves in circumstances vastly different from those we experienced when we were house officers. Many of them have substantial debts from financing their medical school education. Although the salaries of the house staff are better now, many take outside ("moonlight") jobs because of their debts and a desire for a higher standard of living. Most work in emergency rooms, and few, if any, do physical examinations for life-insurance companies. Moonlighting is not the forbidden subject it used to be, and most program directors give tacit approval or simply turn the other way.

The days of working every other night are gone. Most house officers work every third or fourth night while they are on ward services. Because they work fewer nights, however, more patients are assigned to them when they do work. They become very adept at triage and at caring for many sick patients, but they have little time to read and even less to sleep. They are under enormous pressure to discharge patients, both because of pressures to contain costs from third-party payers and the DRG system, and because they have no control over the admission process.

Teaching hospitals are also moneymaking hospitals. The faculty has little time and often little inclination to teach. Attending rounds are made to ensure third-party payments. There are no monetary rewards for teaching, and teaching won't get faculty members promoted. Many big city hospitals, the former bastions of house-staff training, either have closed or are in difficult financial straits. Academic and clinical faculty members don't have time to give to these foundering behemoths. The house-staff members are given, and assume, more and more responsibility. As a result of this increased responsibility and of the decrease in the faculty's time for and interest in teaching, the house staff has become more and more independent. The faculty and the house staff have become estranged. Everyone is busy taking care of patients or doing research. House officers have role models but few heroes.

There is now much more to do for and to patients. We expect house officers to learn all the procedures we learned and many more. We expect them to be equally competent in caring for ambulatory patients and critically ill patients in intensive care units. We keep stressing the history and physical examination as the source of the most important data we gather, but everyone, faculty and house staff alike, is relying more and more on tests and procedures. You need a gimmick to make it in private practice. Because of the pressure to get their work done, the house-staff members seldom, or only reluctantly, attend conferences. When they do attend, they bring their lunches, and the speaker strives to be heard over crackling cellophane, the crunch of potato chips, the rattle of ice cubes, and a cacophony of beepers. An hour spent in conference is an hour taken from time off. House officers today have many interests other than medicine. They want to enjoy these while they are still young.

It is impossible to keep up with medicine today. Knowledge is accumulating and changing so fast that you can't be sure that what is fact today will be true tomorrow. House officers, with little time to read, instead photocopy or tear out enormous numbers of articles from journals and, like squirrels hiding acorns, bury them in ingenious filing systems in the hope that the articles will still be pertinent when they finally get around to reading them some day.

House officers and practicing physicians are under attack from the public, the legal profession, and the government. Subspecialty programs are reducing the numbers of fellowship positions, and future funding is in question. Many will lose autonomy because, by choice or necessity, they accept salaried positions. Competition for patients will create tension among colleagues. Moral, ethical, and medicolegal issues that arise because of technology, greed, and public awareness consume enormous amounts of time, resources, and energy. There is evidence that emotional impairment is increasing in today's house staff. Sleep deprivation, the responsibilities of being a new physician, and rigorous training are cited as causes of the increased strain. These stresses, however, have been present for as long as there have been training programs. Another factor may be that the medicine that today's house officers dreamed about, which they went to college and medical school and deep into debt for, no longer exists. Our young physicians are bemused and beleaguered, and they feel they have been betrayed.

I suppose it is natural for those of us who are nearer the end of a career than the beginning to extol the virtues of our house-staff training over the training of today. Each generation seems to believe it suffered more hardships and did things better than the next. House officers today have enough to worry about without hearing about how hard we worked and how dedicated we were. We accuse them of being the "me generation," of being incapable of delaying gratification. It is difficult, however, to enjoy life today when you are $30,000 in debt and haven't yet begun to earn a living. Medicine has changed drastically since we were house officers. Comparing medicine then and now is like comparing horse-and-buggy days with interplanetary travel. It is impossible to know who worked harder and learned more, and it doesn't matter. There is, however, no question about who has more to learn and more to do. House officers are not responsible for what has happened to medicine, but we are responsible for what happens to our house officers. They are intelligent, diligent, responsible, and compassionate people, and they usually end up being well trained. They deserve our support, appreciation, and affection.

MARY OLIVER

MARY OLIVER (1935–). *American poet. Winner of the Pulitzer Prize in poetry (1984), Mary Oliver often turns to nature to examine the mysteries of life, death, and transformation. She has an acknowledged ability to describe complex issues with clarity and simplicity, and critics have found her ways of describing ordinary matters "breathtaking" and "startlingly fresh." Frequently her lyrical writing conveys a sense of acceptance of the world as a brutal place where the forces of life and death have been set into motion as an ongoing, capricious process. In the poem "In Blackwater Woods," the narrator advises, "To live in this world / you must be able . . . to love what is mortal / to hold it . . . and, when the time comes to let it go, / let it go." Oliver's writings include* No Voyage and Other Poems, American Primitive, A Poetry Handbook, *and* White Pine: Poems and Prose Poems.

UNIVERSITY HOSPITAL, BOSTON

The trees on the hospital lawn
are lush and thriving. They too
are getting the best of care,
like you, and the anonymous many,
in the clean rooms high above this city,
where day and night the doctors keep
arriving, where intricate machines
chart with cool devotion
the murmur of the blood,
the slow patching-up of bone,
the despair of the mind.

When I come to visit and we walk out
into the light of a summer day,
we sit under the trees—
buckeyes, a sycamore and one
black walnut brooding
high over a hedge of lilacs
as old as the red-brick building
behind them, the original
hospital built before the Civil War.

We sit on the lawn together, holding hands
while you tell me: you are better.

How many young men, I wonder,
came here, wheeled on cots off the slow trains
from the red and hideous battlefields
to lie all summer in the small and stuffy chambers
while doctors did what they could, longing
for tools still unimagined, medicines still unfound,
wisdoms still unguessed at, and how many died
staring at the leaves of the trees, blind
to the terrible effort around them to keep them alive?
I look into your eyes

which are sometimes green and sometimes gray,
and sometimes full of humor, but often not,
and tell myself, you are better,
because my life without you would be
a place of parched and broken trees.
Later, walking the corridors down to the street,
I turn and step inside an empty room.
Yesterday someone was here with a gasping face.
Now the bed is made all new,
the machines have been rolled away. The silence
continues, deep and neutral,
as I stand there, loving you.

THE BLACK SNAKE

When the black snake
flashed onto the morning road,
and the truck could not swerve—
death, that is how it happens.

Now he lies looped and useless
as an old bicycle tire.
I stop the car
and carry him into the bushes.

He is as cool and gleaming
as a braided whip, he is as beautiful and quiet
as a dead brother.
I leave him under the leaves

and drive on, thinking
about *death:* its suddenness,
its terrible weight,
its certain coming. Yet under

reason burns a brighter fire, which the bones
have always preferred.
It is the story of endless good fortune.
It says to oblivion: not me!

It is the light at the center of every cell.
It is what sent the snake coiling and flowing forward
happily all spring through the green leaves before
he came to the road.

BEAVER MOON—THE SUICIDE OF A FRIEND

When somewhere life
breaks like a pane of glass,
and from every direction casual
voices are bringing you the news,
you say: I should have known.
You say: I should have been aware.
That last Friday he looked
so ill, like an old mountain-climber
lost on the white trails, listening
to the ice breaking upward, under
his worn-out shoes. You say:
I heard rumors of trouble, but after all
we all have that. You say:
what could I have done? and you go
with the rest, to bury him.

That night, you turn in your bed
to watch the moon rise, and once more
see what a small coin it is
against the darkness, and how everything else
is a mystery, and you know
nothing at all except
the moonlight is beautiful—
white rivers running together
along the bare boughs of the trees—
and somewhere, for someone, life
is becoming moment by moment
unbearable.

JOHN STONE

JOHN STONE (1936–). *American physician, poet, essayist, lecturer, and educator. Born in Jackson, Mississippi, Dr. Stone received his B.A. from Millsaps College, his M.D. from Washington University in St. Louis, and did postgraduate training at the University of Rochester and Emory University. He is the author of* In the Country of Hearts, *essays and stories about his life in cardiology, and has also published four books of poetry, most recently* Where Water Begins: New Poems and Prose.

GAUDEAMUS IGITUR

Gaudeamus Igitur *was delivered as the Valediction Address at Emory University School of Medicine, Atlanta, in July 1982. The Latin title is the first line of a medieval song that became, over the centuries, a drinking song, a song of celebration, in the universities of Europe. The Latin words of the first verse are these:*

> Gaudeamus igitur,
> Iuvenes dum sumus;
> Gaudeamus igitur,
> Iuvenes dum sumus;
> Post iucundam iuventutem,
> Post molestam senectutem,
> Nos habebit humus,
> Nos habebit humus.

The verse translates, roughly: "Therefore let us rejoice / While we are young; / After a delightful youth, / After an irksome old age, / The grave will contain us." The words and the tune to which they were sung have special significance for an academic occasion such as Commencement: Johannes Brahms, years later, incorporated the song into the climactic portion of his "Academic Festival Overture."

The form of the poem, in which every line begins with the word For, *was suggested by a portion of the long poem* Jubilate Agno, *written by the eighteenth-century poet Christopher Smart (1722–1771). The specific portion referred to was written by Smart in praise of his cat Jeoffrey.*

For this is the day of joy
   which has been fourteen hundred and sixty days in coming
   and fourteen hundred and fifty-nine nights
For today in the breathing name of Brahms
   and the cat of Christopher Smart
   through the unbroken line of language and all the nouns
   stored in the angular gyrus
   today is a commencing
For this is the day you know too little
   against the day when you will know too much
For you will be invincible
   and vulnerable in the same breath
   which is the breath of your patients
For their breath is our breathing and our reason
For the patient will know the answer
   and you will ask him
   ask her
For the family may know the answer
For there may be no answer
   and you will know too little again
   or there *will* be an answer and you will know too much
   forever
For you will look smart and feel ignorant
   and the patient will not know which day it is for you
   and you will pretend to be smart out of ignorance
For you must fear ignorance more than cyanosis
For whole days will move in the direction of rain
For you will cry and there will be no one to talk to
   or no one but yourself
For you will be lonely
For you will be alone
For there is a difference
For there is no seriousness like joy
For there is no joy like seriousness
For the days will run together in gallops and the years
   go by as fast as the speed of thought
   which is faster than the speed of light
   or Superman
   or Superwoman
For you will not be Superman
For you will not be Superwoman

For you will not be Solomon
    but you will be asked the question nevertheless*
For after you learn what to do, how and when to do it
    the question will be *whether*
For there will be addictions: whiskey, tobacco, love
For they will be difficult to cure
For you yourself will pass the kidney stone of pain
    and be joyful
For this is the end of examinations
For this is the beginning of testing
For Death will give the final examination
    and everyone will pass
For the sun is always right on time
    and even that may be reason for a kind of joy
For there are all kinds of
    all degrees of joy
For love is the highest joy
For which reason the best hospital is a house of joy
    even with rooms of pain and loss
    exits of misunderstanding
For there is the mortar of faith
For it helps to believe
For Mozart can heal and no one knows where he is buried
For penicillin can heal
    and the word
    and the knife
For the placebo will work and you will think you know why
For the placebo will have side effects and you will know
    you do not know why
For none of these may heal
For joy is nothing if not mysterious
For your patients will test you for spleen
    and for the four humors
For they will know the answer
For they have the disease
For disease will peer up over the hedge
    of health, with only its eyes showing
For the T waves will be peaked and you will not know why
For there will be computers

*I Kings 3:16–27.

283

For there will be hard data and they will be hard
    to understand
For the trivial will trap you and the important escape you
For the Committee will be unable to resolve the question
For there will be the arts
    and some will call them
    soft data
    whereas in fact they are the hard data
    by which our lives are lived
For everyone comes to the arts too late
For you can be trained to listen only for the oboe
    out of the whole orchestra
For you may need to strain to hear the voice of the
    patient
    in the thin reed of his crying
For you will learn to see most acutely out of
    the corner of your eye
    to hear best with your inner ear
For there are late signs and early signs
For the patient's story will come to you
    like hunger, like thirst
For you will know the answer
    like second nature, like first
For the patient will live
    and you will try to understand
For you will be amazed
    or the patient will not live
    and you will try to understand
For you will be baffled
For you will try to explain both, either, to the family
For there will be laying on of hands
    and the letting go
For love is what death would always intend if it had the
    choice
For the fever will drop, the bone remold along its lines of
    force
    the speech return
    the mind remember itself
For there will be days of joy
For there will be elevators of elation
    and you will walk triumphantly
    in purest joy

along the halls of the hospital
and say *Yes* to all the dark corners
where no one is listening
For the heart will lead
For the head will explain
but the final common pathway is the heart
whatever kingdom may come
For what matters finally is how the human spirit is spent
For this is the day of joy
For this is the morning to rejoice
For this is the beginning
Therefore, let us rejoice
Gaudeamus igitur.

TALKING TO THE FAMILY

My white coat waits in the corner
like a father.
I will wear it to meet the sister
in her white shoes and organza dress
in the live of winter,

the milkless husband
holding the baby.

I will tell them.

They will put it together
and take it apart.
Their voices will buzz.
The cut ends of their nerves
will curl.

I will take off the coat,
drive home,
and replace the light bulb in the hall.

LUCILLE CLIFTON

LUCILLE CLIFTON (1936–). *African-American poet. Clifton's collections of poetry include* Good Times *(1969),* Good News About the Earth *(1972),* An Ordinary Woman *(1974), and* Two-Headed Woman, *winner of the Juniper Award in 1980. The* Book of Light *(1993) is a collection of family portraits imbued with Clifton's warmth and wisdom and marked by her fierce unsentimentality. She is also the author of a memoir,* Generations *(1976), and more than a dozen books of poetry and fiction for children.* Blessing the Boats: New and Selected Poems 1988–2000 *was published in April 2000.*

the lost baby poem

the time i dropped your almost body down
down to meet the waters under the city
and run one with the sewage to the sea
what did i know about waters rushing back
what did i know about drowning
or being drowned

you would have been born into winter
in the year of the disconnected gas
and no car   we would have made the thin
walk over Genesee hill into the Canada wind
to watch you slip like ice into strangers' hands
you would have fallen naked as snow into winter
if you were here i could tell you these
and some other things

if i am ever less than a mountain
for your definite brothers and sisters
let the rivers pour over my head
let the sea take me for a spiller
of seas   let black men call me stranger
always   for your never named sake

LUCILLE CLIFTON

poem to my uterus

you   uterus
you have been patient
as a sock
while i have slippered into you
my dead and living children
now
they want to cut you out
stocking i will not need
where i am going
where am i going
old girl
without you
uterus
my bloody print
my estrogen kitchen
my black bag of desire
where i can go
barefoot
without you
where can you go
without me

LAWRENCE K. ALTMAN

LAWRENCE K. ALTMAN (1937–). *American physician and writer. Dr. Altman was the first physician to work full-time as a newspaper reporter. For many years, he has been senior medical correspondent and "The Doctor's World" columnist for* The New York Times. *He has provided memorable coverage of, among other stories, the artificial-heart insertion (performed on Dr. Barney Clark) and the AIDS epidemic. Altman has won the Polk Award for international reporting, and he is cowinner of the Victor Cohn Prize for excellence in medical science reporting. The selection that follows is from his book* Who Goes First? The Story of Self-Experimentation in Medicine.

DON'T TOUCH THE HEART

Civilization has discarded many of the taboos of primitive societies, but some have survived into modern times. As late as the 1920s, for example, it was taboo for a doctor to touch the living human heart. By that time surgeons, aided by advances in anesthesiology, had invaded most areas of the body. They had begun to operate routinely on the abdominal organs, limbs, the face, even the brain—but not the heart. In the few instances in the preceding centuries when, in emergencies, surgeons had entered the chest to cut and sew the heart, the patient generally had died.

Well into the twentieth century, to touch the heart was to molest a sacred area of the body, its spiritual center, and most doctors feared to tamper with it. Even if they had not been afraid of incurring God's wrath, there were seemingly unsolvable physical problems. The heart constantly pumped blood; when cut, it bled profusely. How could anyone survive such a hemorrhage?

Furthermore, the heart seemed inaccessible. It lies at most three inches beneath the skin, but it is enclosed by a bony cage of ribs that protects both it and the lungs. Were a surgeon to open the chest cage to operate on the lungs or heart, air could suddenly rush in, collapsing one lung and possibly both.

By World War II, knowledge of the heart's functions and the physiology of the lungs was still rudimentary, much of the intimate physiological relationship between the two yet to be revealed. In 1628, when William Harvey discovered the circulatory system, he taught us that the heart pumps blood over and over again through a closed system of arteries and veins. But for hundreds of years that was all doctors knew. Even three centuries after Harvey's discovery, few doctors could consistently diagnose a heart condition. Physicians could rely on little more than their hands and ears as diagnostic aids. Too often, the correct diagnosis emerged only after an autopsy.

With the discovery of anesthesia in the mid-nineteenth century, surgeons experimented and devised new operations, but touching the heart remained taboo. In 1880 Dr. Theodor Billroth, the most influential European surgeon of his time, said: "A surgeon who tries to suture a heart wound deserves to lose the esteem of his colleagues." The medical profession adopted an attitude about heart surgery so fatalistic that in 1896 Dr. Stephen Paget, a noted English physician, wrote: "Surgery of the heart has probably reached the limits set by Nature to all surgery: no new method, and no new discovery, can overcome the natural difficulties that attend a wound of the heart."

By the turn of the twentieth century, surgeons had opened the chest, but not the heart. Then, in 1903, Dr. Ferdinand Sauerbruch, a famous German surgeon, performed an operation that was to make history—and it came about accidentally. One of Sauerbruch's patients was a woman with heart failure, and Sauerbruch believed it was due to constriction of the pericardium, the membrane that covers the heart. He decided to relieve this constriction. Sauerbruch, a great teacher, operated in an amphitheater before a group of observant doctors. When he cut open the woman's chest, he saw what he thought was a cyst in her pericardium and he began to cut it out. Suddenly blood spurted. Sauerbruch realized immediately that it was not a cyst in the membrane but a ballooning of the heart wall itself, known as an aneurysm, and the pericardium had become attached to it. This brutally bold, fearless surgeon quickly repaired the aneurysm and sewed the heart. The patient recovered.

Others must have tried, but failed, to duplicate Sauerbruch's success. Although these presumed failures were not reported in medical journals (surgeons prefer to report successful operations), the failures must have been known through the medical grapevine and they must have perpetuated Billroth's and Paget's earlier warnings. It would take twenty-six more years and the courage of a twenty-five-year-old surgical intern to change things.

Werner Forssmann received his medical degree from the University of

Berlin in 1929, and that summer he began his internship in surgery at the Auguste Viktoria Home, a small Red Cross hospital in Eberswalde, Germany, fifty miles outside Berlin.

During his studies, Forssmann had been deeply impressed by a sketch in his physiology textbook that showed French physiologists standing in front of a horse, holding a thin tube that had been put into the jugular vein in the animal's neck and then guided into the heart. An inflated rubber balloon recorded the changes in pressure inside one of the heart chambers. The horse's heart was not disturbed by the procedure. Forssmann became obsessed with the potential value of putting a tube into the human heart. He thought that the technique could be used as an emergency measure to speed delivery of drugs to the heart of a dying patient and as a means to further understanding of the diseases of the heart and circulatory system. He could not understand why this simple technique, which would avoid the complications of opening the chest, had not already been tried on humans.

The more Forssmann thought about the horse experiment, the more he became convinced that it would work on humans as well. But he believed that neck veins would be unsuitable; patients might object because the incision would leave a scar. For cosmetic reasons, then, he focused on the veins in the elbow crease as the point of entry for the tube that would reach the heart.

Forssmann decided to wait a few weeks before asking his superior for permission to try his experiment. He would need a little time to get to know the other doctors at Auguste Viktoria, and to learn the routine.

In the 1920s, the German medical system favored those with independent financial means, and Forssmann, from a middle-class background, was at a disadvantage. His father had been killed in World War I, and he had been raised by his mother and grandmother. When Forssmann decided to emulate a physician-uncle and become a doctor, his mother worked to pay for his medical studies.

In Forssmann's time, paid medical training jobs for postgraduate medical students were rare. But Forssmann was lucky; he found a job for $50 a month—a pittance even then—as an apprentice to Dr. Richard Schneider, a general surgeon at the Auguste Viktoria Home and a friend of the Forssmann family. Then as now, the internship is an intensive training period designed to teach the accepted techniques of medicine or surgery with little or no time for devising or executing experiments. Nevertheless, not long after joining Schneider's staff as an apprentice, Forssmann approached the elder doctor and asked permission to insert a tube through the arm of a human in an effort to reach the human heart. He carefully explained to his superior that since it was too dangerous to touch the beating heart directly, perhaps a less dangerous approach would be to put a tube inside the heart.

How would he reach this vital organ that was so well protected by the ribs?

The same way the French physiologists had reached the horse's heart—through the veins. Forssmann showed Dr. Schneider the sketch from his physiology textbook. Schneider was sympathetic to Forssmann's proposal but advised the young doctor to experiment on animals first. Forssmann countered that the animal experiments by the French physiologists had already proved the technique safe. But he admitted to Schneider he did not know what would happen when the tip of the rubber tube touched the sensitive inside lining of the human heart. So he offered to do it on himself first. "I was convinced that when the problems in an experiment are not very clear, you should do it on yourself and not on another person," Forssmann recalled years later.

But Schneider refused. Forssmann then suggested doing the experiment on a dying patient. Schneider rejected this as well. He forbade Forssmann to do the experiment at all on any person, including himself. As a friend of the family, Schneider feared that Forssmann's widowed mother would have no means of supporting herself if something happened to her only child. The risk was too great, not only to Forssmann but also to Schneider's reputation. An accident would create a scandal.

Forssmann decided to do the experiment anyway—in secret. He would need equipment: sterile scalpels, sutures, and a painkiller to anesthetize the area in the elbow crease he would pierce. He would also need a long piece of sterile rubber tubing, and he knew that only the ureteral catheter, the thin tubing urologists use to drain urine from the kidneys, was long enough for his purpose. This crucial equipment was kept locked in the operating room under the care of Gerda Ditzen, a nurse of about forty-five who had a keen interest in medicine. Forssmann would need her assistance.

"I started to prowl around Gerda like a sweet-toothed cat around the cream jug," he said. He lent her medical books about anatomy and physiology and dropped by the cafeteria after she had finished lunch, ready to talk about what she had read. And each time they met, Forssmann would tell her a little more about his idea. He showed her the picture of the tube in the horse's heart and explained how the same technique could be performed on humans. She was captivated. Forssmann took her to dinner, and during the evening she asked more and more questions about his experiment. She liked the vision and passionate conviction of this young doctor, and, yes, she could clearly understand the importance of his idea. When Forssmann told her he was forbidden to do the experiment, she immediately suggested that they do it together; she would be his human guinea pig.

Forssmann had something else in mind.

A few days later, sweating from the summer heat as well as from his own excitement, he visited Nurse Ditzen in the small operating room. It was the noon break, and she was alone. He asked her to unlock the cabinet and get him a set of sterile surgical instruments—a scalpel, a hollow needle, sutures, and a ureteral catheter. Knowing no operations were scheduled for that afternoon, she asked Forssmann why he needed them. Then she realized what he was going to do. Convinced that she would be the first human to have a tube in her heart and excited by the knowledge that she would be making medical history, Gerda prepared everything Forssmann needed and willingly followed his command to climb onto the surgical table.

Forssmann strapped her arms and legs to the table, then stepped out of her view, toward the surgical workbench. He peeled the white towel from the instrument tray and examined the scalpel, the thin rubber ureteral tube, and the sutures Nurse Ditzen had sterilized. He glanced briefly across the room at the back of Gerda's head. She rested comfortably, expecting him to return at any moment with the novocaine.

Forssmann turned back to the surgical tray and briefly studied the ureteral tube. It was sixty-five centimeters long, just shy of thirty inches. Long enough, he estimated, to push through the hole in the vein in the elbow crease, slide up the arm, and twist across the shoulder, down a large vein in the chest, and into the venous connection to his heart.

His heart, not Gerda Ditzen's.

As the nurse adjusted her body to the tight-fitting straps, Forssmann worked confidently. He dabbed iodine over his left elbow crease and injected the novocaine to numb his skin. While he waited for the local anesthetic to take effect, he returned to the surgical table. Slowly and ceremoniously, he rubbed Nurse Ditzen's arm with iodine. He smiled reassuringly at Gerda, patted her arm gently and returned to the workbench, out of her sight.

Forssmann picked up the scalpel and cut through his skin. When he reached a large vein, he put down the scalpel, picked up the hollow needle, gently pushed it into the vein and left it in place. A small amount of blood spilled over his arm. Forssmann reached for the rubber tubing and pushed its tip through the hollow needle to guide it into the vein. The tube slithered along. There are valves in the veins that close when blood flows away from the heart, but because the tube was moving in the direction of the blood flow, the valves opened naturally and offered no resistance to Forssmann's tube. As he pushed the tube along the course of the vein in his upper arm, he felt a slight warmth, but no pain. Forssmann was learning that nature keeps the veins devoid of pain fibers.

When the tube reached the level of his shoulder, he stopped. Once it got to his heart, he would need documentation, an X ray of his chest to show the tube's precise location. The X-ray machine was in the basement of the hospital. He would need Nurse Ditzen's assistance.

Just then she called to him from across the room. Was anything wrong? When would he begin?

Forssmann went over to the table. As he loosened the straps, he replied, "It's done."

Gerda pushed herself off the table and stared at the tube in Forssmann's arm. She realized immediately that she had been duped.

"She was furious," Forssmann recalled. "I told her to relax and asked her to put a handkerchief around my arm and call the X-ray technician. Then we walked together down a flight of stairs to the X-ray department in the cellar."

There, Forssmann went behind the fluoroscopic X-ray screen and ordered Nurse Ditzen to hold up a mirror so he could look over the screen and see the position of the catheter on the fluoroscope. The two were silent, completely engrossed, as they watched the tube move through Forssmann's vein. Neither noticed the X-ray technician slip out of the room.

Forssmann jiggled the catheter and inched it toward his heart; still there was no pain, only the continued feeling of warmth. On one occasion the tube hit something sensitive, for he had an urge to cough. He restrained himself.

The stillness was abruptly broken when Dr. Peter Romeis and the X-ray technician burst into the room. The frightened X-ray technician had woken Dr. Romeis from a nap. Romeis was Forssmann's friend and colleague and had expressed support for Forssmann's idea when Forssmann had first confided it to him. Now, to Forssmann's dismay, a bleary-eyed Romeis was yelling at him, telling him he was crazy.

"Romeis tried to pull the catheter from my arm," Forssmann recalled. "I fought him off, yelling, 'Nein, Nein. I must push it forward.' I kicked his shins and pushed the catheter until the mirror showed that the tip had reached my heart. Take a picture, I ordered. I knew that the main point was to get radiographic proof that the catheter was indeed in the heart, not in a vein."

The X-ray technician snapped the picture. When it was developed a few minutes later, Forssmann had his proof. The catheter was in his right auricle, the first heart chamber that he could reach through the arm vein. The tube was too short to be pushed further into the heart.

Satisfied that he had the X-ray documentation he needed, Forssmann pulled the tube out of his heart, slid it back through the veins in his chest and arm and out of his elbow crease. A few drops of blood oozed out of the hole where the tube had pierced the vein, and Forssmann put a suture or two into the wound to stop the bleeding. Then he bandaged his elbow. The incision would turn red a few days later from a mild infection. But no further complications developed.

Forssmann was luckier than he could have known. Because so little was understood about the functions of the heart, he was oblivious to the dangers that can occur when anything touches the sensitive endocardium, or inside lining of the heart wall. Abnormal, potentially fatal heart rhythms can develop. Forssmann could have died suddenly, on the spot.

Oblivious to all this, Forssmann faced a more immediate problem: Dr. Schneider. The chief surgeon summoned the young intern to his office and started to give him a lecture about disobedience.

Forssmann was deeply concerned. He knew his career was at stake. Then Schneider asked to see the X ray.

As he told me the story years later, Forssmann burst into a roaring laugh. "When Schneider saw the X-ray pictures," Forssmann said, "he agreed the experiment was a good one and decided to celebrate. That evening we went to Kretchmer's, an old-fashioned, low-ceilinged wine tavern where the waiters wore formal evening dress. We had a good dinner and several bottles of fine wine." Forssmann repeated his experiment on himself five more times over the next four weeks. Each time, he went through the same procedure, and each time he successfully pushed the catheter through his arm to his heart.

Schneider urged Forssmann to write a scientific paper describing his experiments. The older doctor knew that Forssmann's technique was revolutionary, and as the word spread he feared others would steal the idea and claim credit. Schneider also anticipated the furor that would come when the medical profession learned of the daring experiments. He told Forssmann to stress the potential therapeutic applications of catheterization and its perceived usefulness for the emergency administration of drugs to the heart, and to minimize its usefulness for research purposes. "As a method of investigation, it is too revolutionary for doctors to understand," Schneider pointed out to his young apprentice. "Say that you tried it on cadavers before you did it on yourself. The reader of your paper must have the impression that it is not too revolutionary and that it was not made without a lot of forethought. Otherwise, the critics will tear you to pieces."

Decades later, Forssmann was criticized by those who said he had pursued the catheter technique for unmerited impractical ideas and not as the valuable physiological tool it came to be. Nevertheless, Forssmann did report some of the research potential he foresaw from his experiment. In his paper, he wrote, "The method opens up numerous prospects for new possibilities in the investigation of metabolism and of cardiac function." To counterbalance this and in an effort to comply with Schneider's suggestions, Forssmann invented a story. He claimed in his report that a colleague had been with him for the experiment and had, in fact, inserted the catheter into Forssmann's arm. At that point, according to Forssmann's report, the colleague became so frightened by the whole procedure that he ran away, leaving Forssmann alone, the catheter dangling from his arm. Forssmann went on to say that he did not continue with the experiment at that time, but a few days later he decided to do it again, alone. Forssmann also claimed in his report that he had tried the technique first on a cadaver. But, as he told me much later, he catheterized a cadaver only *after* he had put the tube into his own heart. Even today, textbooks describe the fictitious, aborted first effort and the nonexistent preliminary test on the corpse.

On September 13, 1929, Forssmann sent his paper to the *Klinische Wochenschrift*, the leading German medical journal. When it appeared in November, it caused the furor that Schneider had feared. Newspaper accounts sensationalized and distorted the technique. A Berlin paper offered Forssmann a thousand marks to publish pictures of the X rays showing the catheter in his heart. Forssmann declined.

Then, Forssmann's priority in performing the experiment was challenged by Dr. Ernst Unger, the senior surgeon at another, more prestigious German hospital. In 1912, seventeen years before Forssmann's paper appeared, Unger and Fritz Bleichroeder and another colleague had published a series of papers in *Klinische Wochenschrift* in which they had reported inserting tubes into the arm and leg veins of four human volunteers. Unger now claimed that in one experiment he had pushed the catheter through an artery into Bleichroeder's heart. Bleichroeder backed him up, arguing that the stabbing pain in his chest indicated that the tube had reached his heart. But if indeed it had, they had not mentioned it in their report. Furthermore, they had taken no X rays. Without them, there was no proof.

Unger wrote to the *Klinische Wochenschrift*, charging that its editor had shirked his journalistic duties in failing to note the previous claim. Forssmann explained that because the titles of the previous papers had given no hint that they were related in any way to his project, he had not read them before publishing his own paper. The editor printed a brief note from Forssmann that explained the situation but did not yield priority.

On October 1, 1929, a month before his report would be published, Forssmann moved from Eberswalde to Dr. Ferdinand Sauerbruch's clinic at the Charité Hospital in Berlin, where he took an unpaid position in the expectation of working closely with the renowned surgeon. Sauerbruch's clinic had become the mecca of German surgery, but from the start Forssmann was unhappy. He seldom had a chance to operate on patients, and he rarely saw Sauerbruch. When he did manage to corner him for a few minutes to outline his plans for further experiments, Sauerbruch rejected them. Sauerbruch, the great teacher and the surgeon who had performed pioneering heart operations, failed to appreciate the potential benefits of cardiac catheterization. When Forssmann's paper was published, his superiors at Charité accused him of seeking publicity. A little more than a month after he had started work, Sauerbruch summoned Forssmann to his office and fired him.

Happily for Forssmann, his old position with Schneider was vacant, and he returned to Eberswalde. There he outlined a second experiment with implications as revolutionary as his first. It was an experiment in angiocardiography, a technique in which a radiopaque substance that blocks X rays is injected into an artery or a vein so that the circulatory system can be outlined on the pictures. The areas in which the substance is present appear white on the X-ray film.

Forssmann's proposed technique not only was different but also involved considerable risk. Instead of squirting contrast material into the arm vein so that it would disperse into the blood, Forssmann wanted to put a tube directly into the heart and squirt a different type of contrast material through it. He hoped that the contrast material would outline the anatomy of the chambers of the right side of the heart. Unlike his first experiment, this one required prior work with animals. Because the facilities at the hospital in Eberswalde were too small for this type of research, Forssmann arranged to do the studies with Dr. Willy Felix at Neukölln Hospital in Berlin. He began with rabbits, but they proved unsuitable. When Forssmann's thin catheters touched the animals' hearts, abnormal heart rhythms developed and the rabbits died.

Forssmann then tried dogs. At that time hospitals were not equipped, as they are now, with special quarters for experimental animals. Forssmann's mother cared for the dogs at her apartment. There he would inject a dog with morphine, put the sleepy animal into a potato sack and take it by motorcycle to the hospital. In experiments that recalled those of the French physiologists, Forssmann would push a catheter through a vein in the dog's neck and into its heart.

Radiopaque chemicals were just beginning to be used to help X-ray the urinary system and the stomach. Forssmann knew it would be much more difficult to use the technique with the heart, because the heart moves so rapidly. The X-ray exposure would have to be made quickly and at the precise moment. Forssmann chose an arbitrary dose of one of the radiopaque chemicals and injected it into the dogs. He took X rays, hoping that by luck he would catch a flash of the chemical rushing through one of the chambers of the heart. The first chemical he used killed several dogs, and he switched to another, sodium iodide. This proved to be safe and he managed to get the X rays he wanted. By putting about thirty of them in sequence, he showed that the heart actions could be demonstrated radiographically. Now, at least, he knew that the technique was feasible. But would it be safe on humans?

Forssmann wasn't sure. "I didn't know what the reaction of the intima [the inner lining of blood vessels] would be when the chemical was injected," he said. "I was a little anxious, more nervous than I was before the first self-experiment. You can pull a catheter out of the body, but what is injected into the heart stays in. So I experimented for a few days. I pressed the solutions of sodium iodide against my buccal mucosa [the inside of the mouth] for several hours. I also tested it with samples of blood in the laboratory. There were no reactions. Then I thought: Now I can do it on man." There was never any question in his mind who that man would be.

On the first attempt, a bent catheter tip caused the tube to deviate into a neck vein instead of going into the heart. When the tip reached the middle of the neck, it produced a dull pain in his ear. He tried again. This time the tube went smoothly to the heart. He injected the sodium iodide and felt only a mild irritation of the nasal membranes, an unpleasant transient taste in his mouth, and a slight feeling of dizziness, which passed quickly. Disappointingly, the X rays were unsatisfactory.

Forssmann repeated the experiment. At this point, he was no longer threading the catheter through the veins in his elbow crease because the most readily accessible of these blood vessels had been sewn closed after his previous catheterization experiments. Instead, he was injecting a local anesthetic into the skin around his groin and inserting the catheter into a vein in his upper leg. He would then push it up along the veins in his thigh to the abdomen and further into the main vein that drains blood from the lower half of the body and on into its connection with the heart.

Fifty years later the experience was still vivid in Forssmann's mind. As he watched one of his grandchildren crawl across the living room floor, he explained to me why he had had to be the subject of such a messy and technically difficult experiment: "Nobody else," he said, "would dirty his fingers with such experiments."

On that second try, he experienced the same fleeting light-headed feeling and a warm sensation in his mouth. Once again, the X rays were of poor quality. All that could be seen was a little cloud at the end of the catheter. The pictures were useless for diagnostic purposes. By this time Forssmann had put a tube into his heart *nine* times.

Shortly before Forssmann's report of his angiographic experiments appeared in a medical journal, he presented his findings at a scientific meeting in Berlin. Ferdinand Sauerbruch heard his paper and invited him to return to his clinic. Forssmann, believing that Sauerbruch would now encourage his research, accepted and returned to the Charité Hospital, still as an unpaid assistant. The year was 1931.

Unfortunately, it was more of the same. In the next sixteen months, Forssmann performed just three operations, about as many as he might do with Schneider in a week in Eberswalde. Sauerbruch delegated the running of his clinic to a group of subordinates who neither accepted Forssmann nor believed that he was cut out for scientific research. Forssmann was fired again. As a medical friend told him many years later, "Be happy Sauerbruch and his staff did not understand. Had they, they would have won the Nobel Prize, not you."

By 1935 Forssmann was back in Berlin, this time working with another physician, Dr. Karl Heusch, at the Rudolf Virchow Hospital. And he was ready for another self-experiment. Others had reported the technique of aortography (X rays of the aorta, the main vessel leading from the heart), but only under general anesthesia. Forssmann and Heusch wanted to learn if they could perform this technique using a local anesthetic. The two doctors decided to try it on each other. Aiming with a needle for Forssmann's aorta, Heusch pierced an area between his shoulder blade and a vertebra in his spine. Each jab at the aorta caused Forssmann excruciating pain. After the third unsuccessful attempt, Forssmann took to his bed with headaches and a stiff back.

By now Forssmann was married and had small children. When he suggested repeating the experiment, his wife, who was also a doctor, asked him not to go on. This time Forssmann listened. He had performed his last self-experiment.

To support his family, Forssmann decided to specialize in urology and general surgery. But in spite of his research successes, or more accurately because of them, he had great difficulty getting established. In one town, officials who had read his medical papers turned down his application for the job of chief surgeon. They reasoned that if he had done all these experiments on his own heart, what might he do to the hearts of his patients?

Not only did Forssmann's self-experiments create unexpected difficulties, but so would another experience. At Sauerbruch's clinic, Forssmann had been impressed by a senior staff member, a surgeon who now urged him to join the Nazi party. Forssmann's new Nazi affiliations led to an offer of the very thing his medical colleagues would not grant—the best available scientific equipment and plenty of human guinea pigs with which to carry on his research. Forssmann rejected the opportunity. "To use defenseless patients as guinea pigs," he said, "was a price I would never be prepared to pay for the realization of my dreams."

World War II broke out and Forssmann served with the German Army on the Russian front. In 1945 he avoided capture by the Russians by swimming across the Elbe River. On the other side he was taken prisoner by the American Army.

Later, because of his Nazi associations, West German officials forbade him to practice medicine. In the 1950s, when they rescinded the order, Forssmann found work as a urologist in a small German farming community, where his name was not known. It remained for others to apply his revolutionary techniques to the everyday practice of medicine.

Two of the crucial figures in that effort—Dr. André Cournand and Dr. Dickinson Richards—were based in New York City. During the early 1930s they had read Forssmann's papers on cardiac catheterization and angiography. Although they attached little value to his suggestion of using the technique for emergency administration of drugs, they saw enormous potential in catheterization as a technique to obtain blood samples from the heart in order to study the blood concentration of oxygen and carbon dioxide, the chief respiratory gases in the blood. In 1936 they began a series of experiments in which they catheterized the hearts of dogs and a chimpanzee; they discovered that the concentrations of the gases changed drastically as blood passed from the body into the lungs and back into the heart. In order to understand the physiology of the heart and lungs, doctors needed to know how much these concentrations differed in humans.

But it was four more years—1940—before Richards and Cournand felt confident enough to experiment on a human. Their first human catheterization was performed on a patient dying of cancer at Columbia-Presbyterian Medical Center; the attempt failed because cancerous growths obstructed passage of the tube through the veins. Later Richards and Cournand, working at Bellevue Hospital, used the technique experimentally in patients who were suffering from heart failure due to advanced stages of high blood pressure. By 1942 the New York team had perfected the technique for use in measuring blood components in the right side of the heart and later in the pulmonary artery that delivers deoxygenated blood from the heart to the lungs.

Neither Cournand nor Richards did what they knew Forssmann had done—neither put a tube into his own heart.

As a young man, it is true, Cournand had experimented on himself, allowing dozens of blood samples to be taken from an artery in his wrist; he had also breathed nitrogen and other gases. In an interview with me he said his superiors had rejected his offer to have his heart catheterized as a normal volunteer because of his age; he was then approaching fifty. However, a scientific paper published about those experiments, and coauthored by Cournand, lists the age range of the subjects as thirty-eight to seventy-three. That omission was to haunt Cournand for the rest of his life. "My regret," he admitted, "is from a psychological point of view—that people said, well, he did it on other people but not on himself."

In 1956 Forssmann was plucked from obscurity when he, Cournand, and Richards shared the Nobel Prize in Physiology or Medicine. At the Nobel Prize ceremonies in Stockholm, Professor Göran Liljestrand, an official of the Nobel Committee, paid tribute to Forssmann's courage in doing the "by no means harmless" experiments on himself: "It must have required firm conviction of the value of the method to induce self-experimentation of the kind carried out by Forssmann. His later disappointment must have been all the more bitter ... Forssmann was not given the necessary support; he was, on the contrary, subjected to criticism of such exaggerated severity that it robbed him of any inclination to continue. This criticism was based on an unsubstantiated belief in the danger of the intervention, thus affording proof that—even in our enlightened times—a valuable suggestion may remain unexploited on the grounds of a preconceived opinion."

After winning the Nobel Prize, Forssmann was asked to head a German cardiovascular research institute and to perform open-heart surgery. But he recognized that he was not qualified for either position. He returned to his small farming town and continued to practice urology. "I was conscious that the others had made so much progress I could not catch up on the basics," Forssmann told me. Leaning back in a chair in his living room, glancing a little wistfully at the snowdrifts outside his picture window, he continued, "The basic sciences had become so developed that I would have needed ten years to learn the math, chemistry, and physics necessary to run an institute." Forssmann's deep voice gave way to a chuckle as he told me that even experts sometimes forget what they learn. In 1971, he said, he learned that 140 years earlier another German physician, Johann Dieffenbach, had deliberately put a catheter into the heart of a patient near death from cholera. The aim was to drain thick blood from the heart.

A few months before his death in 1979 at age seventy-four, Forssmann said what must have been on his mind for nearly half a century: "It was very painful. I felt that I had planted an apple orchard and other men who had gathered the harvest stood at the wall, laughing at me."

Today the importance of Werner Forssmann's seedling apples is universally recognized. His techniques have become standard in medical practice. Without them, birth defects affecting the heart would be irreparable and there would be no lifesaving operations on patients whose heart valves have been scarred by bouts with rheumatic fever or other diseases. Nor would heart surgeons be able to do coronary bypass operations to relieve the crushing chest pains of angina pectoris or to minimize the chances of a heart attack. Forssmann's techniques are the basis of many tests, now routine, done in coronary care units to monitor the recovery of patients from heart attacks or in cardiac catheterization laboratories to diagnose heart ailments. Without his work, it would be impossible to implant pacemakers to electronically control the beats of a heart whose rhythm is too slow or erratic. His experiments were as courageous—the results as far-reaching—as any in the annals of medicine.

RAYMOND CARVER

RAYMOND CARVER (1939–1988). *American poet and fiction writer. By the late 1970s, Carver's fiction and poetry marked him as one of the most noteworthy talents of his generation. He was a Guggenheim fellow in 1979 and was twice awarded grants by the National Endowment for the Arts. His collections of stories include* Will You Please Be Quiet, Please? *(1978),* What We Talk About When We Talk About Love *(1981),* Cathedral *(1983), and* Where I'm Calling From: New and Selected Stories *(1988). In 1993, the renowned filmmaker Robert Altman directed a major motion picture,* Short Cuts, *based on several of Carver's short stories. Carver also wrote five books of poetry, the last,* A New Path to the Waterfall, *appearing posthumously in 1989. His work has been translated into more than twenty languages.*

WHAT THE DOCTOR SAID

He said it doesn't look good
he said it looks bad in fact real bad
he said I counted thirty-two of them on one lung before
I quit counting them
I said I'm glad I wouldn't want to know
about any more being there than that
he said are you a religious man do you kneel down
in forest groves and let yourself ask for help
when you come to a waterfall
mist blowing against your face and arms
do you stop and ask for understanding at those moments
I said not yet but I intend to start today
he said I'm real sorry he said
I wish I had some other kind of news to give you
I said Amen and he said something else
I didn't catch and not knowing what else to do
and not wanting him to have to repeat it
and me to have to fully digest it
I just looked at him
for a minute and he looked back it was then
I jumped up and shook hands with this man who'd just given me

something no one else on earth had ever given me
I may even have thanked him habit being so strong

MY DEATH

If I'm lucky, I'll be wired every whichway
in a hospital bed. Tubes running into
my nose. But try not to be scared of me, friends!
I'm telling you right now that this is okay.
It's little enough to ask for at the end.
Someone, I hope, will have phoned everyone
to say, "Come quick, he's failing!"
And they will come. And there will be time for me
to bid goodbye to each of my loved ones.
If I'm lucky, they'll step forward
and I'll be able to see them one last time
and take that memory with me.
Sure, they might lay eyes on me and want to run away
and howl. But instead, since they love me,
they'll lift my hand and say "Courage"
or "It's going to be all right."
And they're right. It is all right.
It's just fine. If you only knew how happy you've made me!
I just hope my luck holds, and I can make
some sign of recognition.
Open and close my eyes as if to say,
"Yes, I hear you. I understand you."
I may even manage something like this:
"I love you too. Be happy."
I hope so! But I don't want to ask for too much.
If I'm unlucky, as I deserve, well, I'll just
drop over, like that, without any chance
for farewell, or to press anyone's hand.
Or say how much I cared for you and enjoyed
your company all these years. In any case,
try not to mourn for me too much. I want you to know
I was happy when I was here.
And remember I told you this a while ago—April 1984.
But be glad for me if I can die in the presence
of friends and family. If this happens, believe me,
I came out ahead. I didn't lose this one.

ERRAND

Chekhov. On the evening of March 22, 1897, he went to dinner in Moscow with his friend and confidant Alexei Suvorin. This Suvorin was a very rich newspaper and book publisher, a reactionary, a self-made man whose father was a private at the battle of Borodino. Like Chekhov, he was the grandson of a serf. They had that in common: each had peasant's blood in his veins. Otherwise, politically and temperamentally, they were miles apart. Nevertheless, Suvorin was one of Chekhov's few intimates, and Chekhov enjoyed his company.

Naturally, they went to the best restaurant in the city, a former town house called the Hermitage—a place where it could take hours, half the night even, to get through a ten-course meal that would, of course, include several wines, liqueurs, and coffee. Chekhov was impeccably dressed, as always—a dark suit and waistcoat, his usual pince-nez. He looked that night very much as he looks in the photographs taken of him during this period. He was relaxed, jovial. He shook hands with the maître d', and with a glance took in the large dining room. It was brilliantly illuminated by ornate chandeliers, the tables occupied by elegantly dressed men and women. Waiters came and went ceaselessly. He had just been seated across the table from Suvorin when suddenly, without warning, blood began gushing from his mouth. Suvorin and two waiters helped him to the gentlemen's room and tried to stanch the flow of blood with ice packs. Suvorin saw him back to his own hotel and had a bed prepared for Chekhov in one of the rooms of the suite. Later, after another hemorrhage, Chekhov allowed himself to be moved to a clinic that specialized in the treatment of tuberculosis and related respiratory infections. When Suvorin visited him there, Chekhov apologized for the "scandal" at the restaurant three nights earlier but continued to insist there was nothing seriously wrong. "He laughed and jested as usual," Suvorin noted in his diary, "while spitting blood into a large vessel."

Maria Chekhov, his younger sister, visited Chekhov in the clinic during the last days of March. The weather was miserable; a sleet storm was in progress, and frozen heaps of snow lay everywhere. It was hard for her to wave down a carriage to take her to the hospital. By the time she arrived she was filled with dread and anxiety.

"Anton Pavlovich lay on his back," Maria wrote in her "Memoirs." "He was not allowed to speak. After greeting him, I went over to the table to hide my emotions." There, among bottles of champagne, jars of caviar, bouquets of flowers from well-wishers, she saw something that terrified her: a freehand drawing, obviously done by a specialist in these matters, of Chekhov's lungs. It was the kind of sketch a doctor often makes in order to show his patient what he thinks is taking place. The lungs were outlined in blue, but the upper parts were filled in with red. "I realized they were diseased," Maria wrote.

Leo Tolstoy was another visitor. The hospital staff were awed to find themselves in the presence of the country's greatest writer. The most famous man in Russia? Of course they had to let him in to see Chekhov, even though "nonessential" visitors were forbidden. With much obsequiousness on the part of the nurses and resident doctors, the bearded, fierce-looking old man was shown into Chekhov's room. Despite his low opinion of Chekhov's abilities as a playwright (Tolstoy felt the plays were static and lacking in any moral vision. "Where do your characters take you?" he once demanded of Chekhov. "From the sofa to the junk room and back"), Tolstoy liked Chekhov's short stories. Furthermore, and quite simply, he loved the man. He told Gorky, "What a beautiful, magnificent man: modest and quiet, like a girl. He even walks like a girl. He's simply wonderful." And Tolstoy wrote in his journal (everyone kept a journal or a diary in those days), "I am glad I love . . . Chekhov."

Tolstoy removed his woollen scarf and bearskin coat, then lowered himself into a chair next to Chekhov's bed. Never mind that Chekhov was taking medication and not permitted to talk, much less carry on a conversation. He had to listen, amazedly, as the Count began to discourse on his theories of the immortality of the soul. Concerning that visit, Chekhov later wrote, "Tolstoy assumes that all of us (humans and animals alike) will live on in a principle (such as reason or love) the essence and goals of which are a mystery to us. . . . I have no use for that kind of immortality. I don't understand it, and Lev Nikolayevich was astonished I didn't."

Nevertheless, Chekhov was impressed with the solicitude shown by Tolstoy's visit. But, unlike Tolstoy, Chekhov didn't believe in an afterlife and never had. He didn't believe in anything that couldn't be apprehended by one or more of his five senses. And as far as his outlook on life and writing went, he once told someone that he lacked "a political, religious, and philosophical world view. I change it every month, so I'll have to limit myself to the description of how my heroes love, marry, give birth, die, and how they speak."

Earlier, before his t.b. was diagnosed, Chekhov had remarked, "When a peasant has consumption, he says, 'There's nothing I can do. I'll go off in the spring with the melting of the snows.'" (Chekhov himself died in the summer, during a heat wave.) But once Chekhov's own tuberculosis was discovered he continually tried to minimize the seriousness of his condition. To all appearances, it was as if he felt, right up to the end, that he might be able to throw off the disease as he would a lingering catarrh. Well into his final days, he spoke with seeming conviction of the possibility of an improvement. In fact, in a letter written shortly before his end, he went so far as to tell his sister that he was "putting on a bit of flesh" and felt much better now that he was in Badenweiler.

Badenweiler is a spa and resort city in the western area of the Black Forest, not far from Basel. The Vosges are visible from nearly anywhere in the city, and in those days the air was pure and invigorating. Russians had been going there for years to soak in the hot mineral baths and promenade on the boulevards. In June, 1904, Chekhov went there to die.

Earlier that month, he'd made a difficult journey by train from Moscow to Berlin. He travelled with his wife, the actress Olga Knipper, a woman he'd met in 1898 during rehearsals for "The Seagull." Her contemporaries describe her as an excellent actress. She was talented, pretty, and almost ten years younger than the playwright. Chekhov had been immediately attracted to her, but was slow to act on his feelings. As always, he preferred a flirtation to marriage. Finally, after a three-year courtship involving many separations, letters, and the inevitable misunderstandings, they were at last married, in a private ceremony in Moscow, on May 25, 1901. Chekhov was enormously happy. He called Olga his "pony," and sometimes "dog" or "puppy." He was also fond of addressing her as "little turkey" or simply as "my joy."

In Berlin, Chekhov consulted with a renowned specialist in pulmonary disorders, a Dr. Karl Ewald. But, according to an eyewitness, after the doctor examined Chekhov he threw up his hands and left the room without a word. Chekhov was too far gone for help: this Dr. Ewald was furious with himself for not being able to work miracles, and with Chekhov for being so ill.

A Russian journalist happened to visit the Chekhovs at their hotel and sent back this dispatch to his editor: "Chekhov's days are numbered. He seems mortally ill, is terribly thin, coughs all the time, gasps for breath at the slightest movement, and is running a high temperature." This same journalist saw the Chekhovs off at Potsdam Station when they boarded their train for Badenweiler. According to his account, "Chekhov had trouble making his way up the small staircase at the station. He had to sit down for several minutes to catch his breath." In fact, it was painful for Chekhov to move: his legs ached continually and his insides hurt. The disease had attacked his intestines and spinal cord. At this point he had less than a month to live. When Chekhov spoke of his condition now, it was, according to Olga, "with an almost reckless indifference."

Dr. Schwöhrer was one of the many Badenweiler physicians who earned a good living by treating the well-to-do who came to the spa seeking relief from various maladies. Some of his patients were ill and infirm, others simply old and hypochondriacal. But Chekhov's was a special case: he was clearly beyond help and in his last days. He was also very famous. Even Dr. Schwöhrer knew his name: he'd read some of Chekhov's stories in a German magazine. When he examined the writer early in June, he voiced his appreciation of Chekhov's art but kept his medical opinions to himself. Instead, he prescribed a diet of cocoa, oatmeal drenched in butter, and strawberry tea. This last was supposed to help Chekhov sleep at night.

On June 13th, less than three weeks before he died, Chekhov wrote a letter to his mother in which he told her his health was on the mend. In it he said, "It's likely that I'll be completely cured in a week." Who knows why he said this? What could he have been thinking? He was a doctor himself, and he knew better. He was dying, it was as simple and as unavoidable as that. Nevertheless, he sat out on the balcony of his hotel room and read railway timetables. He asked for information on sailings of boats bound for Odessa from Marseilles. But he *knew*. At this stage he had to have known. Yet in one of the last letters he ever wrote he told his sister he was growing stronger by the day.

He no longer had any appetite for literary work, and hadn't for a long time. In fact, he had very nearly failed to complete "The Cherry Orchard" the year before. Writing that play was the hardest thing he'd ever done in his life. Toward the end, he was able to manage only six or seven lines a day. "I've started losing heart," he wrote Olga. "I feel I'm finished as a writer, and every sentence strikes me as worthless and of no use whatever." But he didn't stop. He finished his play in October, 1903. It was the last thing he ever wrote, except for letters and a few entries in his notebook.

A little after midnight on July 2, 1904, Olga sent someone to fetch Dr. Schwöhrer. It was an emergency: Chekhov was delirious. Two young Russians on holiday happened to have the adjacent room, and Olga hurried next door to explain what was happening. One of the youths was in his bed asleep, but the other was still awake, smoking and reading. He left the hotel at a run to find Dr. Schwöhrer. "I can still hear the sound of the gravel under his shoes in the silence of that stifling July night," Olga wrote later on in her memoirs. Chekhov was hallucinating, talking about sailors, and there were snatches of something about the Japanese. "You don't put ice on an empty stomach," he said when she tried to place an ice pack on his chest.

Dr. Schwöhrer arrived and unpacked his bag, all the while keeping his gaze fastened on Chekhov, who lay gasping in the bed. The sick man's pupils were dilated and his temples glistened with sweat. Dr. Schwöhrer's face didn't register anything. He was not an emotional man, but he knew Chekhov's end was near. Still, he was a doctor, sworn to do his utmost, and Chekhov held on to life, however tenuously. Dr. Schwöhrer prepared a hypodermic and administered an injection of camphor, something that was supposed to speed up the heart. But the injection didn't help—nothing, of course, could have helped. Nevertheless, the doctor made known to Olga his intention of sending for oxygen. Suddenly, Chekhov roused himself, became lucid, and said quietly, "What's the use? Before it arrives I'll be a corpse."

Dr. Schwöhrer pulled on his big mustache and stared at Chekhov. The writer's cheeks were sunken and gray, his complexion waxen; his breath was raspy. Dr. Schwöhrer knew the time could be reckoned in minutes. Without a word, without conferring with Olga, he went over to an alcove where there was a telephone on the wall. He read the instructions for using the device. If he activated it by holding his finger on a button and turning a handle on the side of the phone, he could reach the lower regions of the hotel—the kitchen. He picked up the receiver, held it to his ear, and did as the instructions told him. When someone finally answered, Dr. Schwöhrer ordered a bottle of the hotel's best champagne. "How many glasses?" he was asked. "Three glasses!" the doctor shouted into the mouthpiece. "And hurry, do you hear?" It was one of those rare moments of inspiration that can easily enough be overlooked later on, because the action is so entirely appropriate it seems inevitable.

The champagne was brought to the door by a tired-looking young man whose blond hair was standing up. The trousers of his uniform were wrinkled, the creases gone, and in his haste he'd missed a loop while buttoning his jacket. His appearance was that of someone who'd been resting (slumped in a chair, say, dozing a little), when off in the distance the phone had clamored in the early-morning hours—great God in Heaven!—and the next thing he knew he was being shaken awake by a superior and told to deliver a bottle of Moët to Room 211. "And hurry, do you hear?"

The young man entered the room carrying a silver ice bucket with the champagne in it and a silver tray with three cut-crystal glasses. He found a place on the table for the bucket and glasses, all the while craning his neck, trying to see into the other room, where someone panted ferociously for breath. It was a dreadful, harrowing sound, and the young man lowered his chin into his collar and turned away as the ratchety breathing worsened. Forgetting himself, he stared out the open window toward the darkened city. Then this big imposing man with a thick mustache pressed some coins into his hand—a large tip, by the feel of it—and suddenly the young man saw the door open. He took some steps and found himself on the landing, where he opened his hand and looked at the coins in amazement.

Methodically, the way he did everything, the doctor went about the business of working the cork out of the bottle. He did it in such a way as to minimize, as much as possible, the festive explosion. He poured three glasses and, out of habit, pushed the cork back into the neck of the bottle. He then took the glasses of champagne over to the bed. Olga momentarily released her grip on Chekhov's hand—a hand, she said later, that burned her fingers. She arranged another pillow behind his head. Then she put the cool glass of champagne against Chekhov's palm and made sure his fingers closed around the stem. They exchanged looks—Chekhov, Olga, Dr. Schwöhrer. They didn't touch glasses. There was no toast. What on earth was there to drink to? To death? Chekhov summoned his remaining strength and said, "It's been so long since I've had champagne." He brought the glass to his lips and drank. In a minute or two Olga took the empty glass from his hand and set it on the nightstand. Then Chekhov turned onto his side. He closed his eyes and sighed. A minute later, his breathing stopped.

Dr. Schwöhrer picked up Chekhov's hand from the bedsheet. He held his fingers to Chekhov's wrist and drew a gold watch from his vest pocket, opening the lid of the watch as he did so. The second hand on the watch moved slowly, very slowly. He let it move around the face of the watch three times while he waited for signs of a pulse. It was three o'clock in the morning and still sultry in the room. Badenweiler was in the grip of its worst heat wave in years. All the windows in both rooms stood open, but there was no sign of a breeze. A large, black-winged moth flew through a window and banged wildly against the electric lamp. Dr. Schwöhrer let go of Chekhov's wrist. "It's over," he said. He closed the lid of his watch and returned it to his vest pocket.

At once Olga dried her eyes and set about composing herself. She thanked the doctor for coming. He asked if she wanted some medication—laudanum, perhaps, or a few drops of valerian. She shook her head. She did have one request, though: before the authorities were notified and the newspapers found out, before the time came when Chekhov was no longer in her keeping, she wanted to be alone with him for a while. Could the doctor help with this? Could he withhold, for a while anyway, news of what had just occurred?

Dr. Schwöhrer stroked his mustache with the back of a finger. Why not? After all, what difference would it make to anyone whether this matter became known now or a few hours from now? The only detail that remained was to fill out a death certificate, and this could be done at his office later on in the morning, after he'd slept a few hours. Dr. Schwöhrer nodded his agreement and prepared to leave. He murmured a few words of condolence. Olga inclined her head. "An honor," Dr. Schwöhrer said. He picked up his bag and left the room and, for that matter, history.

It was at this moment that the cork popped out of the champagne bottle; foam spilled down onto the table. Olga went back to Chekhov's bedside. She sat on a footstool, holding his hand, from time to time stroking his face. "There were no human voices, no everyday sounds," she wrote. "There was only beauty, peace, and the grandeur of death."

She stayed with Chekhov until daybreak, when thrushes began to call from the garden below. Then came the sound of tables and chairs being moved about down there. Before long, voices carried up to her. It was then a knock sounded at the door. Of course she thought it must be an official of some sort—the medical examiner, say, or someone from the police who had questions to ask and forms for her to fill out, or maybe, just maybe, it could be Dr. Schwöhrer returning with a mortician to render assistance in embalming and transporting Chekhov's remains back to Russia.

But, instead, it was the same blond young man who'd brought the champagne a few hours earlier. This time, however, his uniform trousers were neatly pressed, with stiff creases in front, and every button on his snug green jacket was fastened. He seemed quite another person. Not only was he wide awake but his plump cheeks were smooth-shaven, his hair was in place, and he appeared anxious to please. He was holding a porcelain vase with three long-stemmed yellow roses. He presented these to Olga with a smart click of his heels. She stepped back and let him into the room. He was there, he said, to collect the glasses, ice bucket, and tray, yes. But he also wanted to say that, because of the extreme heat, breakfast would be served in the garden this morning. He hoped this weather wasn't too bothersome; he apologized for it.

The woman seemed distracted. While he talked, she turned her eyes away and looked down at something in the carpet. She crossed her arms and held her elbows. Meanwhile, still holding his vase, waiting for a sign, the young man took in the details of the room. Bright sunlight flooded through the open windows. The room was tidy and seemed undisturbed, almost untouched. No garments were flung over chairs, no shoes, stockings, braces, or stays were in evidence, no open suitcases. In short, there was no clutter, nothing but the usual heavy pieces of hotel-room furniture. Then, because the woman was still looking down, he looked down, too, and at once spied a cork near the toe of his shoe. The woman did not see it—she was looking somewhere else. The young man wanted to bend over and pick up the cork, but he was still holding the roses and was afraid of seeming to intrude even more by drawing any further attention to himself. Reluctantly, he left the cork where it was and raised his eyes. Everything was in order except for the uncorked, half-empty bottle of champagne that stood alongside two crystal glasses over on the little table. He cast his gaze about once more. Through an open door he saw that the third glass was in the bedroom, on the nightstand. But someone still occupied the bed! He couldn't see a face, but the figure under the covers lay perfectly motionless and quiet. He noted the figure and looked elsewhere. Then, for a reason he couldn't understand, a feeling of uneasiness took hold of him. He cleared his throat and moved his weight to the other leg. The woman still didn't look up or break her silence. The young man felt his cheeks grow warm. It occurred to him, quite without his having thought it through, that he should perhaps suggest an alternative to breakfast in the garden. He coughed, hoping to focus the woman's attention, but she didn't look at him. The distinguished foreign guests could, he said, take breakfast in their rooms this morning if they wished. The young man (his name hasn't survived, and it's likely he perished in the Great War) said he would be happy to bring up a tray. Two trays, he added, glancing uncertainly once again in the direction of the bedroom.

He fell silent and ran a finger around the inside of his collar. He didn't understand. He wasn't even sure the woman had been listening. He didn't know what else to do now; he was still holding the vase. The sweet odor of the roses filled his nostrils and inexplicably caused a pang of regret. The entire time he'd been waiting, the woman had apparently been lost in thought. It was as if all the while he'd been standing there, talking, shifting his weight, holding his flowers, she had been someplace else, somewhere far from Badenweiler. But now she came back to herself, and her face assumed another expression.

She raised her eyes, looked at him, and then shook her head. She seemed to be struggling to understand what on earth this young man could be doing there in the room holding a vase with three yellow roses. Flowers? She hadn't ordered flowers.

The moment passed. She went over to her handbag and scooped up some coins. She drew out a number of banknotes as well. The young man touched his lips with his tongue; another large tip was forthcoming, but for what? What did she want him to do? He'd never before waited on such guests. He cleared his throat once more.

No breakfast, the woman said. Not yet, at any rate. Breakfast wasn't the important thing this morning. She required something else. She needed him to go out and bring back a mortician. Did he understand her? Herr Chekhov was dead, you see. *Comprenez-vous?* Young man? Anton Chekhov was dead. Now listen carefully to me, she said. She wanted him to go downstairs and ask someone at the front desk where he could go to find the most respected mortician in the city. Someone reliable, who took great pains in his work and whose manner was appropriately reserved. A mortician, in short, worthy of a great artist. Here, she said, and pressed the money on him. Tell them downstairs that I have specifically requested you to perform this duty for me. Are you listening? Do you understand what I'm saying to you?

The young man grappled to take in what she was saying. He chose not to look again in the direction of the other room. He had sensed that something was not right. He became aware of his heart beating rapidly under his jacket, and he felt perspiration break out on his forehead. He didn't know where he should turn his eyes. He wanted to put the vase down.

Please do this for me, the woman said. I'll remember you with gratitude. Tell them downstairs that I insist. Say that. But don't call any unnecessary attention to yourself or to the situation. Just say that this is necessary, that I request it—and that's all. Do you hear me? Nod if you understand. Above all, don't raise an alarm. Everything else, all the rest, the commotion—that'll come soon enough. The worst is over. Do we understand each other?

The young man's face had grown pale. He stood rigid, clasping the vase. He managed to nod his head.

After securing permission to leave the hotel he was to proceed quietly and resolutely, though without any unbecoming haste, to the mortician's. He was to behave exactly as if he were engaged on a very important errand, nothing more. He *was* engaged on an important errand, she said. And if it would help keep his movements purposeful he should imagine himself as someone moving down the busy sidewalk carrying in his arms a porcelain vase of roses that he had to deliver to an important man. (She spoke quietly, almost confidentially, as if to a relative or a friend.) He could even tell himself that the man he was going to see was expecting him, was perhaps impatient for him to arrive with his flowers. Nevertheless, the young man was not to become excited and run, or otherwise break his stride. Remember the vase he was carrying! He was to walk briskly, comporting himself at all times in as dignified a manner as possible. He should keep walking until he came to the mortician's house and stood before the door. He would then raise the brass knocker and let it fall, once, twice, three times. In a minute the mortician himself would answer.

This mortician would be in his forties, no doubt, or maybe early fifties—bald, solidly built, wearing steel-frame spectacles set very low on his nose. He would be modest, unassuming, a man who would ask only the most direct and necessary questions. An apron. Probably he would be wearing an apron. He might even be wiping his hands on a dark towel while he listened to what was being said. There'd be a faint whiff of formaldehyde on his clothes. But it was all right, and the young man shouldn't worry. He was nearly a grownup now and shouldn't be frightened or repelled by any of this. The mortician would hear him out. He was a man of restraint and bearing, this mortician, someone who could help allay people's fears in this situation, not increase them. Long ago he'd acquainted himself with death in all its various guises and forms; death held no surprises for him any longer, no hidden secrets. It was this man whose services were required this morning.

The mortician takes the vase of roses. Only once while the young man is speaking does the mortician betray the least flicker of interest, or indicate that he's heard anything out of the ordinary. But the one time the young man mentions the name of the deceased, the mortician's eyebrows rise just a little. Chekhov, you say? Just a minute, and I'll be with you.

Do you understand what I'm saying, Olga said to the young man. Leave the glasses. Don't worry about them. Forget about crystal wineglasses and such. Leave the room as it is. Everything is ready now. We're ready. Will you go?

But at that moment the young man was thinking of the cork still resting near the toe of his shoe. To retrieve it he would have to bend over, still gripping the vase. He would do this. He leaned over. Without looking down, he reached out and closed it into his hand.

MARGARET ATWOOD

MARGARET ATWOOD (1939–). Canadian poet and fiction writer.
Atwood has won numerous prizes for her poetry as well as her fiction,
which critics have dubbed "Atwoodian—for its virtuoso wit and
unmistakable style." She has published eight novels, among them The
Handmaid's Tale *(1986),* Cat's Eye *(1988), and, most recently,* The
Robber Bride *(1993); eleven volumes of poetry; and five collections of*
short fiction, including the critically celebrated Wilderness Tips *(1991)*
and Good Bones and Small Murders *(1994). Her latest novel is* The
Blind Assassin *(2000).*

THE WOMAN WHO COULD NOT LIVE
WITH HER FAULTY HEART

I do not mean the symbol
of love, a candy shape
to decorate cakes with,
the heart that is supposed
to belong or break;

I mean this lump of muscle
that contracts like a flayed biceps,
purple-blue, with its skin of suet,
its skin of gristle, this isolate,
this caved hermit, unshelled
turtle, this one lungful of blood,
no happy plateful.

All hearts float in their own
deep oceans of no light,
wetblack and glimmering,
their four mouths gulping like fish.
Hearts are said to pound:
this is to be expected, the heart's
regular struggle against being drowned.

But most hearts say, I want, I want,
I want, I want. My heart
is more duplicitous,

though no twin as I once thought.
It says, I want, I don't want, I
want, and then a pause.
It forces me to listen,
and at night it is the infra-red
third eye that remains open
while the other two are sleeping
but refuses to say what it has seen.

It is a constant pestering
in my ears, a caught moth, limping drum,
a child's fist beating
itself against the bedsprings:
I want, I don't want.
How can one live with such a heart?

Long ago I gave up singing
to it, it will never be satisfied or lulled.
One night I will say to it:
Heart, be still,
and it will.

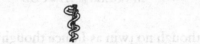

DEREK MAHON

DEREK MAHON (1941–). *Irish poet, playwright, translator, and editor. Mahon was born in Belfast, Northern Ireland, and educated at Trinity College, Dublin. He worked for some years in London as a journalist and screenwriter, working to adapt Irish novels for television. He has worked in editorial positions at the* New Statesman, Vogue, *and the* Irish Times. *He has been a prolific writer: his award-winning books include* The Hudson Letter, Selected Poems, The Hunt by Night, The Yellow Book, *and* Antarctica. *His verse translations include Molière's* The School for Wives *and the* Bacchae *of Euripides. He has edited* The Penguin Book of Contemporary Irish Poetry *and* Modern Irish Poetry. *His work has earned several awards, including the Irish American Foundation Award, a Guggenheim fellowship, the American Ireland Fund Literary Award, and the Eric Gregory Award. The reviewer John Banville has written, "Derek Mahon is one of the finest Irish poets of his generation, graceful, elegiac, and a consummate craftsman."*

EVERYTHING IS GOING TO BE ALL RIGHT

How should I not be glad to contemplate
the clouds clearing beyond the dormer window
and a high tide reflected on the ceiling?
There will be dying, there will be dying,
but there is no need to go into that.
The poems flow from the hand unbidden
and the hidden source is the watchful heart.
The sun rises in spite of everything
and the far cities are beautiful and bright.
I lie here in a riot of sunlight
watching the day break and the clouds flying.
Everything is going to be all right.

MARILYN KRYSL

MARILYN KRYSL (1942–). *American poet and writer. Krysl has published seven books of poetry and two volumes of fiction, the most recent,* How to Accommodate Men. *Her poetry and stories have appeared in such annual anthologies as the* Pushcart Prize Anthology *and* Prize Stories: The O. Henry Awards, *along with many journals and other publications. She is currently director of creative writing at the University of Colorado at Boulder. While her poetry reflects a wide range of her interests, she is particularly interested in health and healing. Some of her poetry grew out of the year she spent as artist in residence at the Center for Human Caring at the University of Colorado School of Nursing, which commissioned her to reflect on and write about the day-to-day experiences of nurses and nursing students and their relationships with patients. Other poetry records her experiences as a volunteer in the Kalighat Home for the Destitute and Dying, administered by Mother Teresa's Missionaries of Charity, or time she spent with* curanderas, Navajo *healers, and alternative healers.*

THERE IS NO SUCH THING AS THE MOMENT OF DEATH

I work nights, and he was awake.
When he saw me, he said, "I'm not going to
make it." Well when they say that
they know. People can tell. You don't

argue with an expert. I wet the cloth
and bathed his face, but it didn't do him
good. So I took his hands in my two
and we held on. No one

was alone in that motion. The way water
is a part of itself, we were the going
until his hands went slack in mine.
Still I held on, some final acknowledgment

317

beginning its climb out of the body,
his skin resilient still, that shine
across a taut thing—then I saw it sag
and go flat. His body had a clearness

about it then, the clean weightlessness
of a crucible completely empty,
in which you hear the air ticking
against the glaze. Then I heard another

sound, like when you're a kid, holding
a shell to your ear, hearing
the ocean. I held on, and then I understood:
it was the sound of my own blood.

SHARON OLDS

SHARON OLDS (1942–). *American poet. Sharon Olds is best known for the candor and eroticism of her poetry, which has been called both "purifying" and "redemptive." Collections of Olds's poetry include* Satan Says *(1980);* The Dead and the Living *(1983), which was the 1983 Lamont Poetry Selection and won the National Book Critics Circle Award in 1984;* The Gold Cell *(1989); and* The Father *(1992). Her most recent books of poetry are* The Wellspring: Poems *(1996) and* Blood, Tin, Straw *(1999).*

35/10

Brushing out my daughter's dark
silken hair before the mirror
I see the grey gleaming on my head,
the silver-haired servant behind her. Why is it
just as we begin to go
they begin to arrive, the fold in my neck
clarifying as the fine bones of her
hips sharpen? As my skin shows
its dry pitting, she opens like a small
pale flower on the tip of a cactus;
as my last chances to bear a child
are falling through my body, the duds among them,
her full purse of eggs, round and
firm as hard-boiled yolks, is about
to snap its clasp. I brush her tangled
fragrant hair at bedtime. It's an old
story—the oldest we have on our planet—
the story of replacement.

MISCARRIAGE

When I was a month pregnant, the great
clots of blood appeared in the pale
green swaying water of the toilet.
Dark red like black in the salty
translucent brine, like forms of life
appearing, jelly-fish with the clear-cut
shapes of fungi.

That was the only appearance made by that
child, the dark, scalloped shapes
falling slowly. A month later
our son was conceived, and I never went back
to mourn the one who came as far as the
sill with its information: that we could
botch something, you and I. All wrapped in
purple it floated away, like a messenger
put to death for bearing bad news.

JACK COULEHAN

JACK COULEHAN (1943–). *American physician, poet, and writer. Born in Pittsburgh, Dr. Coulehan received his B.A. from St. Vincent College and his M.D. and M.P.H. degrees from the University of Pittsburgh. He is now professor of medicine at the State University of New York–Stony Brook. His poetry has been widely published; collections include* The Knitted Glove *(1991) and* First Photographs of Heaven *(1994). With Angela Belli, he edited* Blood and Bone *(1998), a collection of poems by physicians.*

THE KNITTED GLOVE

You come into my office wearing a blue
knitted glove with a ribbon at the wrist.
You remove the glove slowly, painfully,
and dump out the contents, a worthless hand.
What a specimen! It looks much like a regular hand,
warm, pliable, soft, you can move the fingers.

If it's not one thing, it's another.
Last month the fire in your hips had you down
or up mincing across the room with a cane.
When I ask about the hips today, you pass it off
so I can't tell if only the pain
or the memory is gone. The knitted hand
is the long and short of it, pain doesn't exist
in the past any more than this morning does.

This thing, the name for your solitary days,
for the hips, the hand, for the walk of your eyes
away from mine, this thing is coyote, a trickster.
I want to call, "Come out, you son of a dog!"
and wrestle that name to the ground for you,
I want to take its neck between my hands.
But in this world I don't know how to find
the bastard, so we sit. We talk about the pain.

GOOD NEWS

The first bad news is a spot on my lung
when all I came to the doctor for
was a leg that burnt like scalding water.

Then they find a hole in my spine,
right at the place my back kicked out
the day I jumped an aluminum ladder.

But no, my doctor looks at the wall
and says the black egg growing in my back
is not that, it's something new.

Today's scan shows a hole in my liver
and, strangely, though I'm still not sick,
my body begins to die.

There's Drano dripping in my vein
to scour the blood clot, and each day
brings another test and more bad news.

Toward the back of the morning paper,
I read stories of love and reunion,
tales of miraculous cures.

Mothers and children lost in the war,
sons who search, twins parted at birth,
brothers who search . . . at last they meet.

A retired butcher finds a girl
he courted in Palermo, 1946,
and they dance all night in Niles, Ohio.

Good news. That's what I need to hear,
not the next painful step
on the ladder, to the next lower rung.

Good news! If I ever get out of here,
I'll rent a bowling alley
and we'll dance all night in Niles, Ohio.

ALICE WALKER

ALICE WALKER (1944–). *African-American writer. Walker is the author of the critically acclaimed* The Color Purple, *which earned her the American Book Award and the Pulitzer Prize in 1983 and was later made into an Academy Award–winning film. One critic called* The Temple of My Familiar *(1989) "a rich tapestry of human emotion woven with poetry and passion." Other books include* Possessing the Secret of Joy *(1992);* The Third Life of Grange Copeland *(1985); and* Meridian *(1976); two short-story collections,* In Love and Trouble *(1974) and* You Can't Keep a Good Woman Down *(1982); four volumes of poetry; and a biography of Langston Hughes for children. The following selection is from Walker's first book,* Once, *originally published in 1968.*

MEDICINE

Grandma sleeps with
    my sick
              grand-
pa so she
can get him
during the night
medicine
to stop
    the pain

        In
    the morning
        clumsily
        I
    wake
        them

ALICE WALKER

Her eyes
look at me
from under-
     neath
his withered
arm

The
medicine
is all
in
her long
un-
     braided
     hair.

DAVID HILFIKER

DAVID HILFIKER (1945–). *American physician and writer. Dr. Hilfiker graduated from Yale College and the University of Minnesota Medical School. A family practitioner in a small town in Minnesota from 1975 to 1982, he then served as medical director of Columbia Road Health Services in Washington, D.C. His books include* Healing the Wounds: A Physician Looks at His Work *(1985) and* Not All of Us Are Saints: A Doctor's Journey with the Poor *(1994), a painfully honest account of the horrific state of affairs among the poor and ill of Washington, D.C., and of Hilfiker's attempt as a physician to do something about it.*

MISTAKES

On a warm July morning I finish my rounds at the hospital around nine o'clock and walk across the parking lot to the clinic. After greeting Jackie, I look through the list of my day's appointments and notice that Barb Daily will be in for her first prenatal examination. "Wonderful," I think, recalling the joy of helping her deliver her first child two years ago. Barb and her husband, Russ, had been friends of mine before Heather was born, but we grew much closer with the shared experience of her birth. In a rural family practice such as mine, much of every weekday is taken up with disease; I look forward to the prenatal visit with Barb, to the continuing relationship with her over the next months, to the prospect of birth.

At her appointment that afternoon, Barb seems to be in good health, with all the signs and symptoms of pregnancy: slight nausea, some soreness in her breasts, a little weight gain. But when the nurse tests Barb's urine to determine if she is pregnant, the result is negative. The test measures the level of a hormone that is produced by a woman and shows up in her urine when she is pregnant. But occasionally it fails to detect the low levels of the hormone during early pregnancy. I reassure Barb that she is fine and schedule another test for the following week.

Barb leaves a urine sample at the clinic a week later, but the test is negative again. I am troubled. Perhaps she isn't pregnant. Her missed menstrual period and her other symptoms could be a result of a minor hormonal imbalance. Maybe the embryo has died within the uterus and a miscarriage is soon to take place. I could find out by ordering an ultrasound examination. This procedure would give me a "picture" of the uterus and of the embryo. But Barb would have to go to Duluth for the examination. The procedure is also expensive. I know the Dailys well enough to know they have a modest income. Besides, by waiting a few weeks, I should be able to find out for sure without the ultrasound: either the urine test will be positive or Barb will have a miscarriage. I call her and tell her about the negative test result, about the possibility of a miscarriage, and about the necessity of seeing me again if she misses her next menstrual period.

It is, as usual, a hectic summer; I think no more about Barb's troubling state until a month later, when she returns to my office. Nothing has changed: still no menstrual period, still no miscarriage. She is confused and upset. "I feel so pregnant," she tells me. I am bothered, too. Her uterus, upon examination, is slightly enlarged, as it was on the previous visit. But it hasn't grown any larger. Her urine test remains negative. I can think of several possible explanations for her condition, including a hormonal imbalance or even a tumor. But the most likely explanation is that she is carrying a dead embryo. I decide it is time to break the bad news to her.

"I think you have what doctors call a 'missed abortion,'" I tell her. "You were probably pregnant, but the baby appears to have died some weeks ago, before your first examination. Unfortunately, you didn't have a miscarriage to get rid of the dead tissue from the baby and the placenta. If a miscarriage doesn't occur within a few weeks, I'd recommend a re-examination, another pregnancy test, and if nothing shows up, a dilation and curettage procedure to clean out the uterus."

Barb is disappointed; there are tears. She is college-educated, and she understands the scientific and technical aspects of her situation, but that doesn't alleviate the sorrow. We talk at some length and make an appointment for two weeks later.

When Barb returns, Russ is with her. Still no menstrual period; still no miscarriage; still another negative pregnancy test, the fourth. I explain to them what has happened. The dead embryo should be removed or there could be serious complications. Infection could develop; Barb could even become sterile. The conversation is emotionally difficult for all three of us. We schedule the dilation and curettage for later in the week.

Friday morning, Barb is wheeled into the small operating room of the hospital. Barb, the nurses, and I all know one another—it's a small town. The atmosphere is warm and relaxed; we chat before the operation. After Barb is anesthetized, I examine her pelvis again. Her muscles are now completely relaxed, and it is possible to perform a more reliable examination. Her uterus feels bigger than it did two days ago; it is perhaps the size of a small grapefruit. But since all the pregnancy tests were negative and I'm so sure of the diagnosis, I ignore the information from my fingertips and begin the operation.

Dilation and curettage, or D & C, is a relatively simple surgical procedure performed thousands of times each day in this country. First, the cervix is stretched by pushing smooth metal rods of increasing diameter in and out of it. After about five minutes of this, the cervix has expanded enough so that a curette can be inserted through it into the uterus. The curette is another metal rod, at the end of which is an oval ring about an inch at its widest diameter. It is used to scrape the walls of the uterus. The operation is done completely by feel after the cervix has been stretched, since it is still too narrow to see through.

Things do not go easily this morning. There is considerably more blood than usual, and it is only with great difficulty that I am able to extract anything. What should take ten or fifteen minutes stretches into a half-hour. The body parts I remove are much larger than I expected, considering when the embryo died. They are not bits of decomposing tissue. These are parts of a body that was recently alive!

I do my best to suppress my rising panic and try to complete the procedure. Working blindly, I am unable to evacuate the uterus completely; I can feel more parts inside but cannot remove them. Finally I stop, telling myself that the uterus will expel the rest within a few days.

Russ is waiting outside the operating room. I tell him that Barb is fine but that there were some problems with the operation. Since I don't completely understand what happened, I can't be very helpful in answering his questions. I promise to return to the hospital later in the day after Barb has awakened from the anesthesia.

In between seeing other patients that morning, I place several almost frantic phone calls, trying to piece together what happened. Despite reassurances from a pathologist that it is "impossible" for a pregnant woman to have four consequent negative pregnancy tests, the realization is growing that I have aborted Barb's living child. I won't know for sure until the pathologist has examined the fetal parts and determined the baby's age and the cause of death. In a daze, I walk over to the hospital and tell Russ and Barb as much as I know for sure without letting them know all I suspect. I tell them that more tissue may be expelled. I can't face my own suspicions.

Two days later, on Sunday morning, I receive a tearful call from Barb. She has just passed some recognizable body parts; what is she to do? She tells me that the bleeding has stopped now and that she feels better. The abortion I began on Friday is apparently over. I set up an appointment to meet with her and Russ to review the entire situation.

The pathologist's report confirms my worst fears: I aborted a living fetus. It was about eleven weeks old. I can find no one who can explain why Barb had four negative pregnancy tests. My meeting with Barb and Russ later in the week is one of the hardest things I have ever been through. I described in some detail what I did and what my rationale had been. Nothing can obscure the hard reality: I killed their baby.

Politely, almost meekly, Russ asks whether the ultrasound examination would have shown that Barb was carrying a live baby. It almost seems that he is trying to protect my feelings, trying to absolve me of some of the responsibility. "Yes," I answer, "if I had ordered the ultrasound, we would have known the baby was alive." I cannot explain why I didn't recommend it.

Mistakes are an inevitable part of everyone's life. They happen; they hurt—ourselves and others. They demonstrate our fallibility. Shown our mistakes and forgiven them, we can grow, perhaps in some small way become better people. Mistakes, understood this way, are a process, a way we connect with one another and with our deepest selves.

But mistakes seem different for doctors. This has to do with the very nature of our work. A mistake in the intensive care unit, in the emergency room, in the surgery suite, or at the sickbed is different from a mistake on the dock or at the typewriter. A doctor's miscalculation or oversight can prolong an illness, or cause a permanent disability, or kill a patient. Few other mistakes are more costly.

Developments in modern medicine have provided doctors with more knowledge of the human body, more accurate methods of diagnosis, more sophisticated technology to help in examining and monitoring the sick. All of that means more power to intervene in the disease process. But modern medicine, with its invasive tests and potentially lethal drugs, has also given doctors the power to do more harm.

Yet precisely because of its technological wonders and near-miraculous drugs, modern medicine has created for the physician an expectation of perfection. The technology seems so exact that error becomes almost unthinkable. We are not prepared for our mistakes, and we don't know how to cope with them when they occur.

Doctors are not alone in harboring expectations of perfection. Patients, too, expect doctors to be perfect. Perhaps patients have to consider their doctors less prone to error than other people: how else can a sick or injured person, already afraid, come to trust the doctor? Further, modern medicine has taken much of the treatment of illness out of the realm of common sense; a patient must trust a physician to make decisions that he, the patient, only vaguely understands. But the degree of perfection expected by patients is no doubt also a result of what we doctors have come to believe about ourselves, or better, have tried to convince ourselves about ourselves.

This perfection is a grand illusion, of course, a game of mirrors that everyone plays. Doctors hide their mistakes from patients, from other doctors, even from themselves. Open discussion of mistakes is banished from the consultation room, from the operating room, from physicians' meetings. Mistakes become gossip, and are spoken of openly only in court. Unable to admit our mistakes, we physicians are cut off from healing. We cannot ask for forgiveness, and we get none. We are thwarted, stunted; we do not grow.

During the days, and weeks, and months after I aborted Barb's baby, my guilt and anger grew. I did discuss what had happened with my partners, with the pathologist, with obstetric specialists. Some of my mistakes were obvious: I had relied too heavily on one test; I had not been skillful in determining the size of the uterus by pelvic examination; I should have ordered the ultrasound before proceeding to the D & C. There was no way I could justify what I had done. To make matters worse, there were complications following the D & C, and Barb was unable to become pregnant again for two years.

Although I was as honest with the Dailys as I could have been, and although I told them everything they wanted to know, I never shared with them my own agony. I felt they had enough sorrow without having to bear my burden as well. I decided it was my responsibility to deal with my guilt alone. I never asked for their forgiveness.

Doctors' mistakes, of course, come in a variety of packages and stem from a variety of causes. For primary care practitioners, who see every kind of problem from cold sores to cancer, the mistakes are often simply a result of not knowing enough. One evening during my years in Minnesota a local boy was brought into the emergency room after a drunken driver had knocked him off his bicycle. I examined him right away. Aside from swelling and bruising of the left leg and foot, he seemed fine. An x-ray showed what appeared to be a dislocation of the foot from the ankle. I consulted by telephone with an orthopedic specialist in Duluth, and we decided that I could operate on the boy. As was my usual practice, I offered the patient and his mother (who happened to be a nurse with whom I worked regularly) a choice: I could do the operation or they could travel to Duluth to see the specialist. My pride was hurt when she decided to take her son to Duluth.

My feelings changed considerably when the specialist called the next morning to thank me for the referral. He reported that the boy had actually suffered an unusual muscle injury, a posterior compartment syndrome, which had twisted his foot and caused it to appear to be dislocated. I had never even heard of such a syndrome, much less seen or treated it. The boy had required immediate surgery to save the muscles of his lower leg. Had his mother not decided to take him to Duluth, he would have been permanently disabled.

Sometimes a lack of technical skill leads to a mistake. After I had been in town a few years, the doctor who had done most of the surgery at the clinic left to teach at a medical school. Since the clinic was more than a hundred miles from the nearest surgical center, my partners and I decided that I should get some additional training in order to be able to perform emergency surgery. One of my first cases after training was a young man with appendicitis. The surgery proceeded smoothly enough, but the patient did not recover as quickly as he should have, and his hemoglobin level (a measure of the amount of blood in the system) dropped slowly. I referred him to a surgeon in Duluth, who, during a second operation, found a significant amount of old blood in his abdomen. Apparently I had left a small blood vessel leaking into the abdominal cavity. Perhaps I hadn't noticed the oozing blood during surgery; perhaps it had begun to leak only after I had finished. Although the young man was never in serious danger, although the blood vessel would probably have sealed itself without the second surgery, my mistake had caused considerable discomfort and added expense.

Often, I am sure, mistakes are a result of simple carelessness. There was the young girl I treated for what I thought was a minor ankle injury. After looking at her x-rays, I sent her home with what I diagnosed as a sprain. A radiologist did a routine follow-up review of the x-rays and sent me a report. I failed to read it carefully and did not notice that her ankle had been broken. I first learned about my mistake five years later when I was summoned to a court hearing. The fracture I had missed had not healed properly, and the patient had required extensive treatment and difficult surgery. By that time I couldn't even remember her original visit and had to piece together what had happened from my records.

Some mistakes are purely technical; most involve a failure of judgment. Perhaps the worst kind involve what another physician has described to me as "a failure of will." She was referring to those situations in which a doctor knows the right thing to do but doesn't do it because he is distracted, or pressured, or exhausted.

Several years ago, I was rushing down the hall of the hospital to the delivery room. A young woman stopped me. Her mother had been having chest pains all night. Should she be brought to the emergency room? I knew the mother well, had examined her the previous week, and knew of her recurring bouts of chest pains. She suffered from angina; I presumed she was having another attack.

Some part of me knew that anyone with all-night chest pains should be seen right away. But I was under pressure. The delivery would make me an hour late to the office, and I was frayed from a weekend on call, spent mostly in the emergency room. This new demand would mean additional pressure. "No," I said, "take her over to the office, and I'll see her as soon as I'm done here." About twenty minutes later, as I was finishing the delivery, the clinic nurse rushed into the room. Her face was pale. "Come quick! Mrs. Helgeson just collapsed." I sprinted the hundred yards to the office, where I found Mrs. Helgeson in cardiac arrest. Like many doctors' offices at the time, ours did not have the advanced life-support equipment that helps keep patients alive long enough to get them to a hospital. Despite everything we did, Mrs. Helgeson died.

Would she have survived if I had agreed to see her in the emergency room, where the requisite staff and equipment were available? No one will ever know for sure. But I have to live with the possibility that she might not have died if I had not had "a failure of will." There was no way to rationalize it: I had been irresponsible, and a patient had died.

Many situations do not lend themselves to a simple determination of whether a mistake has been made. Seriously ill, hospitalized patients, for instance, require of doctors almost continuous decision-making. Although in most cases no single mistake is obvious, there always seem to be things that could have been done differently or better: administering more of this medication, starting that treatment a little sooner . . . The fact is that when a patient dies, the physician is left wondering whether the care he provided was adequate. There is no way to be certain, for it is impossible to determine what would have happened if things had been done differently. Often it is difficult to get an honest opinion on this even from another physician, most doctors not wanting to be perceived by their colleagues as judgmental—or perhaps fearing similar judgments upon themselves. In the end, the physician has to suppress the guilt and move on to the next patient.

A few years after my mistake with Barb Daily, Maiya Martinen first came to see me halfway through her pregnancy. I did not know her or her husband well, but I knew that they were solid, hard-working people. This was to be their first child. When I examined Maiya, it seemed to me that the fetus was unusually small, and I was uncertain about her due date. I sent her to Duluth for an ultrasound examination—which was by now routine for almost any problem during pregnancy—and an evaluation by an obstetrician. The obstetrician thought the baby would be small, but he thought it could be safely delivered in the local hospital.

Maiya's labor was uneventful, except that it took her longer than usual to push the baby through to delivery. Her baby boy was born blue and floppy, but he responded well to routine newborn resuscitation measures. Fifteen minutes after birth, however, he had a short seizure. We checked his blood sugar level and found it to be low, a common cause of seizures in small babies who take longer than usual to emerge from the birth canal. Fortunately, we were able to put an IV easily into a scalp vein and administer glucose, and baby Marko seemed to improve. He and his mother were discharged from the hospital several days later.

At about two months of age, a few days after I had given him his first set of immunizations, Marko began having short spells. Not long after that he started to have full-blown seizures. Once again the Martinens made the trip to Duluth, and Marko was hospitalized for three days of tests. No cause for the seizures was found, but he was placed on medication. Marko continued to have seizures, however. When he returned for his second set of immunizations, it was clear to me that he was not doing well.

The remainder of Marko's short life was a tribute to the faith and courage of his parents. He proved severely retarded, and the seizures became harder and harder to control. Maiya eventually went East for a few months so Marko could be treated at the National Institutes of Health. But nothing seemed to help, and Maiya and her baby returned home. Marko had to be admitted frequently to the local hospital in order to control his seizures. At two o'clock one morning I was called to the hospital: the baby had had a respiratory arrest. Despite our efforts, Marko died, ending a year-and-a-half struggle with life.

No cause for Marko's condition was ever determined. Did something happen during the birth that briefly cut off oxygen to his brain? Should Maiya have delivered at the high-risk obstetric center in

Duluth, where sophisticated fetal monitoring is available? Should I have sent Marko to the Newborn Intensive Care Unit in Duluth immediately after his first seizure in the delivery room? I subsequently learned that children who have seizures should not routinely be immunized. Would it have made any difference if I had never given Marko the shots? There were many such questions in my mind and, I am sure, in the minds of the Martinens. There was no way to know the answers, no way for me to handle the guilt feelings I experienced, perhaps irrationally, whenever I saw Maiya.

The emotional consequences of mistakes are difficult enough to handle. But soon after I started practicing I realized I had to face another anxiety as well: it is not only in the emergency room, the operating room, the intensive care unit, or the delivery room that a doctor can blunder into tragedy. Errors are always possible, even in the midst of the humdrum routine of daily care. Was that baby with diarrhea more dehydrated than he looked, and should I have hospitalized him? Will that nine-year-old with stomach cramps whose mother I just lectured about psychosomatic illness end up in the operating room tomorrow with a ruptured appendix? Did that Vietnamese refugee have a problem I didn't understand because of the language barrier? A doctor has to confront the possibility of a mistake with every patient visit.

My initial response to the mistakes I did make was to question my competence. Perhaps I just didn't have the necessary intelligence, judgment, and discipline to be a physician. But was I really incompetent? My University of Minnesota Medical School class had voted me one of the two most promising clinicians. My diploma from the National Board of Medical Examiners showed scores well above average. I knew that the townspeople considered me a good physician; I knew that my partners, with whom I worked daily, and the consultants to whom I referred patients considered me a good physician, too. When I looked at it objectively, my competence was not the issue. I would have to learn to live with my mistakes.

A physician is even less prepared to deal with his mistakes than is the average person. Nothing in our training prepares us to respond appropriately. As a student, I was simply not aware that the sort of mistakes I would eventually make in practice actually happened to competent physicians. As far as I can remember from my student experience on the hospital wards, the only doctors who ever made mistakes were the much maligned "LMDs"—local medical doctors. They would transfer their patients who weren't doing well to the University Hospital. At the "U," teams of specialist physicians with their residents, interns, and students would take their turns examining the patient thoroughly, each one delighted to discover (in retrospect, of course) an "obvious" error made by the referring LMD. As students we had the entire day to evaluate and care for our five to ten patients. After we examined them and wrote orders for their care, first the interns and then the residents would also examine them and correct our orders. Finally, the supervising physician would review everything. It was pretty unlikely that a major error would slip by; and if it did, it could always be blamed on someone else on the team. We had very little feeling for what it was like to be the LMD, working alone with perhaps the same number of hospital patients plus an office full of other patients; but we were quite sure we would not be guilty of such grievous errors as we saw coming into the U.

An atmosphere of precision pervaded the teaching hospital. The uncertainty that came to seem inescapable to me in northern Minnesota would shrivel away at the U as teams of specialists pronounced authoritatively upon any subject. And when a hospital physician did make a significant mistake, it was first whispered about the halls as if it were a sin. Much later a conference would be called in which experts who had had weeks to think about the case would discuss the way it should have been handled. The embarrassing mistake was frequently not even mentioned; it had evaporated. One could almost believe that the patient had been treated perfectly. More important, only the technical aspects of the case were considered relevant for discussion. It all seemed so simple, so clear. How could anyone do anything else? There was no mention of the mistake, or of the feelings of the patient or the doctor. It was hardly the sort of environment in which a doctor might feel free to talk about his mistakes or about his emotional responses to them.

Medical school was also a very competitive place, discouraging any sharing of feelings. The favorite pastime, even between classes or at a party, seemed to be sharing with the other medical students the story of the patient who had been presented to one's team, and then describing in detail how the diagnosis had been reached, how the disease worked, and what the treatment was. The storyteller, having spent the day researching every detail of the patient's disease, could, of course, dazzle everyone with the breadth and depth of his knowledge. Even though I knew what was going on, the game still left me feeling incompetent, as it must have many of my colleagues. I never knew for sure, though, since no one had the nerve to say so. It almost seemed that one's peers were the worst possible persons with whom to share those feelings.

Physicians in private practice are no more likely to find errors openly acknowledged or discussed, even though they occur regularly. My own mistakes represent only some of those of which I am aware. I know of one physician who administered a potent drug in a dose ten times that recommended; his patient almost died. Another doctor examined a child in an emergency room late one night and told the parents the problem was only a mild viral infection. Only because the parents did not believe the doctor, only because they consulted another doctor the following morning, did the child survive a life-threatening infection. Still another physician killed a patient while administering a routine test: a needle slipped and lacerated a vital artery. Whether the physician is a rural general practitioner with years of experience but only basic training or a recently graduated, highly trained neurosurgeon working in a sophisticated technological environment, the basic problem is the same.

Because doctors do not discuss their mistakes, I do not know how other physicians come to terms with theirs. But I suspect that many cannot bear to face their mistakes directly. We either deny the misfortune altogether or blame the patient, the nurse, the laboratory, other physicians, the system, fate—anything to avoid our own guilt.

The medical profession seems to have no place for its mistakes. Indeed, one would almost think that mistakes were sins. And if the medical profession has no room for doctors' mistakes, neither does society. The number of malpractice suits filed each year is symptomatic of this. In what other profession are practitioners regularly sued for hundreds of thousands of dollars because of misjudgments? I am sure the Dailys could have successfully sued me for a large amount of money had they chosen to do so.

The drastic consequences of our mistakes, the repeated opportunities to make them, the uncertainty about our culpability, and the professional denial that mistakes happen all work together to create an intolerable dilemma for the physician. We see the horror of our mistakes, yet we cannot deal with their enormous emotional impact.

Perhaps the only way to face our guilt is through confession, restitution, and absolution. Yet within the structure of modern medicine there is no place for such spiritual healing. Although the emotionally mature physician may be able to give the patient or family a full description of what happened, the technical details are often so difficult for the layperson to understand that the nature of the mistake is hidden. If an error is clearly described, it is frequently presented as "natural," "understandable," or "unavoidable" (which, indeed, it often is). But there is seldom a real confession: "This is the mistake I made; I'm sorry." How can one say that to a grieving parent? to a woman who has lost her mother?

If confession is difficult, what are we to say about restitution? The very nature of a physician's work means that there are things that cannot be restored in any meaningful way. What could I do to make good the Dailys' loss?

I have not been successful in dealing with a paradox: I am a healer, yet I sometimes do more harm than good. Obviously, we physicians must do everything we can to keep mistakes to a minimum. But if we are unable to deal openly with those that do occur, we will find neurotic ways to protect ourselves from the pain we feel. Little wonder that physicians are accused of playing God. Little wonder that we are defensive about our judgments, that we blame the patient or the previous physician when things go wrong, that we yell at nurses for their mistakes, that we have such high rates of alcoholism, drug addiction, and suicide.

At some point we must all bring medical mistakes out of the closet. This will be difficult as long as both the profession and society continue to project their desires for perfection onto the doctor. Physicians need permission to admit errors. They need permission to share them with their patients. The practice of medicine is difficult enough without having to bear the yoke of perfection.

MELVIN KONNER

MELVIN KONNER (1946–). *American physician, anthropologist, and writer. Dr. Konner received both his Ph.D. and his M.D. from Harvard, and now teaches in the anthropology department at Emory University. His books include* The Tangled Wing: Biological Constraints on the Human Spirit *(1983),* Becoming a Doctor: A Journey of Initiation in Medical School *(1988),* Why the Reckless Survive *(1991), and* Childhood *(1991), which examines the cultural, biological, and psychological influences on human development from conception through adolescence. In his last two books,* Medicine at the Crossroads *and* Dear America *(1993), Dr. Konner has addressed the health care crisis and the need for reform in America from a physician's critical perspective.*

THE DAWN OF WONDER

The most beautiful experience we can have is the mysterious. It is the fundamental emotion which stands at the cradle of true art and true science.
—ALBERT EINSTEIN, *THE WORLD AS I SEE IT*

One of the most fascinating and least discussed discoveries in the study of the wild chimpanzees was described in a short paper by Harold Bauer. He was following a well-known male chimpanzee through the forest of the Gombe Stream Reserve in Tanzania when the animal stopped beside a waterfall. It seemed possible that he had deliberately gone to the waterfall rather than passing it incidentally, but that was not absolutely clear. In any case, it was an impressive spot: a stream of water cascading down from a twenty-five-foot height, about a mile from the lake, thundering into the pool below and casting mist for sixty or seventy feet; a stunning sight to come upon in the midst of a tropical forest.

The animal seemed lost in contemplation of it. He moved slowly closer, and began to rock, while beginning to give a characteristic round of "pant-hoot" calls. He became more excited, finally beginning to run back and forth while calling, to jump, to call louder, to drum with his fists on trees, to run back again. The behavior was most reminiscent of that observed and described by Jane Goodall in groups of chimpanzees at the start of a rainstorm—the "rain dance," as it has been called. But this was one animal alone, and not surprised as the

337

animals are by sudden rain—even if he had not deliberately sought the waterfall out, he certainly knew where it was and when he would come upon it.

He continued this activity long enough so that it seemed to merit some explanation, and did it again in the same place on other days. Other animals were observed to do it as well. They had no practical interest in the waterfall. The animals did not have to drink from the stream or cross it in that vicinity. To the extent that it might be dangerous, it could be easily avoided, and certainly did not interest every animal. But for these it was something they had to look at, return to, study, watch, become excited about: a thing of beauty, an object of curiosity, a fetish, an imagined creature, a challenge, a communication? We will never know.

But for a very similar animal, perhaps ten million years ago, in the earliest infancy of the human spirit, something in the natural world must have evoked a response like this one—a waterfall, a mountain vista, a sunset, the crater of a volcano, the edge of the sea—something that stopped it in its tracks and made it watch, and move, and watch, and move, and watch again; something that made it return to the spot, though nothing gainful could take place there, no feeding, drinking, reproducing, sleeping, fighting, fleeing, nothing *animal.* In just such a response, in just such a moment, in just such an animal, we may, I think, be permitted to guess, occurred the dawn of awe, of sacred attentiveness, of wonder.

The human infant, for its first few months of life, is all eyes, in a way that no other animal infant quite is. It isn't just that its eyes are good, that it does a lot of looking; it's that it does so little else, really. It can suck, of course, and swallow, but the rest of what it does is very primitive, except for the functions of attentiveness. Even in the adult brain, one-third of all incoming signals come through the eyes. In the infant, looking and seeing are way ahead of most other functions in development, with the possible exception of listening and hearing. The infant is not a passive figure, nor an active one either, but what might be called an actively receptive one—eagerly, hungrily receptive, famished for sights and sounds, no vague, fuzzy intelligence in a blooming, buzzing confusion, but a highly ordered, if simple, mind with a fine sense of novelty, of pattern, even of beauty. The light on a leaf outside the window, the splash of red on a woman's dress, the shadow on the ceiling, the sound of rain—any of these may evoke a rapt attention not, perhaps, unlike that of the chimpanzee at the waterfall.

For most people, as they grow, that sense of wonder diminishes in frequency, becoming at best peripheral to the business of everyday life. For some, it becomes the central fact of existence. These follow two separate paths: Either the sense of wonder leads them down an analytic path, or it leads them to simple contemplation. Either way the sense of wonder is the first fact of life, but the paths are completely different in every other way. The analyst, or scientist, moved to reveal by explaining, breaks apart the image, and the sense of wonder, focusing sequentially on the pieces. The contemplator, or artist, moved to reveal by simply looking, keeps the image and the sense of wonder whole. The artist contrives to keep the attention riveted without fragmentation, by means of high trickery. This trickery involves transmuting the image into human speech—whether a literary, plastic, or musical form of speech—thus fixing in place forever the sense of wonder.

There is a photograph that has by now been seen by most people living in civilized countries. It was taken from an ingenious if crude vehicle traveling many thousands of miles per hour, across a vast expanse of space empty of air, by men who had devoted their lives, courageously and at great personal cost, to the mastery of nature through machinery. This photograph cost perhaps a billion dollars, and in one sense it is worth every penny.

It shows an almost spherical object poised against a backdrop of black. The object is partly colored a deep, warm, pretty blue, with many broken, off-white swirls drawn across it. It looks at first like a mandala, a strange symbol woven on black cloth. It looks whole, somehow, and rather small. But as we study it (it draws us in almost mysteriously), some red-brown shapes obscured among the swirls of white take on before our eyes the unmistakable images we first saw and memorized as children encountering the geography of the continents. If the space program accomplished nothing else (and I am often at pains to discern what it did accomplish), we must be grateful to it for producing that photograph.

"Got the earth right out our front window," said Buzz Aldrin. A medium-size mammal from a middling planet of a middle-aged star in the arm of an average galaxy, gazing at home. There was no excess of poetry on that mission. There was, of course, the stark poetry of aeronautics gobbledygook and the arch, well-prepared, historic *mot* of Neil Armstrong setting foot on the Sea of Tranquility, but "Beautiful, beautiful," "Magnificent sight out here," and "Got the earth right out our front window," was about the level at which these unique first views of the natural world were transmuted to human speech.

This was no fault of Armstrong or Aldrin; they were chosen for other talents, which they had in full measure. But it is intriguing that such spontaneous poetry as there was was evoked by the machinery. "The Eagle has wings," one of them said as the lunar landing vehicle separated, after some difficulty, from the orbiting command station. *The eagle,* bold symbol of human hope on the North American continent and, beyond that, of the hope of humanity in the mission, *has wings,* has the means to transcend technical difficulty and to emerge, having mastered natural law.

But this stepping off the earth is an illusion. The mastery of natural law has proceeded no further than the grasp of some elementary laws of physics. Compared with the uncharted, infinitely more intricate laws of biology and behavior that govern the human spirit, this mastery is trivial, a mere conjurer's trick. The mastery of physical law can no longer save us while we are grounded in a tangle of ignorance of the natural laws that govern our behavior. In this sense, the eagle does not have wings.

When I was a young man in college, a professor took me to the American Museum of Natural History, not to the exhibits, which I had often seen, but into the bowels of the place, among the labyrinths of storage cabinets of bones and skins and rocks and impossibly ancient fossils. I was very much impressed by this chance to see the museum the way insiders, professionals, saw it.

There I met a man who had devoted most of his life to the study of the skeletal remains of archaeopteryx—the earliest tetrapod with feathered wings—embedded in a Mesozoic rock. I was introduced to him, awed by him, impressed with his intelligence and wisdom. It was obvious that he wanted to impart to me some piece of genuine, useful knowledge gained from the countless hours of squinting over that crushed tangle of bone and rock.

What he finally said was that he thought archaeopteryx was very much like people. This of course puzzled me, as it was calculated to do, and when I pressed him to explain, he said, "Well, you know, it's such a transitional creature. It's a piss-poor reptile, and it's not very much of a bird." Apart from the shock of hearing strong language in those relatively hallowed halls, there was an intellectual shock to my young mind that fixed those phrases in it permanently.

The dinosaurs ruled this planet for over a hundred million years, at least a hundred times longer than the brief, awkward tenure of human creatures, and they are gone almost without a trace, leaving nothing but crushed bone as a memento. We can do the same more easily and, in an ecological sense, we would be missed even less. What's the difference? seems an inevitable question, and the best answer I can think of is that we *know*, we are capable of seeing what is happening. We are the only creatures that understand evolution, that, conceivably, can alter its very course. It would be too base of us to simply relinquish this possibility through pride, or ignorance, or laziness.

It seems to me we are losing the sense of wonder, the hallmark of our species and the central feature of the human spirit. Perhaps this is due to the depredations of science and technology against the arts and the humanities, but I doubt it—although this is certainly something to be concerned about. I suspect it is simply that the human spirit is insufficiently developed at this moment in evolution, much like the wing of archaeopteryx. Whether we can free it for further development will depend, I think, on the full reinstatement of the sense of wonder. It must be reinstated in relation not only to the natural world but to the human world as well. At the conclusion of all our studies we must try once again to experience the human soul as soul, and not just as a buzz of bioelectricity; the human will as will, and not just a surge of hormones; the human heart not as a fibrous, sticky pump, but as the metaphoric organ of understanding. We need not believe in them as metaphysical entities—they are as real as the flesh and blood they are made of. But we must believe in them as entities; not as analyzed fragments, but as wholes made real by our contemplation of them, by the words we use to talk of them, by the way we have transmuted them to speech. We must stand in awe of them as unassailable, even though they are dissected before our eyes.

As for the natural world, we must try to restore wonder there too. We could start with that photograph of the earth. It may be our last chance. Even now it is being used in geography lessons, taken for granted by small children. We are the first generation to have seen it, the last generation not to take it for granted. Will we remember what it meant to us? How fine the earth looked, dangled in space? How pretty against the endless black? How round? How very breakable? How small? It is up to us to try to experience a sense of wonder about it that will save it before it is too late. If we cannot, we may do the final damage in our lifetimes. If we can, we may change the course of history and, consequently, the course of evolution, setting the human lineage firmly on a path toward a new evolutionary plateau.

We must choose, and choose soon, either for or against the further evolution of the human spirit. It is for us, in the generation that turns the corner of the millennium, to apply whatever knowledge we have,

in all humility but with all due speed, and to try to learn more as
quickly as possible. It is for us, much more than for any previous generation, to become serious about the human future, and to make
choices that will be weighed not in a decade or a century but in the
balances of geological time. It is for us, with all our stumbling, and in
the midst of our dreadful confusion, to try to disengage the tangled
wing.

JANE KENYON

JANE KENYON (1947–1995). *American poet, translator. Born in Ann Arbor, Michigan, Jane Kenyon grew up in the Midwest. She earned a B.A. from the University of Michigan in 1970 and an M.A. in 1972. She is the author of four books of poetry, including* From Room to Room *(1978),* The Boat of Quiet Hours *(1986),* Let Evening Come *(1990), and* Constance *(1993), and a book of translation,* Twenty Poems of Anna Akhmatova *(1985). She and her husband, poet Donald Hall, moved to Eagle Pond Farm in Wilmot, New Hampshire, where she found the rural New England landscape a subject that allowed her to convey her inner world. A fifth collection of her poetry,* Otherwise: New and Selected Poems, *was published posthumously (1996). Also published after her death was a collection of her translations, interviews, and miscellaneous prose,* A Hundred White Daffodils *(1999). At the time of her death, she was New Hampshire's poet laureate.*

OTHERWISE

I got out of bed
on two strong legs.
It might have been
otherwise. I ate
cereal, sweet
milk, ripe, flawless
peach. It might
have been otherwise.
I took the dog uphill
to the birch wood.
All morning I did
the work I love.

At noon I lay down
with my mate. It might
have been otherwise.
We ate dinner together
at a table with silver
candlesticks. It might
have been otherwise.

I slept in a bed
in a room with paintings
on the walls, and
planned another day
just like this day.
But one day, I know,
it will be otherwise.

LET EVENING COME

Let the light of late afternoon
shine through chinks in the barn, moving
up the bales as the sun moves down.

Let the cricket take up chafing
as a woman takes up her needles
and her yarn. Let evening come.

Let dew collect on the hoe abandoned
in long grass. Let the stars appear
and the moon disclose her silver horn.

Let the fox go back to its sandy den.
Let the wind die down. Let the shed
go black inside. Let evening come.

To the bottle in the ditch, to the scoop
in the oats, to air in the lung
let evening come.

Let it come, as it will, and don't
be afraid. God does not leave us
comfortless, so let evening come.

DAVID RINALDI

DAVID RINALDI (1947–). *American physician. Dr. Rinaldi has been a practicing pediatrician for eleven years; his poetry has been published in the* Pharos *of the* Alpha Omega Alpha Medical Honor Society *and in the* Annals of Behavioral Medicine and Medical Education.

LET'S TALK ABOUT IT

with all the talk
about Dr Death
news-bites sandwiched
between circus and tragedy
hesitantly I say
in my confusion
"I understand him"
but still . . .
as a physician
morally and ethically . . .
and yet . . .
terminal pain . . .
and yet . . .

and surreptitiously
remember
how very secretly
I thought
thought how
Dad's castrated body
lay crooked in
prostatic pain on
his sweaty Tennessee cot
his wife's terminal phone voice
drawling out the daily news . . .
how very secretly
I calculated
how many of
those little pain-killers
it might take . . .

and silently remember
how I put it all
out of my Hippocratic mind
yet felt ashamed
for weakness . . .

and so I waited. . . .

HEATHER MCHUGH

HEATHER MCHUGH (1948–). *American poet, fiction writer, translator. McHugh is the author of many collections of poetry, among them* Dangers *(1977),* A World of Difference *(1981),* To the Quick *(1987), and* Shades *(1988), and of a collection of essays,* Broken English *(1993). Her collection of poems* Hinge and Sign: Poems, 1968–1993 *was a 1994 National Book Award finalist. Her most recent book of poems is* The Father of the Predicaments *(1999). In 1999 she was elected a chancellor of the Academy of American Poets.*

WHAT HELL IS
March 1985

Your father sits inside
his spacious kitchen, corpulent
and powerless. Nobody knows
how your disease is spread; it came
from love, or some
such place. Your father's bought
with forty years of fast talk, door-to-door,
this fancy house you've come home now to die in.
Let me tell you what
hell is, he says: I got this
double fridge all full of food
and I can't let my son go in.

*

Your parents' friends
stop visiting. You are a damper on
their spirits. Every day you feel
more cold (no human being
here can bear
the thought—it's growing
huge, as you grow thin).
Ain't it a bitch, you say, this
getting old? (I'm not sure
I should laugh. No human being
helps, except
suddenly, simply
Jesus: him you hold.)

*

We're not allowed
to touch you if you weep or bleed.
Applying salves to sores that cannot heal
your brother wears a rubber glove.
With equal meaning, cold or kiss
could kill you. Now what do I mean
by love?

*

The man who used
to love his looks
is sunk in bone
and looking out.

Framed by immunities
of telephone and lamp
his mouth is shut,
his eyes are dark.

While we discuss despair
he is it, somewhere
in the house. Increasingly
he's spoken of

not with. In kitchen
conferences we come
to terms that we
can bear. But where is he?

In hell, which is
the living room.
In hell, which has
an easy chair.

SUSAN ONTHANK MATES

SUSAN ONTHANK MATES (1950–). *American physician and writer. Mates studied music and violin at the Juilliard School of Music. She received the B.A. degree from Yale, the M.D. from Albert Einstein College of Medicine. Her honors include the Lenox String Quartet scholarship, a National Institutes for Health Clinical Investigator Award, and the John Simmons Short Fiction Award from the University of Iowa Press for her book of stories,* The Good Doctor *(1994), from which "Laundry" is taken. Her writings often reflect medical training and allied experiences, including the difficulties faced by women physicians caring for patients while carrying out their own family obligations. Her characters struggle to do the right thing in a world marked by loneliness, racial tensions, AIDS, tuberculosis, and death. Mates contributes to literary publications such as* TriQuarterly *and the* Northwest Review.

LAUNDRY

I was folding the baby's diapers—cloth, the kind they make now with a double thickness down the middle—and the phone rang. I was thinking and not thinking; just a second before, the baby had begun to scream that lightning-strike-of-hunger scream, so I was saying to him, wait just a minute let me smooth this crease, and he was shrieking a crescendo and the phone rang. While I was folding and talking to the baby underneath, I was thinking about whether, really, we could afford new bicycles for the girls, the used ones never seem to work quite right, surely it's not such an extravagance, new bikes, but if you've been to Toys "R" Us lately you realize this is a serious issue. On the other hand, I was the fourth child and never had anything new, so I understand that dream, that lust, for something smooth and shiny and unmarked and smelling like paint and not like old garage mildew. So I was thinking: maybe I should try to work another job, after all I am a doctor.

Hi, how are you, yes I'm Dr. Martin, pointing to the name tag that says Dr. Martin on the white coat that says doctor, doctor, doctor. So I hear you're having trouble breathing, pain in your side, a little nausea, the pills bothering you? So sorry to hear about your son, you must take care of yourself, no can tell you for sure that you're going to die, it's a bad disease but there are always exceptions, god, hold my hand god, where in medical school did I miss that course on conviction THIS IS WHAT YOU SHOULD DO MR. DANTIO and me still folding diapers, patting them into squares warm and fresh from the dryer. I don't know Mr. Dantio, the cancer is all over your lungs those cells are eating you, collapsing you, deflating you, your X-ray looks like a drowned man, and each breath drives a spike of pain through your chest. Your wife sits in the corner and hates you and loves you and hates you. I see it in her eyes.

I don't know when can life end, myself I would rather die, but I'm a coward, always have been, I admire your ferocity—I can't help, I can't win this battle, slay the dragon, oh I want to be the hero now, I'll hold your hand Mr. Dantio. I'll watch when you scream and the water in your lungs bubbles up pink like cotton candy from your mouth and nostrils and I'll see the terror in your eyes as you try to pull a breath and your muscles contract and your ribs stand out like a skeleton and no air comes in and your children live three thousand miles away and hate you and love you and your wife is sobbing in the corner. I'm the doctor and I'm supposed to DO SOMETHING, the other doctors say why don't you scope him, biopsy him, give him a hit of chemo, cut him, needle him, anything but don't just let him die and Mr. Dantio I'm not just letting you die, it wasn't my decision, no one asked me should he live or die. But all I can do is watch, I will do that, I will watch even the very end when the air won't come and your fingers claw against the rails on the bed and you said no pain killers doctor, I want to see it coming and I said are you sure oh god.

Do you remember when we first met, and you complained that you itched, and it was flea bites and you had headaches, and it was because your wife yelled at you and you yelled at her, and you would call me in the middle of the night, and I would jump when the phone rang, my husband would groan and roll over in bed, one of the girls would start to cry, and the page operator said with a clothespin clipped on her nose Mr. Salvadore Dantio for you Dr. Martin and I would wake up and you would say, Doctor, that you doctor? Listen, I can't sleep for the itching. And there was nothing wrong with you and I hated you, but in the morning you would say, I'm sorry sorry, things get so bad in the middle of the night and what could I do but laugh, because it's true. The clinic didn't meet every day because I was supposed to do research and teach, I was the first woman doctor at the hospital, I was a role model, I was shiny and new and people whispered, so we met like lovers in the halls and in the lobbies really, you should try to come to your appointments, I said, Mr. Dantio I'll just squeeze you in today meet me on the second floor but next time KEEP YOUR

APPOINTMENT and my friends said you'll never get ahead seeing patients in your research time like that, Mr. Dantio there was nothing wrong with you but your wife and your kids and your boss. You put your bony fingers over my hand and said how's a young girl like you a doctor? and I laughed, you drove me crazy. I'm forty Mr. Dantio forty and I don't know how to live and you finally did get something wrong with you Salvadore, you sure did.

The phone is ringing and the baby is crying and I just want to finish folding the diapers so I can balance them on top of the blue and yellow receiving blankets, which is why I didn't use bleach, which I should have because there is a large brown stain on one of the diapers. How did this happen to me? I swore never a housewife, never, never, I won't fall in that black hole, not me.

You grabbed my hand in that cold white room Mr. Dantio and you said I'm a fighter but only if there's a chance all these doctors want to cut me stick tubes in me I don't really understand I'm just a sales-man now cake decorations, that's something I understand, you tell me what should I do. And I said I can't tell you that Mr. Dantio, Salvadore, I'm not you. And you said honey I need your help and you made your wife sobbing in the corner leave the room and you looked at me and I thought of you lying in the ICU with tubes in your mouth and arms and lungs and penis and nurses ripping the sheet off and turning your stiff blue body and brushing your hair and calling you sweetie while your blank brown eyes look up at the ceiling, you who never wanted a lady doctor who never wanted to be called sweetie, who always wanted to do the honey-sweetie calling and they're adjusting that tube in your penis and your hairless balls are flopping from side to side and no one even bothers to draw the curtain because your eyes are like mirrors: respirator, manometer, IV pump, electro-cardiograph. Your heart keeps going on blip thump, blip thump and your lungs and your liver and your bone marrow filled with infection and your infection is so much like you that we are killing you both together and you asked me what should I do and I couldn't speak. I'm not god. You said well? And you looked out in the hall to make sure your wife wasn't coming in and we were running out of time and I stroked my nine months' pregnant belly and the baby kicked and I said studies show that sometimes if you have this biopsy and we treat you with antibiotics, antifungals, antivirals, you might live longer and you said don't tell me about studies tell me what you would do. And I said studies are important, this is the way doctors know what to do, it's scientific and more systematic than just one doctor's experience, I was good at that stuff even though women aren't supposed to be I knew studies and talked fast clear and incisive and honor society until then I was good at being a doctor. And you said please. I felt my breath clot up somewhere in my throat and I looked at your eyes your ferocious eyes and I said Mr. Dantio, Salvadore I would not do it, don't do it don't let them me do it to you no.

And I couldn't stop the tears, I kissed you and waddled out of the room and stood around the corner so your wife couldn't see me and I cried there right in the middle of the hall with my white coat split down the middle and my belly sticking out, the baby writhing like a snake making ripples in my navy-blue maternity dress with the little red bow on top. The surgeon came up to me, a young man, younger than me, so energetic and clean shaven and he said did you talk him into it? and he ignored the tears and the belly and the baby kicking so unprofessional and I said no.

No! he shouted at me and I said I know as a doctor I should have said do it but as a person I felt no no no and he looked at me and stared at me and finally said there is no difference between how I feel as a doctor and as a person and I saw him with his clean white coat buttoned down his flat front and his neat black hair actually he was a friend of mine I was looking up because he is taller and I said yes I can see that. I should have been angry or distant or something but I wasn't, it would be a lie to say I was—I was feeling no I'm no doctor, I never thickened and rooted and became "Doctor," something's wrong with me, I'm a lost pregnant woman with greasy hair and a discharge in my pants because the baby's coming and I don't know what to do because they never really helped me Plato Aristotle Kant Proust James all I know is this man Salvadore Dantio is dying and I can't do a thing.

I'm still folding the diapers, I have to do a load every day to keep up and the phone is ringing and all I could say Mr. Dantio was that I will be there when your pupils fix and dilate, when your jaw slackens and droops, I'll look though your teeth into the black cavern of your body, I'll smell the diarrhea as your bowels let loose with blood and shit, I'll stay Mr. Dantio, I won't look away. They lied to me about maternity leave and they said well we think you don't really want to be a doctor anyway, you must be conflicted to have a child, want to take two months off, no one sent me flowers they send flowers to all the wives of the doctors but no one sent me anything not even a card when I came back after three weeks still bleeding, I was the only woman doctor in the hospital anyway you never wanted a woman doctor Mr. Dantio, Salvadore, but in the end you looked straight into my eyes, Salvadore and I couldn't lie to you not to you.

I ran into your wife in the supermarket last week over the oranges and she saw me and began to cry and I put my arm around her and tried not to cry myself and she said to me you know when he died that Sunday I tried to call you but they jumped on him and pounded his chest and cut it open and squeezed his heart and he never wanted all of that and she cried and I wondered if she knew that they did it for me, the other doctors, because they knew I didn't want him to die so they couldn't watch him go so they cut him up for me they were embarrassed for me I cared so much I made a spectacle of myself standing in the hall crying. And when they took a piece of his lung, after he died, they found the infection, all I could think of was maybe I was wrong, maybe he could have lived longer if he'd had that biopsy, maybe I never learned this language right, medicine, I feel like I'm a visitor from some other world dressed up like a doctor but they can tell I'm not really one because in moments of great stress I revert to my native tongue. Mrs. Dantio wiped her eyes with the back of her hand and said is that the baby? And she looked at his smooth skin my little son and she smiled and touched the drool on his chin I laughed too.

He's still crying and I pick up the phone and someone says is this the lady of the house? and I don't know what to answer so I think but I still don't know so I hang up and reach for him, he's beginning to make those enunciated baby complaints. I pull up my shirt and my breasts hang out like a cow and just looking at him I feel that sweet pain contraction, the milk spurts and gets us wet. He makes snuffling noises he works his mouth searching for the nipple so I help him wham! he latches on and pulls and the milk is pouring out of both breasts now, I grab a diaper to hold over the other one but it's too late and we're drenched he and I a fecund shower. I know what this means: another load of laundry.

DAVID HELLERSTEIN

DAVID HELLERSTEIN (1953–). *American physician, novelist, and essayist. Born in Cleveland, Dr. Hellerstein received his A.B. from Harvard and his M.D. from Stanford. He trained in psychiatry at New York Hospital/Cornell Medical Center and is now chief of outpatient psychiatry at Beth Israel Medical Center in New York and associate professor of psychiatry at the Albert Einstein College of Medicine. Widely published in periodicals, his books include* Battles of Life and Death *(1987), the novel* Loving Touches *(1988), and* A Family of Doctors *(1993), an autobiographical account that concerns five generations of doctors in the Hellerstein family.*

TOUCHING

"Scoot down to the edge of the table, hon," says Dr. Snarr. The small room is hot, the air stuffy. Our patient winces at the word *hon*. She is a young woman with chronic pelvic pain, the bane of gynecologists, and I can tell she doesn't like Snarr's tone. She does scoot along the table, though, and Snarr kicks a wheeled stool toward me. I sit on it, slide between her legs, ready for my lesson of the day. Feet and calves and thighs surround me, suddenly very close. Snarr positions the lamp before my chest, so light pours on her. I warm the speculum in my gloved hand and, with a twist, insert it.

"Open it up," he says. "Tighten it all the way open. Pull down to keep away from the urethra. You hit the urethra and no patient will ever come back to you."

Snarr is my teacher, a gaunt and narrow-shouldered man with a small potbelly below the belt of his corduroy pants. Before coming in here, he went over the information I had gathered and insisted it was nonsense. She couldn't possibly feel that kind of pain. I must not be asking the right questions. Hadn't I learned anything? Gynecologists traditionally have the reputation of being the dummies of medicine: surgeons laugh at their clumsiness in the operating room, internists at their ignorance of medical fact, psychiatrists at their insensitivity. And so far Snarr had done nothing to dispel that prejudice, which was too bad, considering that I was an impressionable third-year medical student, still trying to decide what field to select.

"Okay," says Snarr. "Now swab it out real well. Get some cells on that."

I swab.

"Pull that speculum out now. Get a good look at those walls."

I see pink folds as I pull, pink, moist walls bulging against the metal of the speculum—aquatic territory, the scalloped forms of submarine life. It's out. Snarr is quick next with lubricating jelly on the first two fingers of my glove. I stand up, push the stool away. I begin the manual exam.

"*Aiee!*" The woman screams and slides up on the table. "God! Oh God!"

"So that's . . . that's where it hurts," I say. I'm sweating. "Just . . . just a second, I'll try more gently."

I feel around again. This time she doesn't scream. She breathes deeply. I can't feel a damn thing, but with Snarr watching I can't pull out right away. For a month I've been spending afternoons in the gynecology clinic with Dr. Snarr—a month of women's bottoms on the edges of tables, of the hot lamp in front of my chest, the examining glove on my hand, powdered inside, the smells of femaleness. And the confidences of women, fascinating and at times overpowering, about their pains, their periods, their fertility, their husbands, their lovers. What gets to me, though, are the exams. The touching. Deep internal touching, feeling for the bulge of the uterus, for those small elusive olives the ovaries, exploring for tenderness, creating sudden moments of pain. Technically I'm reasonably good, as good as can be expected for a third-year medical student rotating through Ob-Gyn. But I still find it strange to be touching intimately but without passion—as a doctor.

I'm not alone in this either; the other medical students on Ob-Gyn seem just as awkward as I. We hang around in the lounge, where the pharmaceutical rep sometimes leaves free coffee and doughnuts, cracking jokes, laughing too much.

It reminds me of another situation, in the second-year physical diagnosis course, where we had to examine each other. The new idea that year was that we'd learn how to be more compassionate doctors if we practiced physical exams on one another first, before going on to patients.

We were divided into small groups, men and women together, and sent to various examining rooms. Our exams began at the head and worked down. You couldn't get too upset about looking into your medical student buddy's eyes, but by the second session, when we got down to the chest, the protests began. First the women complained and refused to be examined, but as it became clear that genital and rectal exams were also part of the required curriculum, men started to protest as well. Finally there was a full-scale revolt. A petition was circulated, meetings were hurriedly arranged with various administrators, protests were loud and vocal. The class was boycotted. We ended up learning the pelvic exam on professional models and doing rectal exams on plastic dummies. No one felt the course should be repeated.

I've always been sort of puzzled why my fellow medical students got so upset. After all, we had done just about everything together— cut open cadavers, crammed for exams, played touch football on the front lawn, dated and flirted and confided and complained. What it comes down to, I think, was that after two years together in med school, we knew each other too well, far too well for touching to be neutral. To palpate, percuss, auscultate, and probe each other's bodies brought out too many undoctorly thoughts.

We were a long way, I realize now, from learning the doctor's dispassionate touch. But the real problem came when our teachers were no better than we—when they were clumsy and awkward, too.

"All right," Dr. Snarr says, "let me try my hand." He steps in. I strip off my glove and wash my hands, ready to observe a deft exam, pinpointing the source of pain, exploring yet reassuring.

But in a second the woman is screaming, writhing on the table. Snarr is reaching way far in, clumsily it seems, pushing so hard her hips rise from the table; and she is crying, grabbing the table with her hands. I feel sick just watching. I have no way of knowing what, if anything, Snarr is finding, since he does not explain.

"All right, hon," he tells her. He pulls off his glove. "Wipe yourself off; we'll come back and see you in a minute."

"I don't know why the heck she hurts," he says when we are outside. "Give her some estrogen cream."

She's dressed when I come back in. She's pale and woozy, and there's still pain in her eyes. I hand her the prescription.

"Come back if it gets worse," I say.

"Than what?" the woman asks.

I am embarrassed. I murmur something, that I'm sorry we didn't come up with anything. Then I hurry out after my teacher.

I find him in the side room, having coffee and doughnuts, courtesy of the pharmaceutical rep. The next patient isn't ready yet.

"Have some," he says.

I decline. I'm too jittery to eat.

"That girl," says Dr. Snarr. "What do you think her problem is?"

I consider the possibilities: pelvic inflammatory disease, endometriosis, cysts. I talk, but I don't say what I really think: that he has no sense of what he put her through. That he's insensitive. Clumsy. A jerk. I'm disappointed, too, but I'm not sure why.

Perhaps it's that I wished he was a better doctor, a better role model. Certainly not all gynecologists are like Dr. Snarr, but at that moment it seemed as though they were. And what I needed so much was to know how to be with patients, how to deal with the feelings they evoked, how to make them feel at ease. If Dr. Snarr had been a better teacher, I might conceivably have gone into his field.

Dr. Snarr washes down the rest of his doughnut.

"So what else have we got out there?" he says.

A young black woman in a white gown looks around nervously as we enter.

"Scoot down to the edge of the table, hon," says Snarr.

Wincing at the word *hon*, the woman nevertheless scoots down.

Snarr kicks the wheeled stool over toward me.

And I begin.

DAVID L. SCHIEDERMAYER

DAVID L. SCHIEDERMAYER (1955–). *American physician, educator, ethicist, poet. Schiedermayer was born in Royal Oak, Michigan, and grew up in Appleton, Wisconsin. He received his bachelor's degree in chemistry* summa cum laude *from St. Olaf College. He attended the Medical College of Wisconsin, from which he received his M.D. in 1981, again with a distinguished record. Schiedermayer trained in internal medicine at the Medical College of Wisconsin, where he is now associate professor of medicine. In 1986–1987, he was Henry J. Kaiser Foundation fellow and National Fund for Medical Education visiting scholar at the Center for Clinical Medical Ethics at the University of Chicago. His poetry writing began well before medical school and has continued. Individual poems have appeared in the* Journal of the American Medical Association, Pharos, Annals of Internal Medicine *and the* Archives of Internal Medicine. *His literary work was published in book form as* House Calls, Rounds, and Healings: A Poetry Casebook *(1996). In teaching, he has a special interest in the interplay between medical ethics and compassion, as well as in the use of literature in addressing clinical issues.*

DUTY

Your husband is obsessed
with your care:
he waits on you.
If he owes you
it is certainly not this much,
not this daily washing
and turning
and feeding.
I think this is duty.
He was a military man.
Perhaps, after all, you are his country now,
maybe this is just patriotic love.

I want you to know
even though you are unable to speak
he talks to you and brushes your hair.

When you began dying
I put an IV just under
the skin of your thigh
to keep you a few days longer.
(It is an old nursing home trick.
Raise a goose egg of normal saline
and prevent dehydration
when you can't find a vein.)

Both he and I knew
it was just an endgame
but we needed time.

It was the reverse of induced childbirth:
a drip to slow down the delivery.
Looking back, I am sorry.

But death came fast anyway
and when it did
we cried
looked down on you together
and he stroked your face.
I went to the kitchen
watched the gray squirrels
run through the snow.

When he shook hands,
your husband always
lifted up my hand
just an inch or two
as if to say
I will take care of it, doctor.

ABRAHAM VERGHESE

ABRAHAM VERGHESE (1955–). *American physician, educator, and author. Abraham Verghese is the author of* My Own Country *(1994), a compelling, heartrending, true-life account of his experience treating AIDS patients in a small Tennessee town. Dr. Verghese is a graduate of the Iowa Writers' Workshop; his writing has appeared in* The New Yorker, Granta, *the* North American Review, *and numerous medical journals. His most recent book is* The Tennis Partner: A Doctor's Story of Friendship and Loss *(1998). He is currently a professor of medicine and chief of infectious diseases at Texas Tech Health Sciences Center in El Paso, Texas.*

Excerpt from MY OWN COUNTRY

Bobby Keller called me in the office as I was about to leave for home. He sounded shrill and alarmed.

"Doc? Ed is *very* sick! He is *very, very* short of breath and running a fever. A hundred and three. Dr. Verghese, he's turning blue on me."

"Bobby, call the emergency ambulance service—tell them to bring you to the Johnson City Medical Center."

Ed Maupin, the diesel mechanic, had had a CD_4 count of 30 the previous week when I had seen him in clinic; Bobby Keller's was 500. At that visit, Ed's oral thrush had cleared up but he was still feeling tired and had been missing work. When I had examined Ed, the lymph nodes in his neck, which had been as big as goose eggs, had suddenly shrunk: I had thought to myself that this was either a good sign or a very bad sign; his immune system had either given up the fight or successfully neutralized the virus. The latter was unlikely.

Bobby, at that visit, had looked well and continued to work in the fashion store. I hoped now that Bobby's description of the gravity of the situation was just histrionics.

I was at the Miracle Center well ahead of the ambulance. Soon it came roaring in, all its lights flashing. When the back door opened, I peeked in: Ed's eyes were rolled back in his head, and he was covered with a fine sheen of sweat. Despite the oxygen mask that the ambulance crew had on, his skin was the color of lead. His chest was making vigorous but ineffective excursions.

Bobby, who had ridden in the front, was scarcely able to stand up. His face was tremulous; he was on the verge of fainting.

"Don't put him on no machines, whatever you do," Bobby begged me. "Please, no machines."

"Why?"

"Because that's what he told me. He doesn't want it."

"When did he tell you? Just now?"

"No. A long time ago."

"Did he put it in writing? Does he have a living will?"

"No . . ."

In the emergency room, I stabilized Ed as best I could without intubating him. I took his oxygen mask off momentarily and looked at his mouth. His mucous membranes were loaded with yeast again—it had blossomed in just a week. But I was examining his mouth to try to decide how difficult it would be to intubate him. His short, receding lower jaw, which the beard concealed well, could make this a tricky intubation. I asked him to say "Aaah." He tried to comply: his uvula and tonsils just barely came into view, another sign that he would be a tough intubation.

Ideally, an anesthetist would have been the best person to perform intubation. But I didn't want to call an anesthetist who, given the patient, might or might not be willing to do this procedure. Time was running out.

Ed was moaning and muttering incomprehensibly; his brain was clearly not getting enough oxygen. His blood pressure was 70 millimeters of mercury systolic over 50 diastolic. This was extremely low for him, because he had baseline hypertension. His cold, clammy extremities told me that the circulation to his arms and legs had shut down in an effort to shunt blood to the brain; even so, what blood got to the brain was not carrying enough oxygen. Ed's chest sounded dull in the bases when I percussed it; on listening with my stethoscope, he was wet and gurgly. The reason he was not oxygenating his blood was clear: his lungs were filled with inflammatory fluid. I ordered a stat chest X-ray and arterial blood gases. I had only a few minutes before I had to either breathe for him, or let him go. I needed more guidance from Bobby as to Ed's wishes.

I had an excellent nurse assisting me; she had already started an IV and brought the "crash cart." The respiratory therapist was administering oxygen and had an Ambu bag ready. I asked them to get goggles and masks in addition to their gloves, and to get a gown, mask, and gloves ready for me. They were to put theirs on and wait for me. The curtains were pulled and Ed's presence was largely unnoticed in the bustle of the ER. An orthopedist was putting a cast on an individual in the next room, and patients were waiting in the other cubicles.

I came out to the waiting room, but Bobby was not there!
I hurried outside.

Bobby and three other men and one woman were near the ambulance entrance, smoking. The men bore a striking resemblance to Ed Maupin—the same sharp features, the slightly receding chin. One of them, the oldest, wore a green work uniform. I recognized his face as a familiar one, someone who worked in an auto parts store where I had ordered a replacement bumper for the rusted one that had fallen off my Z. Bobby Keller, still trembling, introduced me to Ed's brothers, all younger than Ed. The woman was the wife of one of the brothers.

"Bobby," I asked, "can I tell them what's going on?"

"Tell them everything," Bobby said, the tears pouring down uncontrollably, his body shaking with sobs.

I addressed the brothers: "Ed is very sick. A few months ago we found out he has AIDS." (There was no point in trying to make the distinction between HIV infection and AIDS. If Ed had not had AIDS when I saw him in the clinic, he most certainly did now.) "Now he has a bad pneumonia from the AIDS. I need to put him on a breathing machine in the next few minutes or he will die. I have a feeling that the pneumonia he has can be treated. If we put him on the breathing machine, it won't be forever. We have a good chance of getting him off. But Bobby tells me that Ed has expressed a desire *not* to be put on the machine."

The assembled family turned to Bobby who nodded vigorously: "He did! Said he never wanted to be on no machines."

The family was clear-eyed, trying to stay calm. They pulled hard at their cigarettes. The smoke rose quietly around their weathered faces. They looked like a Norman Rockwell portrait—small-town America's citizens in their work-clothes in a hospital parking lot, facing a family crisis. But this situation was one that Norman Rockwell hadn't attempted, one he had never dreamed of. I felt they were fond of their oldest brother, though perhaps disapproving of his relationship with Bobby. Yet judging by how they had all been standing around Bobby when I walked out, I didn't think they had any strong dislike for Bobby—it was almost impossible to dislike him. They had had many years to get used to the idea of Bobby and Ed, the couple, and it was only the idea, I sensed, that they had somehow not accepted.

"We need to discuss this," the older brother said.

"We have no time, I need to go right back in," I said.

They moved a few feet away from Bobby and me. I asked Bobby, "Do you have power-of-attorney or anything like that to make decisions for Ed?" Bobby shook his head.

We looked over to where the family was caucusing. The oldest brother was doing all the talking. They came back.

"We want for you to do everything you can. Put him on the breathing machine, if you have to."

At this a little wail came out of Bobby Keller and then degenerated into sobs. I put my hand on Bobby's shoulder. He shook his head back and forth, back and forth. He wanted to say something but could not find a voice.

The oldest brother spoke again. His tone was matter-of-fact and determined:

"*We* are his family. *We* are legally responsible for him. We want you to do *everything* for him."

We are his family. I watched Bobby's face crumble as he suddenly became a mere observer with no legal right to determine the fate of the man he had loved since he was seven years old. He was finally, despite the years that had passed and whatever acceptance he and Ed found together, an outsider.

I took him aside and said, "Bobby, I have to go on. There is no way for me not to at this point. There's a really good chance that I can rescue Ed from the pneumonia. If I thought it would only make Ed suffer, I wouldn't do it. If this is *Pneumocystis*, it should respond to treatment."

Bobby kept sobbing, shaking his head as I talked, fat tears rolling off his eyes onto the ground, onto his chest. He felt he was betraying Ed. He could not deliver on his promise.

I had no time to pacify Bobby or try to convince him. I rushed back in. Ed looked worse. As I went through the ritual of gowning and masking (it was reassuring to have rituals to fall back on, a ritual for every crisis), it struck me that the entire situation had been in my power to dictate. All I had to do was to come out and say that the pneumonia did not look good, that it looked like the end. *I* mentioned the respirator, *I* offered it as an option. I could have just kept quiet. I had, when it came down to the final moment, given Ed's brothers the power of family. Not Bobby.

But there was no time to look back now.

I leaned down to Ed's ear and explained what I was about to do. He showed no sign of understanding. He was expending tremendous amounts of energy to breathe.

I stood behind Ed with the endotracheal tube in my right hand and the laryngoscope in the other. I put Xylocaine jelly on the tip of the endotracheal tube. We lowered the head of the stretcher, extended Ed's head over the edge.

I had the nurse now give Ed an intravenous bolus of 20 milligrams of Valium. An anesthetist might have used a curarelike paralyzing agent. In a few seconds, Ed's breathing ceased altogether.

The respiratory therapist gave him a few brisk breaths of oxygen from the squeeze bag and stepped away. I inserted the laryngoscope blade into his mouth and heaved up on the tongue. I could not see the vocal cords and could only barely see the epiglottis. I pushed the tube past the epiglottis, giving the tube some torque, hoping to steer it into the voice box and down the trachea. It went in too easily and I knew I had missed.

I pulled out and we bagged him with the squeeze bag again. I was talking to myself. *Come on Abe; hamsters are ten times as difficult as this, and you have intubated 260 hamsters at last count.* Another voice in my head replied: *This ain't no hamster.*

Ed was a deeper shade of blue now. If I didn't do it in the next try, we were going to have to call an anesthetist. Or call a Code Blue. The second time and I still did not see the vocal cords. But this time I felt the tube grate against the tracheal rings, just as with my hamsters. I listened over first one side of the chest and then the other while the respiratory therapist pumped air into the tube. I could hear good breath sounds on both sides; we had secured an airway and the tube was sitting in perfect position, just above the carina, where the trachea divides into the left and right bronchi.

It had been a while since I had intubated anyone myself; usually there were layers of interns and residents and students who fought for and did all the procedures. I was pleased with our success. The nurse patted me on the back.

"Did you know," I asked her, in the glow of my postprocedural success, "that intubation was invented by a physician named O'Dwyer as a lifesaving measure in diphtheria? It's therefore an infectious diseases procedure!"

"Yeah, right," she said, unimpressed. "I'll keep that in mind. Next time we have a trauma case that needs intubation we'll call in an infectious diseases consult."

I went upstairs with Ed to the intensive care unit. Now I wrote orders for the settings on the ventilator that would optimally oxygenate Ed's lungs. I put him on a 100 percent inspired oxygen concentration (in contrast to the 21 percent oxygen concentration we normally breathe) and dialed in the rate and the volume of each breath the ventilator would deliver. I wrote an order to have an arterial blood oxygen measurement made in half an hour to allow me to cut back on the oxygen if at all possible; pure oxygen in high concentrations is damaging in and of itself. I wrote orders for intravenous fluids and for laboratory tests. I felt better about Ed in the ICU than I had with Scotty Daws. I had inherited Scotty Daws and in retrospect it had been a no-win situation. Ed was the best sort of patient to bring to the ICU. Someone who I thought would perhaps walk out of there.

Pneumocystis pneumonia is easy to diagnose if you get a good specimen of sputum. Secretions obtained by washing out a segment of lung during bronchoscopy—so-called bronchoalveolar lavage, or BAL—are ideal, but even an ordinary sputum, as long as it is not grossly contaminated with saliva, can serve almost as well.

Since Ed had a tube going down into his trachea, breathing for him, it was simple enough to squirt some saline down it and then suck it back out with a catheter.

I carried the specimen down to the lab, made some smears of it on glass slides, then looked at them under the microscope after staining them for bacteria and TB. I saw only an outpouring of inflammatory cells and little else. To see *Pneumocystis carinii* requires a special stain called a silver stain. It would take a day for the pathology department to complete the stain and give me the definitive word on what it showed. The fact that I saw nothing but pus cells on my simple stains—no TB, no bacteria—suggested that this was *Pneumocystis*. I began Ed on trimethoprim-sulfamethoxazole, or Bactrim, the drug of choice for this organism.

The only cases of *Pneumocystis* pneumonia I had ever seen were in persons with AIDS. This was unique to my generation of infectious diseases physicians: we had all come of age in the era of AIDS.

But *Pneumocystis* had a long history before AIDS made it a household word. Epidemics of *Pneumocystis* swept through Europe in the 1940s. They occurred primarily in premature infants in orphanages, in the setting of overcrowding and malnutrition.

After the war years, the organism began to manifest only in select patients with immune-compromising conditions such as leukemia or after long-term cortisone administration. St. Jude Children's Hospital in Memphis, at the other end of the state from us, had accrued tremendous experience with this disease by virtue of their patient population—children with leukemias.

How are we to view this organism? As an invader from outside? Or an opportunist from within? To give a rat *Pneumocystis* pneumonia, all you have to do is give the rat cortisone—a potent suppressor of the immune system—and the rat then *spontaneously* develops *Pneumocystis* infection. By contrast, Betty and I had to pour staphylococci in massive doses down the hamster trachea to produce infection with staphylococci. The rat experiment suggests that *Pneumocystis* is present in low numbers in the lung at all times. The *Pneumocystis* that at this moment was filling up Ed's lungs lives in my lungs and in yours. The constant vigilance of the immune system keeps it in check. Immune suppression by steroids or, as in Ed's case, AIDS, results in unchecked multiplication of this organism.

I sought out Bobby Keller in the ICU waiting room. His eyes were red and puffy from crying. I tried to explain what I had done so far. Bobby listened perfunctorily to what I had to say about *Pneumocystis* and the amount of oxygen Ed required. It was clear he felt Ed's time had come and that we had gone beyond a threshold of intervention that Ed had not wanted to cross.

When I got home it was after midnight. Steven was in our bed. Rather than disturb them, I went to Steven's room and crawled into his bed.

It felt as if my head had just touched the pillow when my beeper went off. It was from the ICU at the Miracle Center. An intern was calling to say that Ed's heart had gone into a malignant and chaotic rhythm. A Code Blue was in progress.

"What time is it?" I asked.

"Four-thirty in the morning," he said.

"How long has the code been going on?"

"Five minutes. And there has been no sign of his heartbeat coming back."

"Keep going, I'll be right there. Ask the nurses to call in his lover and the family and have them wait in the quiet room."

In the ICU, a furious Code Blue was in progress. All the bustle and activity *around* Ed was in contrast to the activity *in* Ed's body: there was no heartbeat, and only the forceful chest compression by the intern was sending blood around. I reviewed the code chart: everything I would have done had been tried: calcium, epinephrine, bicarbonate. I waved everyone off, thanked them, and we pulled out the tube from Ed's trachea. Ed now looked peaceful, asleep.

In a few minutes there was no one in the room but an ICU nurse and myself. She was a night nurse I had seen around, but never worked with. She was picking up the debris from the code. She was dressed for a shuttle mission—gloves, gown, mask, goggles. This was not inappropriate, as during the Code Blue there was potential for splashing.

I said to her, by way of small talk, "I'm surprised that his heart should have quit so quickly. I really thought I could cure the pneumonia, wean him off the respirator, get a few more meaningful months or even years of life for him."

She stopped what she was doing, looked at me and said, affecting nonchalance: "Well they're *all* going to die, aren't they? There's not much point to this."

She left the room before I could think of an appropriate reply.

I was furious.

I wanted to ask her what the "point" was in the ninety-year-old patients that they played with in the unit for days until they were brain dead, all the while running up a huge bill that we, the taxpayers, would pay. Right at that moment there was a patient in the ICU whom we were sending up for dialysis three times a week when there was no hope of any other organ in the body recovering.

I wanted to ask her if *she* was in the same boat, would she like an extra year of life, or would she opt to leave the world right away? And for that matter, weren't we ALL going to die one day? Did she think her job was to solely take care of immortals?

I calmed myself. "Pick and choose your battles, Abe," I said to myself. In a way she had been baiting me; anything I said back to her would have been a self-fulfilling prophecy for her. It would prove my lack of objectivity. Besides, I *had* failed in this instance. Ed's corpse was proof of my failure.

When I stepped out of the room, I saw her with some other nurses at the nurses' station. She had surely finished telling them about our little encounter. I bade them all good night.

Bobby Keller and the Maupin family were in the quiet room. It was very difficult for me to go in there and tell them Ed had died. Bobby cried. His sobs were big and wrenching. Ed's brothers covered their eyes or turned their heads away from me. The eldest came over and shook my hand and thanked me. Bobby came out with, "Praise the Lord, his suffering is over," and walked alone toward the door.

The next day the pathology report of the bronchial washing from Ed's lung came back. The specimen had been loaded with the saucer-shaped, dark-staining *Pneumocystis*. At this point, of course, it hardly mattered. Ed was dead.

I thought of funerals I had been to in Johnson City where the grieving widow was escorted to the memorial service by friends and family. Tears and hugs, happy memories, casseroles and condolences. Who would comfort Bobby Keller, I wondered.

PERRI KLASS

PERRI KLASS (1958–). *American physician and writer of short stories and novels. Dr. Klass is a pediatrician in Boston. She has written two novels,* Recombinations *(1991) and* Other Women's Children *(1990), a collection of short stories, and a nonfiction account of her experiences as a medical student,* A Not Entirely Benign Procedure *(1988). Her most recent book,* Baby Doctor *(1992), the sequel to* A Not Entirely Benign Procedure, *recounts Klass's three years of mishaps and adventures as a pediatric intern and resident and the lessons she learned from both her patients and their families.*

INVASIONS

Morning rounds in the hospital. We charge along, the resident leading the way, the interns following, the two medical students last, pushing the cart that holds the patients' charts. The resident pulls up in front of a patient's door, the interns stop as well, and we almost run them over with the chart cart. It's time to present the patient, a man who came into the hospital late last night. I did the workup—interviewed him, got his medical history, examined him, wrote a six-page note in his chart, and (at least in theory) spent a little while in the hospital library, reading up on his problems.

"You have sixty seconds, go!" says the resident, looking at his watch. I am of course thinking rebelliously that the interns take as long as they like with their presentations, that the resident himself is long-winded and full of pointless anecdotes—but at the same time I am swinging into my presentation, talking as fast as I can to remind my listeners that no time is being wasted, using the standard hospital turns of phrase. "Mr. Z. is a seventy-eight-year-old white male who presents with dysuria and intermittent hematuria of one week's duration." In other words, for the past week Mr. Z. has experienced pain with urination, and has occasionally passed blood. I rocket on, thinking only about getting through the presentation without being told off for taking too long, without being reprimanded for including nonessential items—or for leaving out crucial bits of data. Of course, fair is fair, my judgment about what is critical and what is not is very faulty. Should I include in this very short presentation (known as a "bullet") that Mr. Z. had gonorrhea five years ago? Well, yes, I decide, and include it in my sentence, beginning, "Pertinent past medical history includes . . ." I don't even have a second to remember how Mr. Z. told me about his gonorrhea, how he made me repeat the question three times last night, my supposedly casual question dropped in between "Have you ever been exposed to tuberculosis?" and "Have you traveled out of the country recently?"

"Five years ago?" The resident interrupts me. "When he was seventy-three? Well, good for him!"

Feeling almost guilty, I think of last night, of how Mr. Z.'s voice dropped to a whisper when he told me about the gonorrhea, how he then went on, as if he felt he had no choice, to explain that he had gone to a convention and "been with a hooker—excuse me, miss, no offense," and how he had then infected his wife, and so on. I am fairly used to this by now, the impulse people sometimes have to confide everything to the person examining them as they enter the hospital. I don't know whether they are frightened by suggestions of disease and mortality, or just accepting me as a medical professional and using me as a comfortable repository for secrets. I have had people tell me about their childhoods and the deaths of their relatives, about their jobs, about things I have needed to ask about and things that have no conceivable bearing on anything that concerns me.

In we charge to examine Mr. Z. The resident introduces himself and the other members of the team, and then he and the interns listen to Mr. Z.'s chest, feel his stomach. As they pull up Mr. Z.'s gown to examine his genitals, the resident says heartily, "Well now, I understand you had a little trouble with VD not so long ago." And immediately I feel like a traitor; I am sure that Mr. Z. is looking at me reproachfully. I have betrayed the secret he was so hesitant to trust me with.

I am aware that my scruples are ridiculous. It is possibly relevant that Mr. Z. had gonorrhea; it is certainly relevant to know how he was treated, whether he might have been reinfected. And in fact, when I make myself meet his eyes, he does not look nearly as distressed at being examined by three people and asked this question in a loud booming voice as he seemed last night with my would-be-tactful inquiries.

In fact, Mr. Z. is getting used to being in the hospital. And in the hospital, as a patient, you have no privacy. The privacy of your body is of necessity violated constantly by doctors and nurses (and the occasional medical student), and details about your physical condition are discussed by the people taking care of you. And your body is made to give up its secrets with a variety of sophisticated techniques, from blood tests to X rays to biopsies—the whole point is to deny your body the privacy that pathological processes need in order to do their damage. Everything must be brought to light, exposed, analyzed, and noted in the chart. And all this is essential for medical care, and even the most modest patients are usually able to come to terms with it, exempting medical personnel from all the most basic rules of privacy and distance.

So much for the details of the patient's physical condition. But the same thing can happen to details of the patient's life. For the remainder of Mr. Z.'s hospital stay, my resident was fond of saying to other doctors, "Got a guy on our service, seventy-eight, got gonorrhea when he was seventy-three, from a showgirl. Pretty good, huh?" He wouldn't ever have said such a thing to Mr. Z.'s relatives, of course, or to any nondoctor. But when it came to his fellow doctors, he saw nothing wrong with it.

I remember another night, 4:00 A.M. in the hospital and I had finally gone to sleep after working up a young woman with a bad case of stomach cramps and diarrhea. Gratefully, I climbed into the top bunk in the on-call room, leaving the bottom bunk for the intern, who might never get to bed, and who, if she did, would have to be ready to leap up at a moment's notice if there was an emergency. Me, I hoped that, emergency or not, I would be overlooked in the top bunk and allowed to sleep out the next two hours and fifty-five minutes in peace (I reserved five minutes to pull myself together before rounds). I lay down and closed my eyes, and something occurred to me. With typical medical student compulsiveness, I had done what is called a "mega-workup" on this patient, I had asked her every possible question about her history and conscientiously written down all her answers. And suddenly I realized that I had written in her chart careful details of all her drug use, cocaine, amphetamines, hallucinogens, all the things she had said she had once used but didn't anymore. She was about my age and had talked to me easily, cheerfully, once her pain was relatively under control, telling me she used to be really into this and that, but now she didn't even drink. And I had written all the details in her chart. I couldn't go to sleep, thinking about those sentences. There was no reason for them. There was no reason everyone had to know all this. There was no reason it had to be written in her official chart, available for legal subpoena. It was four in the morning and I was weary and by no means clear-headed; I began to fantasize one scenario after another in which my careless remarks in this woman's record cost her a job, got her thrown into jail, discredited her forever. And as I dragged myself out of the top bunk and out to the nurses' station to find her chart and cross out the offending sentences with such heavy black lines that they could never be read, I was conscious of an agreeable sense of self-sacrifice—here I was, smudging my immaculate mega-writeup to protect my patient. On rounds, I would say, "Some past drug use," if it seemed relevant.

Medical records are tricky items legally. Medical students are always being reminded to be discreet about what they write—the patient can demand to see the record, the records can be subpoenaed in a trial. Do not make jokes. If you think a serious mistake has been made, do not write that in the record—that is not for you to judge, and you will be providing ammunition for anyone trying to use the record against the hospital. And gradually, in fact, you learn a set of evasions and euphemisms with which doctors comment in charts on differences of opinion, misdiagnoses, and even errors. "Unfortunate complication of usually benign procedure." That kind of thing. The chart is a potential source of damage; damage to the patient, as I was afraid of doing, or damage to the hospital and the doctor.

Medical students and doctors have a reputation for crude humor; some is merely off-color, which comes naturally to people who deal all day with sick bodies. Other jokes can be more disturbing; I remember a patient whose cancer had destroyed her vocal cords so she could no longer talk. In taking her history from her daughter we happened to find out that she had once been a professional musician, singing and playing the piano in supper clubs. For the rest of her stay in the hospital, the resident always introduced her case, when discussing it with other doctors, by saying, "Do you know Mrs. Q.? She used to sing and play the piano—now she just plays the piano."

As you learn to become a doctor, there is a frequent sense of surprise, a feeling that you are not entitled to the kind of intrusion you are allowed into patients' lives. Without arguing, they permit you to examine them; it is impossible to imagine, when you do your very first physical exam, that someday you will walk in calmly and tell a man your grandfather's age to undress, and then examine him without thinking about it twice. You get used to it all, but every so often you find yourself marveling at the access you are allowed, at the way you are learning from the bodies, the stories, the lives and deaths of perfect strangers. They give up their privacy in exchange for some hope— sometimes strong, sometimes faint—of the alleviation of pain, the curing of disease. And gradually, with medical training, that feeling of amazement, that feeling that you are not entitled, scars over. You begin to identify more thoroughly with the medical profession—of course you are entitled to see everything and know everything; you're a doctor, aren't you? And as you accept this as your right, you move further from your patients, even as you penetrate more meticulously and more confidently into their lives.

ELSPETH CAMERON RITCHIE

ELSPETH CAMERON RITCHIE (1958–). *American physician and military psychologist. Born in San Francisco and raised in Washington, D.C., Dr. Ritchie is a graduate of Harvard University and George Washington Medical School. Her writing has been published in a variety of periodicals including the* Journal of the American Medical Association, Military Medicine, *the* Journal of Clinical Psychology, *as well as literary magazines. A major in the U.S. Army, she is currently the head of psychiatry services at the U.S. Army Hospital in Seoul, Korea.*

HOSPITAL SKETCHBOOK: LIFE ON THE WARD THROUGH AN INTERN'S EYES

On the Ward

I carry three AIDS patients, about the same as any other intern on the medicine service at my hospital. One is a young black male, one a young white female, the third a middle-aged black male. The young man received a lethal blood transfusion three years ago. The black man, married with children, has told us of his homosexual activity. The white female has known no risk factors, but we suspect IV drug use. She may simply have slept with an infected man.

A scant two years ago, in a hospital that has a high proportion of AIDS patients, an intern would average only one AIDS patient. I was a third-year medical student then. I cared for, and became close to, my intern's AIDS patient.

His name was Dave. He was attractive, very thin, and gay. He ran fevers and we could not find the cause. So we drew cultures every night, seeking the bug that shot his temperature up to 104 degrees. He would ask me late at night, while I was setting up the tubes and bottles, why I was planning to hurt him. I never had an answer I believed in. The blood cultures were always negative. We finally treated for pneumocystis pneumonia. Then he spiked fevers in reaction to the antibiotic.

At first I gowned and gloved whenever I entered his room; I hated to draw his blood, fearing needle sticks and contamination. I grew more relaxed; sometimes I almost forgot to put on gloves when I drew blood cultures.

He hated being in the hospital. He could not eat the food and seemed thinner every day. I tried once bringing him his favorite flavor of ice cream, butter pecan, from the cafeteria. He thanked me for it but I think he just let it melt.

I rotated off service. I remember his fantasies of leaving, going home to Florida, and floating downstream in a leaky canoe. I'm sure he is long since dead.

Now, with so many patients to care for, both tragedy and precautions are routine. Any patient is risky. I recently stuck myself with a needle for the first time in my life. Fortunately, the married lady had no risk factors. I sent off hepatitis screen and HTLV-3 (now called HIV) tests anyway. They are due back in two weeks. Should I sleep with my husband until then?

All of my HIV patients are sick, hurting, up here on the medicine ward. Asymptomatic ones wait for disposition on the self-care ward. They also wait for the first signs of real illness: the white thrush over the throat, the purple spots of Kaposi's, and shortness of breath of pneumocystis.

My middle-aged black man will die soon. He has cryptococcal meningitis and pneumocystis pneumonia. The titer of cryptococcus is the highest that this hospital has ever seen. Recently he has become even more short of breath and his tremor has gotten worse. He also has painful rectal herpes. Today his bronchoscopy specimens show an acid-fast bacillus, probably a special form of tuberculosis that immunosuppressed patients get. He is already on four toxic antibiotics. What do we do now?

He finally allowed me to tell his family that he is very sick. They do not know of his AIDS diagnosis. His numerous and respectable family arrived last week. They questioned me as to whether he has cancer. I hedge and talk of his pneumonia. They ask me whether he will come home soon. Not yet, he's very sick, I answer. They suspect the truth, I think, but do not ask. His wife has not called.

Interns see a lot of sickness and death. We build up protective mechanisms: she was old, he drank too much. If somebody our age is dying, our mental dams sway. It could be my best friend (who is gay), it could be my college-age brother. There, but for the grace of God, go I.

My young black male received a blood transfusion after he had a minor accident two years ago. He developed a painful throat ulcer and fevers. He was diagnosed six months ago. He did not tell his family for three more months. He is from a remote town in Kentucky and he did not know how his family would respond. They are angry that he did not tell them sooner. He is about to go home for a convalescent leave. What will his neighbors say? Will they believe the blood transfusion or suspect his morals? Will anybody enter his house?

He is still attractive and personable, if thin. This morning he told me how nice I looked. I replaced his feeding tube; his throat hurts too much to swallow. We are doctor and patient. Two years ago I would have hoped that he would ask me out.

I tell myself severely that it is no good crying for him. He has five sisters who will weep. I have other patients to care for.

The third patient, the young white female, is hostile, remote. She has end-stage renal disease and is on dialysis. You have to coax her into drawing her blood. I don't want to do it either, but the consultants recommend an antibiotic level. Of course, they are not the ones who stick her. I am her intern.

I have other patients, patients with heart, lung, liver, and kidney disease, but they come and go quickly. They die or leave. Except, of course, the elderly waiting for nursing home placement. I hope to send one to a home soon. He has been in the hospital for ninety days.

I also care for healthy HIV-positive patients. They are still working and active and only come to the hospital for staging. While here, they have their blood drawn for T-cell count and their skin pricked to see if they react to allergens. Then they return home to their jobs and families. One recent twenty-nine-year-old admission was diagnosed eight months ago. His wife was initially negative; a month ago she converted. They have two children, six and eight, who have not yet been tested.

In a year or three, they will probably be lying in a hospital bed with pneumocystis and cryptococcus raging through their brains and bodies.

Fortunately I am HIV negative. I feel lucky. My husband cooks me supper when I surface after call. My older brother and his wife just had a healthy baby. I know infected two-year-olds.

I warn my younger unmarried brother. My friends all question me. I have only moralistic-sounding statements to make. Don't sleep around!—or even occasionally. I am glad that I am married and tested negative twice. If I were single, would I insist on a blood test before sleeping with a man? I hate to sound so pessimistic when friends grill me at a cocktail party—but I don't want my friends to die that kind of death.

I wish the families of AIDS patients would come more often. You won't catch it by persuading them to eat! They need their mothers, wives, sons here. They are hurt, sick, dying. They need family. I substitute where I can. It is too little for them and too painful for me.

The Intensive Care Unit
December 25, 1985

The lady lies
surrounded by a court
of alarmed machines.
They record life:
blood pressure, pulse
and respirations.
The lady does not talk
so we read her numbers:
the language of
her failing heart.

Her daughter questions
incessantly,
her husband is mute.
Grandchildren in the waiting room
watch Road Runner.
Over the thicket of IV poles
nurses snatch glimpses
of *M*A*S*H* and *St. Elsewhere*.
Electronic Christmas carols
spew over her bed.

Once she ate, excused herself
to her powder room, breathed on her own.
Now, her body is helpless
and her mind.
Perhaps her soul
wonders at her ruined holiday.
She did not mail her Christmas cards.

I draw the bloods,
apologize for sticking her again.
She does not twitch.
Only the ventilator answers.
The Redskins' field goal
should excite her to wake.
Instead her heart throws a
crazy beat.
Then another—
time for another EKG.

I sigh; no sleep again
tonight, Christmas night.
I nibble microwave popcorn and
stale fruitcake, swig Diet Coke.
A tube bears Osmolyte for her.

The clouded moon through the window
over her busy bed, reminds me of
when I believed in Angels.
Every Christmas, when I was a child,
I searched the orange city skies
for their shining.

I seek again tonight.
No answer.
Winged men triumphantly
should bear her soul to Heaven,
bring me a festival stocking.

Yet, I hope she does not die today
(though my tasks would be fewer).
Her grandchildren should not remember
Christ's birthday and new toys
by her death.

Her blood pressure is dropping.

I will try to keep her
breathing until tomorrow.

Language Barrier

It gets hard to communicate in the old language.

When I started medical school, our courses were basically word lists. The lists were anatomy and microbiology. We memorized the eleven muscles of the thumb, chambers of the heart, classification of diseases of the colon. It was like studying French. All those nouns to memorize!

We all studied how the organs work, of course: the lungs exchange gases, the heart spins blood around, the kidney filters the waste. We peered at purple-painted bacteria, watched antibiotics scour those bugs from the petri dishes. But it was the names that we were tested on, the vocabulary that would isolate us as physicians.

In medical school we were taught never to refer to patients as a disease. To say "the gall bladder down the hall" was demeaning. We resolved always to give our patients due respect.

Back in those pre-war days, they also warned us to continue to communicate with our families, friends, and children. "Spend an hour with your child every day." "Take time out to go running." "It's important to keep up with politics."

Then came third year, the clinical years. The dicta were moot. Even if we had a free half hour it was more important, it seemed, to polish up the history and physical for presentation to our preceptors, to volunteer to hold retractors for another cholecystectomy, to scour the library for articles on esoteric aspects of lupus.

Shakespeare, botany, evolution were lost fantasies. Once, I learned how many petals adorned roses. Now, flower petals are submerged beneath liver enzymes.

The gap widened. How could our husbands know the frustrations of missing a blood draw three times, then have the intern draw pints with ease? When eating with in-laws we could not talk at dinner of the smell of melena (old blood leaking out of the rectum), nor of the skin lesions on our AIDS patients.

As time rolled by, life outside the hospital dwindles. Now I am an intern.

"How was your day, dear?" I politely inquire at home at eight P.M. after a night on call.

"Terrible. The computer went down on a very important project. I was at work from eight this morning to seven tonight. Then the bus broke down. I need a drink. Oh, yes, how was yours?"

I am silent for a minute. "Well, I was lucky last night on call. I slept from one A.M. to four A.M. Then I got a drunk hit from the nursing home with chest pain. But I slept again from six-thirty to seven-thirty. So, almost four hours." Of course that is in a cell-like call room in the bottom of a creaky bunk bed. Meal carts creaking and nurses gossiping loudly outside. Another thirty-seven-hour shift. But I got close to four hours. These days that's cause for celebration. Almost.

So, my sympathies for others' trials are slight. Unfairly, I become impatient with their tribulations. Sometimes I explode.

"Don't tell me about your difficulties with your computer. My favorite patient is dying. And one of my AIDS patients developed pneumocystis pneumonia. And you're whining because you partied too late with friends when I was on call and only got six hours of sleep."

Non-medical friends sympathize. "Oh, you poor dear." They try to help and are puzzled when I am nasty and irritable.

In cocktail conversations acquaintances say: "That's a terrible system. It should not be allowed. I wouldn't want to be cared for by somebody who had been up all night." Noses tilt. Their anger descends on me. I'm a doctor.

Thanks. I don't want to care for them either after I've been up all night. But I can't afford the energy to waste on rage at the system.

After all, it's a privilege to be a doctor.

My fellows on the battlefront become my in-arms comrades, at least until we rotate to a new service. We joke about the drunk hit. We share doughnuts and popcorn. On rounds we talk about the gall bladder down the hall and the valve in Room 4116.

We develop sexual fantasies about those in the trenches with us. At two A.M. your resident is your staff. When a patient is spurting blood out of his tracheostomy and you together insert a central line (an IV in the neck), transfer him to the unit, and save his life (at least for now), then you are brothers. Afterwards you raise Diet Cokes in companionship.

How can your husband compare to him, the man who just helped you save a life?

Marriages are made in medical school and dissolve in internship.

But the deans who pontificated in medical school about the values of outside interests were right. We—the battered products of medical school—know that to be true. It just gets harder. The gap widens.

"She didn't make it. We coded her and shocked her and put a pacemaker into her. It didn't work. Why, I'm not sure. We asked for an autopsy. What should we have for dinner?"

Hospital Spaces

Life is defined by bounds:
here, sickness and health are also sequestered.
We have the isolated rooms of infection,
and social wards of men whose
efforts are limited by chest pain.
They play spades with vigor.

Metal rails surround the beds with
air bubbling up through fluid plastic beads,
confining and relieving the comatose.

The staff have large hectic rooms
with multiple desks and phones ringing.
We report local recoveries and deaths,
call the public health department,
and field calls about AIDS and angina.
Chairs are constantly swiped from one desk
to another, as an intern dashes in to
scribble a note, feet hurting,
or to try to turf a patient to a nursing home.
This one has been in for ninety-seven days.

The hallways link the separate worlds.
Like salt sea barnacles
groups of doctors cling on the walls,
discussing their patients' potassium
(barely out of earshot),
drinking instant coffee, grateful
if a stretcher appears to perch on.
Two hours' sleep last night.
A long day's journey ahead.

The pantry is guarded by fierce ladies
microwaving the trays of hospital food.
Medical students sneak in to steal
leftover chocolate pudding.

Elevators frustrate. Waiting,
pondering my clipboard,
I can hear them ping at every floor.
Rumbling food racks are loaded.
To the lab, to x-ray, then to surgery clinic
to drop off another consult.
I wave to friends on contralateral trips.
How many romances start, and stop,
with the opening and shutting of doors?

Sometimes a patient crashes on the
seventh floor.
With cardiac monitor beeping,
and code drugs on the stretcher,
in case his heart stops,
we transport a patient vomiting blood
to the ICU on the fourth floor,
squeezing past the linen carts
in the narrow hallways,
hoping that we will make it,
before he stops breathing.

So far, so good.
More lines intersect.
The snack bar, the chapel, and barber shop,
the clinics and the morgue.
The library offers a soft chair for sleep.

My beeper is a leash,
jerking me back
to headaches and chest pain.

When I finally break out into the
winter evening,
after 38 hours of the hospital,
it is amazing that
I can remember where the car is,
and that
yellow crocuses are blooming.

JON MUKAND

JON MUKAND (1959–). *American physician, poet, and editor. Dr. Mukand attended the University of Minnesota and received his M.D. from the Medical College of Wisconsin. Midway through medical school, he obtained an M.A. in English literature from Stanford. He did postgraduate training in physical medicine/rehabilitation at Boston University School of Medicine. He subsequently received a Ph.D. in literature from Brown University. He is on the clinical faculties of Boston University, Brown University, and Tufts University. Mukand is the editor of* Articulations: The Body and Illness in Poetry *(1994) and* Vital Lines: Contemporary Fiction About Medicine. *He also edited* Rehabilitation for Patients with HIV Disease.

LULLABY

Each morning I finish my coffee,
And climb the stairs to the charts,
Hoping yours will be filed away.
But you can't hear me,
You can't see yourself clamped
Between this hard plastic binder:
Lab reports and nurses' notes, a sample
In a test tube. I keep reading
These terse comments: stable as before,
Urine output still poor, respiration normal.
And you keep on poisoning
Yourself, your kidneys more useless
Than seawings drenched in an oil spill.
I find my way to your room
And lean over the bedrails
As though I can understand
Your wheezed-out fragments.
What can I do but check
Your tubes, feel your pulse, listen
To your heartbeat insistent
As a spoiled child who goes on begging?

Old man, listen to me:
Let me take you in a wheelchair
To the back room of the records office,
Let me lift you in my arms
And lay you down in the cradle
Of a clean manila folder.

FIRST PAYMENT

In the waiting room, she releases
her white hair from a blue gauze scarf.
Her body has accepted the disease with
no cure, her questions are
empty snail shells. The pain stays,
with the appetite of crabgrass.
She cannot reach
inside, pluck it out by the roots.

Some days, she wants to be only
a gust of winter wind sweeping
the fresh snow
into drifts & whorls on the prairie, filtering
through an apple orchard. She might
linger, wrap herself around
naked branches, wait for spring buds.
She might even learn to be
patient for the orange sun
to drag the bleached skeleton of each day
behind the snow-tinted hills.

The intercom calls. Clenching her
body, she lifts herself up
with a gnarled, polished walking-stick.
In the examining room, her eyes
wander over the fresh table,
the chrome lamp with its fixed gaze.

The student knocks and enters, ready
for her coerced smiles, her
handshake brittle as a curled up leaf.
From her black handbag, a
sealed envelope. *Open it.*
Inside, a new fifty-dollar bill.
To help with school, I know it's expensive.
He can only smile, return her money.
It lies in her palm like a
handful of earth picked up, raised
to the sky
as an offering to the spring wind.

ETHAN CANIN

ETHAN CANIN (1961–). *American physician and writer. Canin received a B.A. in engineering from Stanford, an M.F.A. from the Iowa Writers' Workshop/University of Iowa, and an M.D. from Harvard Medical School. His first book,* Emperor of the Air *(1988), won the prestigious Houghton Mifflin Literary Fellowship. His subsequent books have also won great acclaim:* Blue River *(1991) and* The Palace Thief *(1994). His latest book is* For Kings and Planets *(1998). He is a tenured professor at the Iowa Writers' Workshop.*

WE ARE NIGHTTIME TRAVELERS

Where are we going? Where, I might write, is this path leading us? Francine is asleep and I am standing downstairs in the kitchen with the door closed and the light on and a stack of mostly blank paper on the counter in front of me. My dentures are in a glass by the sink. I clean them with a tablet that bubbles in the water, and although they were clean already I just cleaned them again because the bubbles are agreeable and I thought their effervescence might excite me to action. By action, I mean I thought they might excite me to write. But words fail me.

This is a love story. However, its roots are tangled and involve a good bit of my life, and when I recall my life my mood turns sour and I am reminded that no man makes truly proper use of his time. We are blind and small-minded. We are dumb as snails and as frightened, full of vanity and misinformed about the importance of things. I'm an average man, without great deeds except maybe one, and that has been to love my wife.

I have been more or less faithful to Francine since I married her. There has been one transgression—leaning up against a closet wall with a red-haired purchasing agent at a sales meeting once in Minneapolis twenty years ago; but she was buying auto upholstery and I was selling it and in the eyes of judgment this may bear a key weight. Since then, though, I have ambled on this narrow path of life bound to one woman. This is a triumph and a regret. In our current state of affairs it is a regret because in life a man is either on the uphill or on the downhill, and if he isn't procreating he is on the downhill. It is a steep downhill indeed. These days I am tumbling, falling headlong among the scrub oaks and boulders, tearing my knees and abrading all the bony parts of the body. I have given myself to gravity.

Francine and I are married now forty-six years, and I would be a bamboozler to say that I have loved her for any more than half of these. Let us say that for the last year I haven't; let us say this for the last ten, even. Time has made torments of our small differences and tolerance of our passions. This is our state of affairs. Now I stand by myself in our kitchen in the middle of the night; now I lead a secret life. We wake at different hours now, sleep in different corners of the bed. We like different foods and different music, keep our clothing in different drawers, and if it can be said that either of us has aspirations, I believe that they are to a different bliss. Also, she is healthy and I am ill. And as for conversation—that feast of reason, that flow of the soul—our house is silent as the bone yard.

Last week we did talk. "Frank," she said one evening at the table, "there is something I must tell you."

The New York game was on the radio, snow was falling outside, and the pot of tea she had brewed was steaming on the table between us. Her medicine and my medicine were in little paper cups at our places.

"Frank," she said, jiggling her cup, "what I must tell you is that someone was around the house last night."

I tilted my pills onto my hand. "Around the house?"

"Someone was at the window."

On my palm the pills were white, blue, beige, pink: Lasix, Diabinese, Slow-K, Lopressor. "What do you mean?"

She rolled her pills onto the tablecloth and fidgeted with them, made them into a line, then into a circle, then into a line again. I don't know her medicine so well. She's healthy, except for little things. "I mean," she said, "there was someone in the yard last night."

"How do you know?"

"Frank, will you really, please?"

"I'm asking how you know."

"I heard him," she said. She looked down. "I was sitting in the front room and I heard him outside the window."

"You heard him?"

"Yes."

"The front window?"

She got up and went to the sink. This is a trick of hers. At that distance I can't see her face.

"The front window is ten feet off the ground," I said.

"What I know is that there was a man out there last night, right outside the glass." She walked out of the kitchen.

"Let's check," I called after her. I walked into the living room, and when I got there she was looking out the window.

"What is it?"

She was peering out at an angle. All I could see was snow, blue-white.

"Footprints," she said.

I built the house we live in with my two hands. That was forty-nine years ago, when, in my foolishness and crude want of learning, everything I didn't know seemed like a promise. I learned to build a house and then I built one. There are copper fixtures on the pipes, sanded edges on the struts and queen posts. Now, a half-century later, the floors are flat as a billiard table but the man who laid them needs two hands to pick up a woodscrew. This is the diabetes. My feet are gone also. I look down at them and see two black shapes when I walk, things I can't feel. Black clubs. No connection with the ground. If I didn't look, I could go to sleep with my shoes on.

Life takes its toll, and soon the body gives up completely. But it gives up the parts first. This sugar in the blood: God says to me: "Frank Manlius—codger, man of prevarication and half-truth—I shall take your life from you, as from all men. But first—" But first! Clouds in the eyeball, a heart that makes noise, feet cold as uncooked roast. And Francine, beauty that she was—now I see not much more than the dark line of her brow and the intersections of her body: mouth and nose, neck and shoulders. Her smells have changed over the years so that I don't know what's her own anymore and what's powder.

We have two children, but they're gone now too, with children of their own. We have a house, some furniture, small savings to speak of. How Francine spends her day I don't know. This is the sad truth, my confession. I am gone past nightfall. She wakes early with me and is awake when I return, but beyond this I know almost nothing of her life.

I myself spend my days at the aquarium. I've told Francine something else, of course, that I'm part of a volunteer service of retired men, that we spend our days setting young businesses afoot: "Immigrants," I told her early on, "newcomers to the land." I said it was difficult work. In the evenings I could invent stories, but I don't, and Francine doesn't ask.

I am home by nine or ten. Ticket stubs from the aquarium fill my coat pocket. Most of the day I watch the big sea animals—porpoises, sharks, a manatee—turn their saltwater loops. I come late morning and move a chair up close. They are waiting to eat then. Their bodies skim the cool glass, full of strange magnifications. I think, if it is possible, that they are beginning to know me: this man—hunched at the shoulder, cataractic of eye, breathing through water himself—this man who sits and watches. I do not pity them. At lunchtime I buy coffee and sit in one of the hotel lobbies or in the cafeteria next door, and I read poems. Browning, Whitman, Eliot. This is my secret. It is night when I return home. Francine is at the table, four feet across from my seat, the width of two dropleaves. Our medicine is in cups. There have been three Presidents since I held her in my arms.

The cafeteria moves the men along, old or young, who come to get away from the cold. A half-hour for a cup, they let me sit. Then the manager is at my table. He is nothing but polite. I buy a pastry then, something small. He knows me—I have seen him nearly every day for months now—and by his slight limp I know he is a man of mercy. But business is business.

"What are you reading?" he asks me as he wipes the table with a wet cloth. He touches the saltshaker, nudges the napkins in their holder. I know what this means.

"I'll take a cranberry roll," I say. He flicks the cloth and turns back to the counter.

This is what:

> Shall I say, I have gone at dusk through narrow streets
> And watched the smoke that rises from the pipes
> Of lonely men in shirt-sleeves, leaning out of windows?

Through the magnifier glass the words come forward, huge, two by two. With spectacles, everything is twice enlarged. Still, though, I am slow to read it. In a half-hour I am finished, could not read more, even if I bought another roll. The boy at the register greets me, smiles when I reach him. "What are you reading today?" he asks, counting out the change.

The books themselves are small and fit in the inside pockets of my coat. I put one in front of each breast, then walk back to see the fish some more. These are the fish I know: the gafftopsail pompano, sixgill shark, the starry flounder with its upturned eyes, queerly migrated. He rests half-submerged in sand. His scales are platey and flat-hued. Of everything upward he is wary, of the silvery seabass and the bluefin tuna that pass above him in the region of light and open water.

For a life he lies on the bottom of the tank. I look at him. His eyes are dull. They are ugly and an aberration. Above us the bony fishes wheel at the tank's corners. I lean forward to the glass. *"Platichthys stellatus,"* I say to him. The caudal fin stirs. Sand moves and resettles, and I see the black and yellow stripes. "Flatfish," I whisper, "we are, you and I, observers of this life."

"A man on our lawn," I say a few nights later in bed.
"Not just that."
I breathe in, breathe out, look up at the ceiling. "What else?"
"When you were out last night he came back."
"He came back."
"Yes."
"What did he do?"
"Looked in at me."
Later, in the early night, when the lights of cars are still passing and the walked dogs still jingle their collar chains out front, I get up quickly from bed and step into the hall. I move fast because this is still possible in short bursts and with concentration. The bed sinks once, then rises. I am on the landing and then downstairs without Francine waking. I stay close to the staircase joists.

In the kitchen I take out my almost blank sheets and set them on the counter. I write standing up because I want to take more than an animal's pose. For me this is futile, but I stand anyway. The page will be blank when I finish. This I know. The dreams I compose are the dreams of others, remembered bits of verse. Songs of greater men than I. In months I have written few more than a hundred words. The pages are stacked, sheets of different sizes.

If I could

one says.

It has never seemed

says another. I stand and shift them in and out. They are mostly blank, sheets from months of nights. But this doesn't bother me. What I have is patience.

Francine knows nothing of the poetry. She's a simple girl, toast and butter. I myself am hardly the man for it: forty years selling (anything—steel piping, heater elements, dried bananas). Didn't read a book except one on sales. Think victory, the book said. Think *sale.* It's a young man's bag of apples, though; young men in pants that nip at the waist. Ten years ago I left the Buick in the company lot and walked home, dye in my hair, cotton rectangles in the shoulders of my coat. Francine was in the house that afternoon also, the way she is now. When I retired we bought a camper and went on a trip. A traveling salesman retires, so he goes on a trip. Forty miles out of town the folly appeared to me, big as a balloon. To Francine, too. "Frank," she said in the middle of a bend, a prophet turning to me, the camper pushing sixty and rocking in the wind, trucks to our left and right big as trains—"Frank," she said, "these roads must be familiar to you."

So we sold the camper at a loss and a man who'd spent forty years at highway speed looked around for something to do before he died. The first poem I read was in a book on a table in a waiting room. My eyeglasses made half-sense of things.

> These
> are the desolate, dark weeks

I read

> when nature in its barrenness
> equals the stupidity of man.

Gloom, I thought, and nothing more, but then I reread the words, and suddenly there I was, hunched and wheezing, bald as a trout, and tears were in my eye. I don't know where they came from.

In the morning an officer visits. He has muscles, mustache, skin red from the cold. He leans against the door frame.

"Can you describe him?" he says.

"It's always dark," says Francine.

"Anything about him?"

"I'm an old woman. I can see that he wears glasses."

"What kind of glasses?"

"Black."

"Dark glasses?"

"Black glasses."

"At a particular time?"

"Always when Frank is away."

"Your husband has never been here when he's come?"

"Never."

"I see." He looks at me. This look can mean several things, perhaps that he thinks Francine is imagining. "But never at a particular time?"

"No."

"Well," he says. Outside on the porch his partner is stamping his feet. "Well," he says again. "We'll have a look." He turns, replaces his cap, heads out to the snowy steps. The door closes. I hear him say something outside.

"Last night—" Francine says. She speaks in the dark. "Last night I heard him on the side of the house."

We are in bed. Outside, on the sill, snow has been building since morning.

"You heard the wind."

"Frank." She sits up, switches on the lamp, tilts her head toward the window. Through a ceiling and two walls I can hear the ticking of our kitchen clock.

"I heard him climbing," she says. She has wrapped her arms about her own waist. "He was on the house. I heard him. He went up the drainpipe." She shivers as she says this. "There was no wind. He went up the drainpipe and then I heard him on the porch roof."

"Houses make noise."

"I heard him. There's gravel there."

I imagine the sounds, amplified by hollow walls, rubber heels on timber. I don't say anything. There is an arm's length between us, a cold sheet, a space uncrossed since I can remember.

"I have made the mistake in my life of not being interested in enough people," she says then. "If I'd been interested in more people, I wouldn't be alone now."

"Nobody's alone," I say.

"I mean that if I'd made more of an effort with people I would have friends now. I would know the postman and the Giffords and the Kohlers, and we'd be together in this, all of us. We'd sit in each other's living rooms on rainy days and talk about the children. Instead we've kept to ourselves. Now I'm alone."

"You're not alone," I say.

"Yes, I am." She turns the light off and we are in the dark again. "You're alone, too."

My health has gotten worse. It's slow to set in at this age, not the violent shaking grip of death; instead—a slow leak, nothing more. A bicycle tire: rimless, thready, worn treadless already and now losing its fatness. A war of attrition. The tall camels of the spirit steering for the desert. One morning I realized I hadn't been warm in a year.

And there are other things that go, too. For instance, I recall with certainty that it was on the 23rd of April, 1945, that, despite German counteroffensives in the Ardennes, Eisenhower's men reached the

Elbe; but I cannot remember whether I have visited the savings and loan this week. Also, I am unable to produce the name of my neighbor, though I greeted him yesterday in the street. And take, for example, this: I am at a loss to explain whole decades of my life. We have children and photographs, and there is an understanding between Francine and me that bears the weight of nothing less than half a century, but when I gather my memories they seem to fill no more than an hour. Where has my life gone?

It has gone partway to shoddy accumulations. In my wallet are credit cards, a license ten years expired, twenty-three dollars in cash. There is a photograph but it depresses me to look at it, and a poem, half-copied and folded into the billfold. The leather is pocked and has taken on the curve of my thigh. The poem is from Walt Whitman. I copy only what I need.

But of all things to do last, poetry is a barren choice. Deciphering other men's riddles while the world is full of procreation and war. A man should go out swinging an axe. Instead, I shall go out in a coffee shop.

But how can any man leave this world with honor? Despite anything he does, it grows corrupt around him. It fills with locks and sirens. A man walks into a store now and the microwaves announce his entry; when he leaves, they make electronic peeks into his coat pockets, his trousers. Who doesn't feel like a thief? I see a policeman now, any policeman, and I feel a fright. And the things I've done wrong in my life haven't been crimes. Crimes of the heart perhaps, but nothing against the state. My soul may turn black but I can wear white trousers at any meeting of men. Have I loved my wife? At one time, yes—in rages and torrents. I've been covered by the pimples of ecstasy and have rooted in the mud of despair; and I've lived for months, for whole years now, as mindless of Francine as a tree of its mosses.

And this is what kills us, this mindlessness. We sit across the tablecloth now with our medicines between us, little balls and oblongs. We sit, sit. This has become our view of each other, a tableboard apart. We sit.

"Again?" I say.

"Last night."

We are at the table. Francine is making a twisting motion with her fingers. She coughs, brushes her cheek with her forearm, stands suddenly so that the table bumps and my medicines move in the cup.

"Francine," I say.

The half-light of dawn is showing me things outside the window:

silhouettes, our maple, the eaves of our neighbor's garage. Francine moves and stands against the glass, hugging her shoulders.

"You're not telling me something," I say.

She sits and makes her pills into a circle again, then into a line. Then she is crying.

I come around the table, but she gets up before I reach her and leaves the kitchen. I stand there. In a moment I hear a drawer open in the living room. She moves things around, then shuts it again. When she returns she sits at the other side of the table. "Sit down," she says. She puts two folded sheets of paper onto the table. "I wasn't hiding them," she says.

"What weren't you hiding?"

"These," she says. "He leaves them."

"He leaves them?"

"They say he loves me."

"Francine."

"They're inside the windows in the morning." She picks one up, unfolds it. Then she reads:

> Ah, I remember well (and how can I
> But evermore remember well) when first

She pauses, squint-eyed, working her lips. It is a pause of only faint understanding. Then she continues:

> Our flame began, when scarce we knew what was
> The flame we felt.

When she finishes she refolds the paper precisely. "That's it," she says. "That's one of them."

At the aquarium I sit, circled by glass and, behind it, the senseless eyes of fish. I have never written a word of my own poetry but can recite the verse of others. This is the culmination of a life. *Coryphaena hippurus*, says the plaque on the dolphin's tank, words more beautiful than any of my own. The dolphin circles, circles, approaches with alarming speed, but takes no notice of, if he even sees, my hands. I wave them in front of his tank. What must he think has become of the sea? He turns and his slippery proboscis nudges the glass. I am every part sore from life.

> Ah, silver shrine, here will I take my rest
> After so many hours of toil and quest,
> A famished pilgrim—saved by miracle.

There is nothing noble for either of us here, nothing between us, and no miracles. I am better off drinking coffee. Any fluid refills the blood. The counter boy knows me and later at the café he pours the cup, most of a dollar's worth. Refills are free but my heart hurts if I drink more than one. It hurts no different from a bone, bruised or cracked. This amazes me.

Francine is amazed by other things. She is mystified, thrown beam ends by the romance. She reads me the poems now at breakfast, one by one. I sit. I roll my pills. "Another came last night," she says, and I see her eyebrows rise. "Another this morning." She reads them as if every word is a surprise. Her tongue touches teeth, shows between lips. These lips are dry. She reads:

> Kiss me as if you made believe
> You were not sure, this eve,
> How my face, your flower, had pursed
> Its petals up

That night she shows me the windowsill, second story, rimmed with snow, where she finds the poems. We open the glass. We lean into the air. There is ice below us, sheets of it on the trellis, needles hanging from the drainwork.

"Where do you find them?"

"Outside," she says. "Folded, on the lip."

"In the morning?"

"Always in the morning."

"The police should know about this."

"What will they be able to do?"

I step away from the sill. She leans out again, surveying her lands, which are the yard's-width spit of crusted ice along our neighbor's chain link and the three maples out front, now lost their leaves. She peers as if she expects this man to appear. An icy wind comes inside. "Think," she says. "Think. He could come from anywhere."

One night in February, a month after this began, she asks me to stay awake and stand guard until the morning. It is almost spring. The earth has reappeared in patches. During the day, at the borders of yards and driveways, I see glimpses of brown—though I know I could be mistaken. I come home early that night, before dusk, and when darkness falls I move a chair by the window downstairs. I draw apart the outer curtain and raise the shade. Francine brings me a pot of tea. She turns out the light and pauses next to me, and as she does, her hand on the chair's backbrace, I am so struck by the proximity of elements—of the night, of the teapot's heat, of the sounds of water outside—that I consider speaking. I want to ask her what has become of us, what has made our breathed air so sorry now, and loveless. But the timing is wrong and in a moment she turns and climbs the stairs. I look out into the night. Later, I hear the closet shut, then our bed creak.

There is nothing to see outside, nothing to hear. This I know. I let hours pass. Behind the window I imagine fish moving down to greet me: broomtail grouper, surfperch, sturgeon with their prehistoric rows of scutes. It is almost possible to see them. The night is full of shapes and bits of light. In it the moon rises, losing the colors of the horizon, so that by early morning it is high and pale. Frost has made a ring around it.

A ringed moon above, and I am thinking back on things. What have I regretted in my life? Plenty of things, mistakes enough to fill the car showroom, then a good deal of the back lot. I've been a man of gains and losses. What gains? My marriage, certainly, though it has been no knee-buckling windfall but more like a split decision in the end, a stock risen a few points since bought. I've certainly enjoyed certain things about the world, too. These are things gone over and over again by the writers and probably enjoyed by everybody who ever lived. Most of them involve air. Early morning air, air after a rainstorm, air through a car window. Sometimes I think the cerebrum is wasted and all we really need is the lower brain, which I've been told is what makes the lungs breathe and the heart beat and what lets us smell pleasant things. What about the poetry? That's another split decision, maybe going the other way if I really made a tally. It's made me melancholy in old age, sad when if I'd stuck with motor homes and the National League standings I don't think I would have been rooting around in regret and doubt at this point. Nothing wrong with sadness, but this is not the real thing—not the death of a child but the feelings of a college student reading *Don Quixote* on a warm afternoon before going out to the lake.

Now, with Francine upstairs, I wait for a night prowler. He will not appear. This I know, but the window glass is ill-blown and makes moving shadows anyway, shapes that change in the wind's rattle. I look out and despite myself am afraid.

Before me, the night unrolls. Now the tree leaves turn yellow in moonshine. By two or three, Francine sleeps, but I get up anyway and change into my coat and hat. The books weigh against my chest. I don gloves, scarf, galoshes. Then I climb the stairs and go into our bedroom, where she is sleeping. On the far side of the bed I see her white hair and beneath the blankets the uneven heave of her chest. I watch the bedcovers rise. She is probably dreaming at this moment. Though we have shared this bed for most of a lifetime I cannot guess what her dreams are about. I step next to her and touch the sheets where they lie across her neck.

"Wake up," I whisper. I touch her cheek, and her eyes open. I know this though I cannot really see them, just the darkness of their sockets.

"Is he there?"

"No."

"Then what's the matter?"

"Nothing's the matter," I say. "But I'd like to go for a walk."

"You've been outside," she says. "You saw him, didn't you?"

"I've been at the window."

"Did you see him?"

"No. There's no one there."

"Then why do you want to walk?" In a moment she is sitting aside the bed, her feet in slippers. "We don't ever walk," she says.

I am warm in all my clothing. "I know we don't," I answer. I turn my arms out, open my hands toward her. "But I would like to. I would like to walk in air that is so new and cold."

She peers up at me. "I haven't been drinking," I say. I bend at the waist, and though my head spins, I lean forward enough so that the effect is of a bow. "Will you come with me?" I whisper. "Will you be queen of this crystal night?" I recover from my bow, and when I look up again she has risen from the bed, and in another moment she has dressed herself in her wool robe and is walking ahead of me to the stairs.

Outside, the ice is treacherous. Snow has begun to fall and our galoshes squeak and slide, but we stay on the plowed walkway long enough to leave our block and enter a part of the neighborhood where I have never been. Ice hangs from the lamps. We pass unfamiliar houses and unfamiliar trees, street signs I have never seen, and as we walk the night begins to change. It is becoming liquor. The snow is banked on either side of the walk, plowed into hillocks at the corners. My hands are warming from the exertion. They are the hands of a younger man now, someone else's fingers in my gloves. They tingle. We take ten minutes to cover a block but as we move through this neighborhood my ardor mounts. A car approaches and I wave, a boatman's salute, because here we are together on these rare and empty seas. We are nighttime travelers. He flashes his headlamps as he passes, and this fills me to the gullet with celebration and bravery. The night sings to us. I am Bluebeard now, Lindbergh, Genghis Khan.

No, I am not.

I am an old man. My blood is dark from hypoxia, my breaths singsong from disease. It is only the frozen night that is splendid. In it we walk, stepping slowly, bent forward. We take steps the length of table forks. Francine holds my elbow.

I have mean secrets and small dreams, no plans greater than where to buy groceries and what rhymes to read next, and by the time we reach our porch again my foolishness has subsided. My knees and elbows ache. They ache with a mortal ache, tired flesh, the cartilage gone sandy with time. I don't have the heart for dreams. We undress in the hallway, ice in the ends of our hair, our coats stiff from cold. Francine turns down the thermostat. Then we go upstairs and she gets into her side of the bed and I get into mine.

It is dark. We lie there for some time, and then, before dawn, I know she is asleep. It is cold in our bedroom. As I listen to her breathing I know my life is coming to an end. I cannot warm myself. What I would like to tell my wife is this:

> What the
> imagination
> seizes
> as beauty must be truth. What holds you
> to what you see of me is
> that grasp alone.

But I do not say anything. Instead I roll in the bed, reach across, and touch her, and because she is surprised she turns to me.

When I kiss her the lips are dry, cracking against mine, unfamiliar as the ocean floor. But then the lips give. They part. I am inside her mouth, and there, still, hidden from the word, as if ruin had forgotten a part, it is wet—Lord! I have the feeling of a miracle. Her tongue comes forward. I do not know myself then, what man I am, who I lie with in embrace. I can barely remember her beauty. She touches my chest and I bite lightly on her lip, spread moisture to her cheek, and then kiss there. She makes something like a sigh. "Frank," she says. "Frank." We are lost now in seas and deserts. My hand holds her fingers and grips them, bone and tendon, fragile things.

RAFAEL CAMPO

RAFAEL CAMPO (1964–). *American physician, poet. Rafael Campo was born in Dover, New Jersey. After attending college at Amherst, he went to Harvard Medical School, where he currently teaches and practices general internal medicine. He is the author of three books of poetry, including* The Other Man Was Me: A Voyage to the New World *(1994), winner of the National Poetry Series 1993 Open Competition;* What the Body Told *(1996), winner of a Lambda Literary Award; and* Diva *(1999), a finalist for the National Book Critics Circle Award. His 1996 book,* The Poetry of Healing, *also received a Lambda Literary Award in the memoir category. His poetry often focuses on family, particularly his immigrant family's roots in Spain and Cuba; on his work as a physician; on his patients, many of whom have AIDS; and on his identity as a gay Latino.*

EL CURANDERO

I am bathing. All my greyness—
The hospital, the incurable illnesses,
This headache—is slowly given over
To bathwater, deepening it to where

I lose sight of my limbs. The fragrance,
Twenty different herbs at first (dill, spices
From the Caribbean, aloe vera)
Settles, and becomes the single, warm air

Of my sweat, of the warmth deep in my hair—
I recognize it, it's the smell of my pillow
And of my sheets, the closest things to me.
Now one with the bathroom, every oily tile

A different picture of me, every square
One in which I'm given the power of curves,
Distorted, captured in some less shallow
Dimension—now I can pray. I can cry, and he'll

Come. He is my shoulder, maybe, above
The grey water. He is in the steam,
So he can touch my face. Rafael,
He says, I am your saint. So I paint

For him the story of the day: the wife
Whose husband beat purples into her skin,
The jaundiced man (who calls me Ralph, still,
Because that's more American), faint

Yellows, his eyes especially—then,
Still crying, the bright red a collision
Brought out of its perfect vessel, this girl,
This life attached to, working, the wrong thing

Of a tricycle. I saw pain—
Primitive, I could see it, through her split
Chest, in her crushed ribs—white-hot. Now,
I can stop. He has listened, he is silent.

When he finally speaks, touching my face,
It sounds herbal, or African, like drums
Or the pure, tiny bells her child's cries
Must have been made of. Then, somehow,

I'm carried to my bed, the pillow, the sheets
Fragrant, infinite, cool, and I recognize
His voice. In the end, just as sleep takes
The world away, I know it is my own.

WHAT THE BODY TOLD

Not long ago, I studied medicine.
It was terrible, what the body told.
I'd look inside another person's mouth,
And see the desolation of the world.
I'd see his genitals and think of sin.

Because my body speaks the stranger's language,
I've never understood those nods and stares.
My parents held me in their arms, and still
I think I've disappointed them; they care,
They stare and nod, they make their pilgrimage

To somewhere distant in my heart, they cry.
I look inside their other-person's mouths
And see the sleek interior of souls.
It's warm and red in there—like love, with teeth.
I've studied medicine until I cried

All night. Through certain books, a truth unfolds.
Anatomy and physiology,
The tiny sensing organs of the tongue—
Each nameless cell contributing its needs.
It was fabulous, what the body told.

GREGORY EDWARDS

GREGORY EDWARDS (1990–). *American student, poet. When he wrote "The Shot," Gregory was in Ms. Carole Dunn's fourth-grade class at Robert Shaw Elementary School in Scottdale, Dekalb County, Georgia. He plans to become either a physician or a writer.*

THE SHOT

Going to the doctor
With my father.

The scary, scary doctor!

Dad's gonna get a shot.
He's as stiff as a robot!

The scary, scary doctor!

We are getting closer.
We are in.

The scary, scary doctor!

He got his shot.
All that was left was a dot.

HANS ZINSSER

HANS ZINSSER (1878–1940). *American physician, bacteriologist, writer. Hans Zinsser was born in New York City and received both his B.A. (1899) and M.D. (1903) degrees from Columbia University. Beginning in 1911, he served successively as professor of bacteriology at Stanford, Columbia, and Harvard University, to which he came in 1923 and where he completed his career. A noted epidemiologist, his most famous work was on typhus: he isolated the bacterium that causes the disease and, with his colleagues at Harvard, developed a way to mass-produce the vaccine. He served with the American Red Cross Sanitary Commission during the 1915 typhus epidemic in Serbia and with the League of Nations Sanitary Commission (1923) in the U.S.S.R. His best known book,* Rats, Lice, and History *(1935), describes the impact on civilization of epidemics from typhus to the black plague. The selection below is from the autobiographical* As I Remember Him *(1940).*

Excerpt from AS I REMEMBER HIM

I remember one dark, rainy day when we buried a Russian doctor. A ragged band of Serbian reservists stood in the mud and played the Russian and Serbian anthems out of tune. The horses on the truck slipped as it was being loaded, and the coffin fell off. When the chanting procession finally disappeared over the hill, I was glad that the rain on my face obscured the tears that I could not hold back. I felt in my heart, then, that I never could or would be an observer, and that, whatever Fate had in store for me, I would always wish to be in the ranks, however humbly or obscurely; and it came upon me suddenly that I was profoundly happy in my profession, in which I would never aspire to administrative power or prominence so long as I could remain close, heart and hands, to the problems of disease.

SUGGESTIONS FOR FURTHER READING

The following list, in random order, is a partial one drawn from teachers of literature and medicine at medical schools across the country. The list is not an exhaustive one, but we hope it conveys something of the wide variety of readings that commend themselves to your further study and reading for pleasure.

Albert Camus, *The Plague*
William Carlos Williams, poems, *The Doctor Stories, Autobiography*
Anton Chekhov, "Ward Six," other stories, *Uncle Vanya*, other plays
Leo Tolstoy, "The Death of Ivan Ilych"
Richard Selzer, *Mortal Lessons*, other books of his prose
Franz Kafka, *The Metamorphosis*
Thomas Mann, *Death in Venice*
Sinclair Lewis, *Arrowsmith*
Tillie Olsen, "Tell Me a Riddle" (short story)
George Bernard Shaw, *The Doctor's Dilemma* (play)
Abraham Verghese, *My Own Country*
Bernard Pomerance, *The Elephant Man* (play)
Oliver Sacks, *Awakenings*
Mary Shelley, *Frankenstein*
Susan Sontag, *Illness As Metaphor*
Lewis Thomas, *Lives of a Cell*
Ken Kesey, *One Flew Over the Cuckoo's Nest*
Perri Klass, *A Not Entirely Benign Procedure*, other works
Mitch Albom, *Tuesdays with Morrie*
Frank Gonzales-Crussi, *The Day of the Dead and Other Mortal Reflections*
Ferroll Sams, novels, stories, *When All the World Was Young* (medical school)
George Eliot, *Middlemarch*
A. J. Cronin, *The Citadel*
Arthur Conan Doyle, stories
Henrik Ibsen, *Enemy of the People* (play)
Gerald Weissmann, *The Woods Hole Cantata*, other prose
Flannery O'Connor, "Everything That Rises Must Converge," "The Enduring Chill"
L. J. Schneiderman, *Sea Nymphs by the Hour*, short stories, plays
William Shakespeare, *King Lear* (play)

Alexander Solzhenitsyn, *Cancer Ward*
Molière, *The Physician in Spite of Himself,* other plays
W. Somerset Maugham, *Of Human Bondage*
Albert Schweitzer, *Out of My Life and Thought*
Jon Mukand, *Articulations: The Body and Illness in Poetry*
Walker Percy, *Lancelot, Love in the Ruins,* other novels
Sherwin Nuland, *How We Die*

ADDITIONAL RESOURCES

Literature and Medicine: An Annotated Bibliography, ed. by Joanne Trautmann and Carol Pollard. University of Pittsburgh Press, 1982. An excellent compendium of information about the subject, with concise annotations of hundreds of literary works, divided into time periods (Classical, Medieval, 20th Century, etc.); with cross-references to subject matter (Disease and Health, Women as Healers, The Body, Doctors, etc.).

Journal: *Literature and Medicine,* Johns Hopkins University Press, edited by Suzanne Poirier. A scholarly journal complete with well-written articles, book reviews, and theme issues.

Web site: New York University, Literature and Medicine Database, edited by Felice Aull. This site is a resource that is growing rapidly; invaluable annotations of various works, with provocative insights into all kinds of interactions between art and medicine—with links to related resources. The Web address is:

<http://endeavor.med.nyu.edu/lit-med/>

THE EDITORS

PERMISSIONS

ILLUSTRATION CREDITS

Costume of a seventeenth-century plague physician. Engraving from J. J. Manget: *Traite de la peste* . . . Geneva, 1721. Frontis to vol. I.

Thomas Eakins, *The Gross Clinic*. Jefferson Medical College of Thomas Jefferson University, Philadelphia, Pennsylvania.

Edvard Munch, *The Sick Child*. The Tate Gallery, London.

Pieter Brueghel, *Landscape with the Fall of Icarus*. Musées Royaux des Beaux-Arts de Belgique, Brussels.

Photo of Dr. Ernest Ceriani: W. Eugene Smith, *Life* magazine © Time Warner Inc.

The Doctor, painting by Luke Fildes. The Tate Gallery, London.

INDEX OF AUTHORS

ABOUT THE EDITORS

RICHARD REYNOLDS was born in Saugerties, New York, and educated at Rutgers University (B.S.) and Johns Hopkins School of Medicine (M.D.). His postgraduate training in internal medicine was done at Johns Hopkins Hospital. For a number of years Dr. Reynolds was in private practice in Frederick, Maryland. His academic career includes appointments as chair of the department of community health and family medicine at the University of Florida College of Medicine; dean of the Robert Wood Johnson Medical School, a unit of the University of Medicine and Dentistry of New Jersey, where he also served as senior vice president for academic affairs. He then became executive vice president of the Robert Wood Johnson Foundation. Dr. Reynolds has written many papers and held leadership positions in several regional and national medical organizations. Currently he is courtesy professor of medicine at the University of Florida.

JOHN STONE was born in Jackson, Mississippi, and educated at Millsaps College (B.A.) and Washington University in St. Louis (M.D.). His postgraduate training in internal medicine and cardiology was done at Strong Memorial Hospital/University of Rochester School of Medicine and Emory University School of Medicine. He is now professor of medicine (cardiology) and associate dean at Emory. Dr. Stone was coeditor of *Principles and Practice of Emergency Medicine,* the first comprehensive textbook of that discipline. His writings include four books of poetry, all from LSU Press: *The Smell of Matches, In All This Rain, Renaming the Streets,* and *Where Water Begins: New Poems and Prose. In the Country of Hearts: Journeys in the Art of Medicine* is a collection of essays and stories about his life in cardiology.

LOIS LACIVITA NIXON received her A.B. degree from the University of Miami (literature and nursing) and holds master's degrees from Middlebury College and Rollins College; her M.P.H. is from the University of South Florida, as is her Ph.D. in English literature. Dr. Nixon is now associate professor of medicine at the University of South Florida School of Medicine, where she teaches in the division of medical ethics and humanities. She is also chair of the Hillsborough County Hospital Authority.

DELESE WEAR was born in Louisiana, Missouri, but has spent most of her life in northeast Ohio. Since finishing her Ph.D. at Kent State University in 1981, she has taught at the Northeastern Ohio Universities College of Medicine, where she is now professor of behavioral sciences. In addition to numerous articles, she is the author (with Lois Nixon) of *Literary Anatomies: Women's Bodies and Health in Literature* (1994) and *Privilege in the Medical Academy: A Feminist Looks at Race, Gender, and Power* (1997). She has also edited several books, most recently (with Janet Bickel) *Educating for Professionalism: Creating a Climate of Humanism in Medical Education* (2000). Her academic interests are in literature and medicine, pedagogical issues in the medical humanities, and the professional development of medical students.